Pain Medicine
Board Review

Pain Medicine Board Review

SECOND EDITION

Anna Woodbury, MD, MSCR, C.Ac
Associate Program Director, Emory Multidisciplinary Pain Fellowship
Associate Professor, Department of Anesthesiology, Division of Pain Medicine
Emory University School of Medicine
Atlanta Veterans Affairs Healthcare System
Atlanta, Georgia

Boris Spektor, MD
Program Director, Emory Multidisciplinary Pain Fellowship
Associate Professor, Department of Anesthesiology, Division of Pain Medicine
Emory University School of Medicine
Atlanta, Georgia

Vinita Singh, MD
Director of Cancer Pain
Assistant Professor, Department of Anesthesiology Division of Pain Medicine
Emory University School of Medicine
Atlanta, Georgia

Brian Bobzien, MD
Pain Clinic Director, Grady Health System
Assistant Professor, Department of Anesthesiology, Division of Pain Medicine
Emory University School of Medicine
Atlanta, Georgia

Trusharth Patel, MD
Assistant Professor, Department of Anesthesiology, Division of Pain Medicine
Emory University School of Medicine
Atlanta, Georgia

Jerry Kalangara, MD
Interventional Pain Division Chief, Atlanta Veterans Affairs Healthcare System
Assistant Professor, Department of Anesthesiology, Division of Pain Medicine
Emory University School of Medicine
Atlanta, Georgia

ELSEVIER

Elsevier
1600 John F. Kennedy Blvd.
Ste 1800
Philadelphia, PA 19103-2899

PAIN MEDICINE BOARD REVIEW, SECOND EDITION

ISBN: 978-0-323-77586-1

Copyright © 2022 by Elsevier, Inc. All rights reserved.

Notice

Previous editions copyrighted 2018

Library of Congress Control Number: 2021935855

Executive Content Strategist: Michael Houston
Content Development Specialist: Erika Ninsin
Publishing Services Manager: Shereen Jameel
Project Manager: Aparna Venkatachalam
Design Direction: Patrick Ferguson

Printed in the United States of America

Last digit is the print number: 9   8   7   6   5   4   3   2

 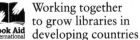

In loving memory of my father, pain physician and patient advocate, who inspired me to heal.
To my many trainees, who have stimulated me to grow with thoughtful and provocative questions.
Boris Spektor, MD

Preface

The field of pain medicine is an ever-developing and expanding field with an inherently multidisciplinary nature. The field continues to advance with research into newer, safer, and more comprehensive techniques for the management of pain. In the face of a widespread opioid epidemic, physicians from a variety of fields have become intensely interested in nonnarcotic management of acute and chronic pain conditions, and learning how to appropriately assess opioid risk. As those who study pain know, there are many varieties of pain and many ways to target these individual pain sources and interrupt their mechanisms of development.

This second edition question book continues to highlight key concepts in the pathophysiology and treatment of pain and has undergone more thorough editing. It was compiled by physicians from specialties and subspecialties including Anesthesiology, Emergency Medicine, Pain Medicine, Palliative Care, Physical Medicine and Rehabilitation, Regional Anesthesia/Acute Pain, and also includes editors with expertise and special interests in Cancer Pain, Integrative Medicine, and Pediatric Pain. Questions were written primarily by fellows during their subspecialty training at Emory University School of Medicine and reviewed/edited by faculty. Editors represent four separate institutions associated with Emory, bringing with them a wide range of backgrounds and expertise with diverse patient populations.

This question book is not intended as a standalone resource, but as an aid to guide studying and highlight key points in pain management. It is a companion book to *Practical Management of Pain*, edited by Honorio Benzon et al. *Practical Management of Pain* stands out as a comprehensive resource for those interested in the study of pain; it is appropriate both for those seeking board certification as well as for those who simply wish to gain a deeper understanding of pain and its various treatments. Healthcare practitioners from a variety of fields would benefit from information found in these books. In assessing currently available books regarding pain medicine for our fellows to use for self-study and board review, we found that most books on the market were inadequate and inherently flawed. We therefore encouraged them to read *Practical Management of Pain* and, as a group interested in furthering education and understanding regarding pain medicine, came together (fellows and faculty) to develop a question book based on this comprehensive text. As such, this question book should be used as an adjunct to specifically target areas in need of further study, whether for board preparation or simply as a "test your knowledge" guide to accompany *Practical Management of Pain*.

Acknowledgments

The editors would like to acknowledge helpful discussions and input from their colleagues and trainees in multiple departments at Emory University School of Medicine. The multidisciplinary pain fellowship at Emory and the development of this book could not exist without the willingness and enthusiasm to teach that has come from the cohesive groups of individuals within these departments. These departments include Anesthesiology, Emergency Medicine, Hematology & Oncology, Interventional Radiology, Neurology, Palliative Care, Physical Medicine and Rehabilitation, Primary Care, Psychiatry, Psychology, Radiology, and many others. Specific individuals deserving of thanks for their support and their commitment to medical education include Andrew Patterson (chair, Department of Anesthesiology), Anne Marie McKenzie-Brown (director, Center for Pain), Colette Curtis (Acute Pain), Tammie Quest (Emergency Medicine & Palliative Care), Paul Desandre (Emergency Medicine & Palliative Care), Lynn O'Neill (Geriatrics, Internal Medicine & Palliative Care), Michael Silver (Neurology), Taylor Harrison (Neurology & Electrodiagnostics), Nadine Kaslow (Pain Psychology), Howard Levy (Physical Medicine & Rehabilitation), William Beckworth (Physical Medicine & Rehabilitation), Jose Garcia (Physical Medicine & Rehabilitation), Randy Katz (Occupational Medicine & Physical Medicine & Rehabilitation), Scott Firestone (Psychiatry), and Walter Carpenter (Radiology).

Anna Woodbury, MD, MSCR, C.Ac

Contents

PHARMACOLOGIC, PSYCHOLOGICAL, AND PHYSICAL MEDICINE TREATMENTS

PART 6   NERVE BLOCK TECHNIQUES

PART 7   INTERVENTIONAL TECHNIQUES

PAIN MANAGEMENT IN SPECIAL SITUATIONS AND SPECIAL TOPICS

PART 9 **RESEARCH, ETHICS, AND REIMBURSEMENT IN PAIN**

PART 1

GENERAL CONSIDERATIONS

The History of Pain Medicine 1

QUESTIONS

1. Which of the following anesthetics was administered for labor pain to Queen Victoria in 1874 and subsequently legitimized the need for analgesia during labor?
   A. Chloroform
   B. Nitrous oxide
   C. Cocaine
   D. Morphine
   E. Procaine

2. Which of the following theories combines both physical and psychological aspects of pain perception and is credited with revolutionizing pain research?
   A. Pattern Theory
   B. Sensory Interaction Theory
   C. Gate Control Theory
   D. The Fourth Theory of Pain
   E. Specificity Theory

3. Which of the following organizations is the largest, with multidisciplinary members including but not limited to physicians, dentists, psychologists, nurses, and physical therapists?
   A. The American Academy of Pain Medicine (AAPM)
   B. The International Association for the Study of Pain (IASP)
   C. The International Spine Intervention Society (SIS, formally ISIS)
   D. The American Society of Interventional Pain Physicians (ASIPP)
   E. The American Society of Regional Anesthesia (ASRA)

ANSWERS

1. **A.** Queen Victoria was given chloroform by James Simpson in 1847 for the delivery of her eighth child, at which point it became widely accepted that labor pain should be medically managed. Prior to this, it was considered against Christian beliefs to provide or accept analgesia during labor.

2. **C.** The Gate Control Theory, developed by Melzack and Wall in 1965, states that non-nociceptive signals can override nociceptive signals, and, as a result, the perception of pain is reduced or eliminated. Interventions such as peripheral nerve stimulators, TENS units, and spinal cord stimulators, as well as

biofeedback techniques, are based on the Gate Control Theory. This theory is cited as ending the debate regarding whether or not the cerebral cortex plays a role in pain. Development of imaging such as PET, fMRI, and SPECT later added credibility to this theory by demonstrating the activation of the cerebral cortex in response to pain.

3. **B.** The International Association for the Study of Pain (IASP) is the largest multidisciplinary international association, with a goal of furthering pain research by integrating professionals with different backgrounds and disciplines.

2 Taxonomy and Classification of Chronic Pain Syndromes

QUESTIONS

1. The International Association for the Study of Pain (IASP) classification focuses on chronic pain; however, it includes syndromes that are not acute in nature, including which of the following?
   A. Acute herpes zoster
   B. Burns with spasm
   C. Pancreatitis
   D. Prolapsed intervertebral disk
   E. All of the above

2. The classification of chronic pain specifies five axes for describing pain. The second axis is the *system* most related to the cause of the pain. Which of the following are identified systems?
   A. Central, peripheral, and autonomic nervous systems and special senses
   B. Psychological and social function of the nervous system
   C. Respiratory and vascular systems
   D. Musculoskeletal system and connective tissue
   E. All of the above

3. Which of the following is **NOT** part of the diagnosis of complex somatic symptom disorder?
   A. Emotional disturbances
   B. Health anxiety
   C. Excessive amount of time devoted to health concerns
   D. Symptoms and concerns must have lasted 12 months
   E. None of the above

4. Based on the ICD-10 classification, a predominant complaint that is persistent, severe, and distressing that cannot be explained fully by a physiologic process or physical disorder is categorized as:
   A. Pain Disorder, Somatoform Persistent
   B. Pain Disorder, Psychological Origin
   C. Pain Disorder, Malingering
   D. Pain Disorder, Neuropathic
   E. Psychological or Behavioral Factor Associated with Disorders or Disease Classified Elsewhere

5. The definition of complex regional pain syndrome (type 1):
   A. Is related to the sympathetic nervous system
   B. Is defined by its clinical phenomena
   C. Is defined solely for research purposes
   D. Serves to exclude new syndromes such as those involving painful legs and moving toes
   E. Is entirely psychogenic in nature

6. Tension headaches fall under which of the following diagnostic categories?
   A. Pain Disorder, Somatoform Persistent
   B. Pain Disorder, Psychological Origin
   C. Pain Disorder, Malingering
   D. Pain Disorder, Neuropathic
   E. Psychological or Behavioral Factor Associated with Disorders or Disease Classified Elsewhere

7. While defining pain, it is important to recognize that pain is always a subjective state related to which of the following?
   A. Emotional state
   B. Physical state
   C. Psychiatric state
   D. Psychological state
   E. Social state

8. According to the IASP Taxonomy Committee, *chronic pain* is defined as pain that has been present for what length of time?
   A. 3 months
   B. 12 months
   C. 6 months
   D. 24 months
   E. None of the above

9. Consensus generally exists on the meaning or definition of which of the following terms?
   A. Condition
   B. Disease
   C. Disorder
   D. Symptom
   E. Syndrome

10. All of the following are listed by the IASP as relatively generalized pain syndromes except:
    A. Fibromyalgia
    B. Phantom Pain
    C. Complex Regional Pain Syndrome
    D. Pain of Psychological Origin
    E. Radicular Pain

ANSWERS

1. **E.** The IASP (International Association for the Study of Pain) focuses on the classification of chronic pain syndrome, but includes some acute syndromes that can often become chronic. Acute herpes zoster, burns with spasm, pancreatitis, and prolapsed intervertebral disk are all examples of acute pain syndromes that are included.

2. **E.** The classifications are divided into five axes: (1) anatomic, (2) system, (3) temporal characteristics and pattern, (4) intensity, (5) etiology. The second axis systems include (a) central, peripheral, and autonomic nervous and special senses; (b) psychological and social function; (c) respiratory and vascular; (d) musculoskeletal and connective tissue; (e) cutaneous and subcutaneous tissue and glands, gastrointestinal, genitourinary, and other organs/viscera; and (g) unknown systems.

3. **D.** To be diagnosed with complex somatic symptom disorder by DSM-IV criteria, patients must report at least one distressing somatic symptom as well as at least one of "emotional/cognitive/behavioral disturbances: high levels of health anxiety, disproportionate and persistent concerns about the medical seriousness of the 'symptoms' and an excessive amount of time and energy devoted to the symptoms and health concerns," for at least 6 months' duration. It is not required to last 12 months.

4. **A.** Persistent Somatoform Pain Disorder is persistent, severe, distressing pain that cannot be explained fully by physiologic mechanisms. Pain during schizophrenia or depression is not included.

5. **B.** The name of complex regional pain syndrome (CRPS) was changed from reflex sympathetic dystrophy (RSD) based on the advice of a special subcommittee. Steps taken have (1) defined CRPS type 1 by its clinical phenomena and (2) developed identifying diagnostic criteria for clinical agreement as well as for more stringent research purposes.

The classification has also helped in understanding relatively new syndromes. The old name, RSD, was based on a theoretical relationship to the sympathetic nervous system.

6. **E.** Pain that is due to known or inferred psychophysiological mechanisms, such as muscle tension pain or migraines, but is believed to have a psychogenic cause falls under the ICD-10 classification of Psychological or Behavioral Factor Associated with Disorders or Disease Classified Elsewhere.

7. **D.** The definition of pain by the IASP is "an unpleasant sensory and emotional experience associated with actual or potential tissue damage or described in terms of such damage." This addresses the situation of patients who appear to have pain but do not have obvious tissue damage, and acknowledges that pain is always subjective and psychological, regardless of tissue damage.

8. **C.** Chronic pain is pain that persists beyond the normal healing process. Although the timeframe for this may differ in practice and many types of pain become chronic or persistent at 3 months, the 6-month division was chosen for scientific purposes by the IASP as a good entry to the patient population treated by pain physicians.

9. **D.** The words "disorder," "syndrome," and "disease" are all in dispute regarding whether they reflect the true phenomena that physicians treat. However, the word "symptom" is not in dispute.

10. **E.** Relatively generalized syndromes include diffuse or widespread pain that is poorly localized, such as rheumatoid arthritis, fibromyalgia, polymyalgia rheumatica, pain of psychological origin, syringomyelia, central pain, CRPS, phantom pain, stump pain, and peripheral neuropathy. Localized syndromes are divided by the area affected (head, neck, limbs, thorax, abdomen, spinal/radicular).

3 Organizing an Inpatient Acute Pain Service

1. Which of the following factors is likely to influence postoperative opioid requirements?
   A. Preoperative pain sensitivity
   B. Presurgical opioid tolerance or a history of drug abuse
   C. Psychological factors, including catastrophizing and anxiety
   D. Age
   E. All of the above

2. Which is the best intervention for inhibition of surgical stress responses?
   A. Neuraxial steroids
   B. Neuraxial local anesthetics
   C. Perineural local anesthetics
   D. Systemic steroids
   E. None of the above

3. What percentage of patients undergoing surgery consider postoperative pain to be their primary fear?
   A. 30%–40%
   B. 40%–50%
   C. 50%–60%
   D. 60%–70%
   E. 80%–90%

4. All of the following are examples of multimodal analgesia **EXCEPT**:
   A. Neuraxial block and music therapy
   B. IV morphine and fentanyl patch
   C. PCA morphine and thoracic epidural
   D. Acupuncture and TENS
   E. Femoral nerve block and stress reduction

5. Which is an important first step in organizing an inpatient acute pain service?
   A. Enlisting the support of hospital administration and defining resources
   B. Assessment of need
   C. Definition of service
   D. Financing and business plan
   E. Nursing education

ANSWERS

1. **E.** Achieving satisfactory acute pain management can be challenging. It is often difficult to estimate a patient's postoperative analgesic requirements. The following factors may influence postoperative opioid requirements: preoperative pain sensitivity, coexisting medical conditions and associated multiple drug administration, presurgical opioid tolerance or a history of drug abuse, psychological factors (including catastrophizing and anxiety), age, and type of surgery.

2. **B.** Surgical stress responses are best inhibited by neuraxial administration of local anesthetics; the administration of other agents—systemically, neuraxially, or perineurally—appear to contribute little additional reduction of the endocrine (metabolic and catabolic) stress response following operative procedures.

3. **C.** Inadequacy of pain relief has been highlighted as a quality-of-care measure and a focus of patients' concerns. In a questionnaire survey, approximately 57% of patients identified pain after surgery as their primary fear.

4. **B.** A time-, energy-, and cost-effective acute pain program should optimally provide multimodal and multidisciplinary interventions, including systemic and regional pharmacologic treatments, stress reduction, transcutaneous electrical nerve stimulation, music therapy, and acupuncture. Extracting and integrating the relevant expertise from multiple healthcare disciplines often allows individualized and optimized pain management. Disciplines commonly involved include psychology, pharmacy, physical therapy, and nutrition.

5. **A.** Enlisting the support of hospital administration and defining resources are a vital first step in organizing an inpatient acute pain service. Once the challenge of organizing an acute pain service is accepted, assessment of need is mandatory. Once the mission statement has been formulated in response to the perceived institutional and community needs, it is necessary to define the resources that will be required. The next step in the process of organizing an inpatient acute pain service is to construct the business plan.

Measurement-Based Stepped Care Approach to Interdisciplinary Chronic Pain Management

QUESTIONS

1. Which of the following is **FALSE** regarding the World Health Organization cancer pain analgesic ladder?
   A. It is focused on the relief of intensity of cancer pain.
   B. It incorporates relief of suffering of the cancer pain patient.
   C. It emphasizes treating the intensity of pain even at the expense of function.
   D. It includes three steps in its analgesic strategy.
   E. The goal of the ladder is complete freedom from pain.

2. Which of the following pain treatment domains should ideally be included in a measurement-based stepped care pain treatment algorithm?
   A. Physical and emotional function
   B. Quality of sleep
   C. Risk for chemical dependency
   D. Self-reported quality of life
   E. All of the above

3. The Patient Health Questionnaire 4 (PHQ-4) is a screening tool for depression and anxiety. Which of the following is **NOT** assessed on this questionnaire?
   A. Feeling nervous, anxious, or on edge
   B. Not being able to stop or control worrying
   C. Feeling down, depressed, or hopeless
   D. Having little interest or pleasure in doing things
   E. Feeling better off dead

4. Which of the following is true about daily morphine equivalent dose (MED) and relative risk of mortality in patients on chronic opioid therapy?
   A. As daily morphine equivalent dose increases, mortality risk increases in tandem.
   B. As daily morphine equivalent dose increases, mortality risk tends to plateau.
   C. As daily morphine equivalent dose increases, mortality risk decreases.
   D. The 50–100 mg morphine equivalent dose has the highest risk of mortality.
   E. Using between 20 and 50 mg morphine equivalents per day does not increase mortality risk relative to less than 20 mg daily.

5. All of the following are aberrant drug behaviors **EXCEPT**:
   A. Self-induced oversedation
   B. Continuing medication despite report of feeling intoxicated
   C. Early refill requests
   D. Calling the office to report worsening pain
   E. Self-directed dose increase

6. The 2006 Trends and Risks of Opioid Use for Pain (TROUP) study found opioid use to be higher in patients with mental health disorders and what other health problem?
   A. Chronic pelvic pain
   B. Substance use disorders
   C. Chronic back pain
   D. Postsurgical patients
   E. Patients with whiplash history

7. All of the following are validated opioid risk scales **EXCEPT**:
   A. ORT
   B. COMM
   C. SOAPP-R
   D. DIRE
   E. DOLOPLUS

8. Which of the following is true about patient access to pain specialists?
   A. There is an overabundance of pain care providers in the United States today.
   B. There is currently a significant shortage in pain providers relative to the number of people with chronic pain.
   C. The number of patients with chronic pain is currently well matched to the number of board-certified providers in pain care.
   D. In the United States, fewer than 1000 physicians were board certified in pain care between 2000 and 2009.
   E. The current shortage in pain care expertise leaves more than 100,000 people with chronic pain for every pain specialist in the United States.

9. Obstructive sleep apnea risk is thought to increase with the dose of opioid used. Which of the following is **NOT** an additional risk factor for obstructive sleep apnea based on STOP-BANG criteria?
   A. Hypertension
   B. Snoring
   C. BMI greater than 35
   D. Age less than 50 years
   E. Male gender

10. According to the model of measurement-based stepped care, referral to a behavioral health specialist is indicated when all of the following are present **EXCEPT**:
   A. PHQ-9 ≥ 15
   B. PHQ-4 ≥ 5
   C. Suicidal ideation
   D. PTSD
   E. Anxiety

11. A 28-year-old male with chronic pain presents to your clinic. Opioid risk screening reveals a personal and family history of cocaine use as well as a psychological history of anxiety. According to the stepped care model, he should be referred to see:
   A. Pain physician
   B. Physiatrist
   C. Behavioral health specialist
   D. Addiction medicine specialist
   E. Sleep medicine specialist

12. A primary care physician is treating a 26-year-old female with chronic diffuse pain of unclear etiology, unresponsive to 3 months of conservative management including opioid escalation. According to the stepped care model, she should be referred to see:
   A. Pain physician
   B. Physiatrist

C. Behavioral health specialist
   D. Addiction medicine specialist
   E. Sleep medicine specialist

13. The concept of "adverse selection" in relation to substance use disorders and chronic pain opioid prescribing argues which of the following:
   A. The patients at highest opioid risk are being prescribed the highest opioid doses.
   B. The patients with highest socioeconomic status are being prescribed the highest opioid doses.
   C. The patients with lowest opioid needs are being prescribed the lowest opioid doses.
   D. The patients at highest opioid risk are being prescribed the lowest opioid doses.
   E. The patients at lowest opioid risk are being prescribed the highest opioid doses.

14. What is the morphine equivalent dose (MED) that prompts a referral to a pain specialist according to the stepped care model?
   A. 0–19 mg MED
   B. 20–49 mg MED
   C. 50–79 mg MED
   D. 80–119 mg MED
   E. Greater than 120 mg MED

15. Physical medicine and rehabilitation referral is prompted by all of the following **EXCEPT**:
   A. Disability greater than 4 weeks
   B. On-the-job pain interference
   C. Ineffective return-to-work plan
   D. Roland Morris > 12/24
   E. Obesity

ANSWERS

1. **B.** The WHO cancer pain analgesic ladder is focused strictly on alleviating the intensity of pain and does not incorporate suffering of the cancer pain patient in its analgesic strategy. Other answer choices listed are true statements regarding the ladder.

2. **E.** All of the listed pain treatment domains should ideally be included in a stepped care pain treatment algorithm.

3. **E.** The question regarding suicidality comes from the PHQ-9 screening tool rather than the simpler PHQ-4 questionnaire.

4. **A.** Relative risk of mortality with chronic opioid therapy increases in parallel with escalating morphine equivalent dose.

5. **D.** Contacting the office to report worsening pain is considered appropriate behavior meriting reevaluation.

6. **B.** Presence of substance use disorder in addition to mental health disorders predisposed patients to higher opioid use in the TROUP study.

7. **E.** The first four options are validated opioid risk screening tools: Opioid Risk Tool (ORT), the Screener and Opioid Assessment for Patients with Pain-Revised (SOAPP-R); the Current Opioid Misuse Measure (COMM); and the Diagnosis, Intractability, Risk, and Efficacy (DIRE). The DOLOPLUS scale, though validated, is used for behavioral pain assessment in elderly patients with verbal communication problems, not for opioid risk screening.

8. **B.** There is currently a significant shortage of board-certified pain physicians in the United States relative to the number of patients with chronic pain.

9. **D.** Age greater than 50 years is a risk factor for OSA per the STOP-BANG criteria.

10. **E.** Although anxiety is often associated with chronic pain, its presence alone is not considered sufficient for psychiatrist referral according to the stepped care model unless deemed poorly controlled despite conservative measures.

11. **D.** This patient has an opioid risk tool score ≥8 and thus merits referral to an addiction medicine specialist.

12. **A.** This patient merits referral to a pain medicine specialist for further evaluation.

13. **A.** The patients at highest opioid risk are being prescribed the highest opioid doses.

14. **E.** Greater than 120 mg MED.

15. **E.** All are true except obesity, which is one of the risk factors for sleep medicine referral.

5 The Health Care Policy of Pain Management

QUESTIONS

1. Which of these statements is part of the International Association for the Study of Pain (IASP) *Declaration of Montreal*?
   A. Only pain that has been objectively verified must be treated.
   B. Pain must be treated by a medical doctor specialty-trained in pain management.
   C. Patients should receive analgesia based on their ability to pay.
   D. Access to effective pain management is a basic human right.
   E. Patients must have a history negative for substance abuse to qualify for opioids.

2. Which of the following phases of the Food and Drug Administration Center for Drug Evaluation and Research (FDA CDER) approval process focuses on the basic safety profile and pharmacokinetics of the drug in human subjects?
   A. Preclinical Investigational New Drug (IND) application
   B. Phase I
   C. Phase II
   D. Phase III
   E. Phase IV

3. Which of the following is **NOT** identified as a barrier to access to pain treatment around the world?
   A. Education of patient population
   B. High cost of treatment
   C. Lack of government policy on pain treatment and drug supply
   D. Poor training of health care workers
   E. Fear among health care workers of legal action

ANSWERS

1. **D.** The *Declaration of Montreal*, published in 2010, states that effective pain management is a basic human right. It underscores the importance of government to enact legislature that promotes access to pain management for all. It consists of three articles, including:
   - Article 1: The right of all people to have access to pain management without discrimination.
   - Article 2: The right of people in pain to have their pain acknowledged and to be informed about how it can be assessed and managed.
   - Article 3: The right of all people with pain to have access to appropriate assessment and treatment of the pain by adequately trained health care professionals.

2. **B.** The phases of the FDA CDER approval process are tiered as follows:
   - Preclinical IND application: Animal data used to justify testing of the drug in humans.
   - Phase I: Basic safety profile and pharmacokinetics of the drug in 50–100 human subjects.
   - Phase II: Drug dosage, efficacy, and safety in 100–500 human subjects.
   - Phase III: Confirmation of the safety and effectiveness of the drug, its dosages, and drug interactions in 1000–4000 human subjects.
   - Phase IV: New or expanded use for patient population and long-term risks versus benefits.

3. **A.** Access to appropriate pain management worldwide remains largely inadequate. Seventy-eight percent of morphine consumed in 2010 went to only six countries. Inexpensive oral medications are unobtainable in many countries. Reasons cited include:
   - Failure of governments to put functioning drug supply systems in place.
   - Failure to enact policies on pain treatment and palliative care.
   - Poor training of health care workers.
   - Existence of unnecessarily restrictive drug control regulations and practices.
   - Fear among health care workers of legal sanctions for legitimate medical practice.
   - Unnecessarily high cost of pain treatment.

Quality Assessment and Improvement and Patient Safety in the Pain Clinic

6

QUESTIONS

1. The majority of errors that take place in health care are a result of which of the following?
   A. Patient factors
   B. System defects
   C. Provider carelessness
   D. Equipment malfunction
   E. Resource misallocation

2. Which of the following is identified as the biggest hurdle to establishing Continuous Quality Improvement (CQI) in pain medicine?
   A. Lack of additional reimbursement to justify higher quality care
   B. Lack of support from hospital administration
   C. Lack of evidence-based benchmarks or national "best practices"
   D. Lack of cooperation from patients
   E. Lack of government regulation to support such programs

3. Which of the following tools has been shown to lower the death rate significantly, to reduce patient complications, and to be especially helpful in emergencies?
   A. E-conferencing/telecommuting
   B. Speech recognition software
   C. Electronic prescriptions
   D. Safety checklist
   E. Patient portals

ANSWERS

1. **B.** According to the Institute of Medicine (IOM), a majority of errors in health care are more likely attributable to system defects (as opposed to individual errors).

2. **C.** Because evidence available in the peer-reviewed literature is insufficient for chronic pain interventions, establishing a CQI in the field of pain medicine largely relies on consensus expert opinion instead.

3. **D.** Using a checklist has been shown to reduce patient complications, which is thought to be a result of decreases in human error. Data show that merely implementing a safety checklist can substantially reduce patient mortality. Checklists are critical in emergencies, such as local anesthetic toxicity, where a checklist/protocol should be readily available.

Education, Training, and Certification in Pain Medicine

QUESTIONS

1. Which of the following describes the design of current pain medicine training programs?
   A. Comprehensive and multidisciplinary
   B. Emphasis on pharmacologic-only treatment
   C. Centered around principles from anesthesiology
   D. Incorporating multidisciplinary principles from three specialties including anesthesiology, psychiatry, and neurology
   E. Focus on objective physical exam findings

2. Which of the following is a consequence of the Food and Drug Administration's (FDA) 510(k) "substantially similar device" process?
   A. There must be data from > 1000 patients demonstrating device efficacy.
   B. There must be data from > 1000 patients demonstrating device safety.
   C. Guideline stringency hinders device innovation.
   D. Introduction of devices to the market often outpaces practitioner familiarity.
   E. Creation of new devices becomes cost prohibitive for manufacturers.

3. Which of the following is a problem in using interventional techniques in pain medicine?
   A. The procedures are only suitable for a small subset of patients.
   B. Randomized, controlled clinical trials are still lacking for many interventional treatments.
   C. There is a lack of patient cooperation with adhering to the schedule of frequency required.
   D. The complications from most of the procedures are such that the risk outweighs the benefit.
   E. Patients are unwilling to try novel procedures.

ANSWERS

1. **A.** The original fellowship training programs in pain medicine were extensions of the department of anesthesiology. Since that time, there has been a broadening of specialties seeking training in pain medicine. In an effort to standardize and ensure quality of pain medicine training programs, four specialties have agreed to ACGME requirements for fellowship programs, including anesthesiology, neurology, physical medicine and rehabilitation, and psychiatry, since 2007. This collaboration between specialties echoes the views of the American Academy of Pain Medicine and the American Board of Pain Medicine, emphasizing a multidisciplinary and multimodal approach to pain medicine.

2. **D.** In order to expedite innovation and the introduction of new technology, devices can be cleared for market if the FDA deems the risks and benefits are comparable to a device that has been previously approved. The FDA's 510(k) "substantially similar device" process can require little additional efficacy data. In some cases, practitioners are overwhelmed with new technology available and are not able to keep pace with the skills and knowledge required to use the device.

3. **B.** The trend in medicine favoring evidence-based therapy has highlighted a relative lack of randomized controlled trials in the pain medicine subspecialty to validate treatments. At the same time, patients with chronic pain require treatment and are often willing to try novel procedures. Practitioners must monitor their own outcomes to aid in making decisions in patient care as well as use best judgment of risk versus benefit for each individual patient.

8

Pain Pathways: Peripheral, Spinal, Ascending, and Descending Pathways

QUESTIONS

1. What is the primary termination site for sensory integration in the pain pathway?
   A. Thalamus
   B. Medulla
   C. Basal ganglia
   D. Dorsal columns
   E. Frontal cortex

2. What are the small unmyelinated axonal fibers with slow conduction velocities that relay noxious input from the skin and other tissues to the central nervous system?
   A. A-delta fibers
   B. A-beta fibers
   C. C fibers
   D. Free nerve endings
   E. Dorsal root ganglia

3. The dorsal horn is anatomically organized in laminae. Small unmyelinated fibers terminate in laminae_____, while large myelinated fibers terminate in laminae_____.
   A. II–III, IV–V
   B. I–II, III–V
   C. III–V, I–II
   D. II–IV, I–III
   E. V, I–II

4. The substantia gelatinosa is associated with which of the following lamina?
   A. Lamina I
   B. Lamina II
   C. Lamina III
   D. Lamina IV
   E. Lamina V

5. Prolonged membrane hyperpolarization has what effect on the role of GABA-B receptors?
   A. Change from inhibition to more inhibition
   B. Change from inhibition to excitation
   C. Change from excitation to inhibition
   D. Increased threshold for depolarization
   E. No effect

6. Which of the following is the primary afferent excitatory neurotransmitter?
   A. Substance P
   B. CGRP
   C. IL-1
   D. Glutamate
   E. Norepinephrine

7. Noxious cutaneous input is relayed by which of the following lamina projection neurons as the crossed spinothalamic tract pathway traveling in the lateral and ventrolateral white matter en route to the VPL?
   A. II
   B. III
   C. IV
   D. X
   E. IX

8. The gray matter of the dorsal horn includes the following Rexed laminae:
   A. I–IV
   B. I–VI
   C. II–IV
   D. II–VI
   E. I–X

9. All of the following are considered ascending medial pain pathways **EXCEPT**:
   A. Spinoamygdalar
   B. Spinohypothalamic
   C. Spinoreticular
   D. Spinothalamic
   E. Medial spinothalamic

10. Which of the following structures most likely contribute to memory and learning related to painful stimuli as indicated by fMRI imaging studies?
    A. The VPL thalamus, SI, and SII cortices
    B. The ACC, cerebellum, and lentiform nucleus
    C. The insula, cerebellum, and frontal cortex
    D. The ACC, PCC, SI, and SII cortices
    E. The insula, lentiform nucleus, and periaqueductal gray

ANSWERS

1. **A.** The primary termination site for sensory integration is the thalamus. Peripheral nociceptors transmit noxious information to second-order neurons at the spinal cord and brainstem levels, which are then sent by projection neurons of the pain system to integration sites in the brainstem. Although the primary site for integrating sensory information is the thalamus, many other brain structures are also involved.

2. **C.** C fibers (group IV) are small unmyelinated nociceptors with conduction velocities less than 2.5 m/s. A-delta fibers (group III) are small fibers with a conduction velocity of 4–30 m/s and conduct faster because of a thin myelin sheath produced by Schwann cells. Both of these axonal fibers carry noxious input from tissue to the CNS.

3. **B.** Small unmyelinated C-fiber nociceptor endings for somatic sensation are distributed mainly in focused areas of laminae **I** and **II**, although visceral afferents can extend multiple segments and are widely dispersed in ipsilateral laminae I, II, V, and X, or contralateral V and X. Large myelinated A-beta fibers carrying non-nociceptive input terminate in laminae **III–V** of the dorsal horn.

4. **B.** Interneurons of lamina II (substantia gelatinosa) synthesize inhibitory (GABA) and excitatory (glutamate) neurotransmitters. Opioid receptors are also found on these nerve cells.

5. **B.** GABA (γ-aminobutyric acid) primarily reduces neuronal excitability and provides pre-synaptic inhibition, though with prolonged hyperpolarization/nociceptive input, GABA-B receptors can change their role from inhibition to excitation, leading to a positive feedback loop that can establish chronic pain.

6. **D.** Glutamate is an excitatory amino acid and plays key roles in neural activation throughout the nervous system. It is the primary neurotransmitter in afferent nociception.

7. **C.** Noxious cutaneous input from lamina I, IV, and V is relayed by projection neurons along the crossed spinothalamic tract (STT) in the lateral and ventrolateral white matter to the ventral posterolateral (VPL) and posterior thalamus.

8. **B.** Laminae I–X are all considered gray matter, but the dorsal horn includes only laminae I–VI. Some deeper laminae are also involved in nociceptive processing.

9. **D.** The spinoamygdalar, spinohypothalamic, *medial spinothalamic* and spinoreticular pathways, and connections to the anterior cingulate and prefrontal and insular limbic cortices are all *medial* pain pathways. The spinothalamic tract is a non-overlapping but parallel *lateral* pathway.

10. **C.** Centers for higher processing can modulate awareness of and responses to pain as well as regulate emotional, autonomic, and motor responses. The insula, cerebellum, and frontal cortex contribute to avoidance behaviors and other types of *memory and learning* related to the painful stimulus. The VPL thalamus and SI and SII cortices are *somatosensory-processing* regions. The ACC (anterior cingulate cortex) may be involved in interpreting *emotional significance* of pain via the limbic system.

A Review of Pain-Processing Pharmacology

9

1. What are the two key inhibitory neurotransmitters?
   A. NMDA, glycine
   B. Somatostatin, substance P
   C. AMPA, glutamate
   D. GABA, glycine
   E. Somatostatin, NMDA

2. Following a peripheral nerve injury, ongoing pain from ectopic activity is caused by the up-regulation of which type of channels?
   A. Calcium
   B. Sodium
   C. Potassium
   D. Chloride
   E. Fluoride

3. All of the following are effects of substance P binding **EXCEPT:**
   A. Mast cell degranulation
   B. Swelling of skin
   C. Local erythema
   D. Vomiting
   E. Vasoconstriction

4. After nerve injury, there is an increase in axonal excitability that is associated with which of the following?
   A. Up-regulation of potassium channels and down-regulation of sodium channels
   B. Up-regulation of sodium channels and down-regulation of potassium channels
   C. Down-regulation of sodium and potassium channels
   D. Up-regulation of sodium and potassium channels
   E. Up-regulation of calcium channels and down-regulation of sodium channels

5. All of the following mediators are released with tissue injury and depolarize and sensitize primary afferent terminals **EXCEPT:**
   A. TNF-alpha
   B. Substance P
   C. Bradykinin
   D. Histamine
   E. Glycine

6. Which of the following receptors are activated by cold or menthol?
   A. TRPM8
   B. TRPV1
   C. ASIC
   D. TRPV2
   E. TRPV3

7. Which of the following protein kinases phosphorylates the NMDA receptor to lower its threshold for activation?
   A. PKA
   B. PKC
   C. MAPK
   D. AMPA
   E. All of the above

8. Blockage of the facilitated state called "wind-up" has been reported with the use of:
   A. Opioids
   B. Prostaglandins
   C. Nitric oxide
   D. NMDA antagonists
   E. 5-HT3 inhibitors

9. Chemical injury to a nerve is **MOST LIKELY** to be characterized by:
   A. Reddening at the site of the stimulus
   B. An initial burst of afferent firing
   C. Increased capillary permeability
   D. Local arterial dilation
   E. Regional hyperalgesia

10. Which of the following occurs after nerve injury?
    A. Increased local catecholamine release
    B. Alpha-adrenergic antagonists increase excitation of the injured axon
    C. Down-regulation of alpha-1-adrenergic receptor expression
    D. Decreased local catecholamine release
    E. Decreased activity at the DRG or injured neuroma

ANSWERS

1. **D.** Glycine and γ-aminobutyric acid (GABA) act on glycine, GABA-A, and GABA-B receptors, reducing excitation. Glycine is an inhibitory amino acid. Somatostatin is classified as an inhibitory hormone with a range of functions throughout the body including modulating peripheral inflammation, the gastrointestinal tract, and the brain. The N-methyl-D-aspartate (NMDA) receptor requires glutamate or aspartate binding for activation. Substance P contributes to enhanced nociception. Receptors for α-amino-3-hydroxy-5-methyl-4-isoxazolepropionate (AMPA), like NMDA receptors, are activated by glutamate. Glutamate is a main excitatory neurotransmitter. GABA primarily reduces neuronal excitability and provides presynaptic inhibition, although with prolonged hyperpolarization/nociceptive input, GABA-B receptors can change their role from inhibition to excitation, leading to a positive feedback loop that can establish chronic pain.

2. **B.** Sodium channel expression is increased in neuromas and dorsal root ganglia following nerve injury. Lidocaine can block ectopic activity and attenuate hyperpathic states after nerve injury because of its action on the sodium channels. There are a variety of sodium channels in primary afferent neurons (Nav1.6–Nav1.9). Nav1.8 and Nav1.9 are resistant to sodium channel blocker TTX and found primarily in C fibers. Variants such as Nav1.8 are important because, for example, Nav1.8 reverses nerve-injury-evoked pain states in animal models. Mutations in Nav1.7 in humans can cause extremely painful conditions, while loss-of-function mutations can lead to prominent insensitivity. Gain of function mutations (i.e., to the sodium ion channel alpha subunit gene SCN9A) can result in syndromes such as erythromelalgia, characterized by severe periodic pain from blocked blood vessels.

3. **E.** Substance P acts on the neurokinin-1 (NK-1) receptor and is involved in inflammation, pain perception (along with glutamate), and the vomiting centers. Substance P is also a potent vasodilator in conjunction with nitric oxide.

4. **B.** Following nerve injury, sodium channel expression has been found to be significantly increased, while potassium (K+) currents have been shown to be reduced.

5. **E.** Following tissue injury, a variety of cytokines and inflammatory neurotransmitters are released, leading to sensitization. Glycine, however, is an inhibitory neurotransmitter and has not been shown to result in increased afferent sensitization.

6. **A.** Transducer channels on afferent terminals have different sensitivities to specific stimuli. Some channels transducing a physical sensation are also activated by chemicals and can reproduce the physical sensation when exposed to the chemical. For example, the TRPV1 ($> 43°C$) vanilloid receptor is activated by capsaicin (heat sensation), while the TRPM8 ($25–28°C$) receptor is activated by menthol (cold sensation), and the TRPA ($< 17°C$) receptor is activated by mustard oil.

7. **B.** It has been shown that protein kinase C (PKC) phosphorylates sites on NMDA and AMPA receptors, which can lower threshold for activation and increase membrane permeability.

8. **E.** Through the bulbospinal pathway, C fibers make contact with neurons that project into the brainstem contacting serotonergic neurons, which then project to the spinal dorsal horn contacting lamina V neurons. Cells of lamina V in the deep dorsal horn are noted for their ability to display a state known as "wind-up." Blockage of this pathway using 5-HT3 inhibitors has been reported to reduce "wind-up" facilitation.

9. **B.** Following nerve injury, afferent axons display an initial burst of afferent firing followed by electrical silence for hours to days and finally the appearance of spontaneous bursting activity. This is correlated to an initial degeneration of the injured nerve followed by new sprouting. Answer choices A, C, D, and E are associated with tissue injury.

10. **A.** Stimulation of these postganglionic axons and increased catecholamine release can excite the injured axon and DRG following injury, but this activation can be blocked by alpha-adrenergic antagonism.

Pain and Brain Changes

10

QUESTIONS

1. The TRPV1 receptor differentiates which type(s) of pain?
   A. Noxious heat
   B. Acidity
   C. Capsaicin
   D. All of the above
   E. None of the above

2. The dominant excitatory neurotransmitter in all nociceptors is:
   A. Substance P
   B. Serotonin
   C. Acetylcholine
   D. Glutamate
   E. Norepinephrine

3. Intracranial recordings show that the earliest pain-induced brain activity occurs where?
   A. SI cortex
   B. SII cortex
   C. Thalamus
   D. Hypothalamus
   E. Dorsal horn

4. Enhanced sensation and neural transmission at sites remote from the site of injury is referred to as:
   A. Hyperalgesia
   B. Primary sensitization
   C. Secondary sensitization
   D. Desensitization
   E. Allodynia

5. Which of the following is considered a non-nociceptive touch afferent receptor that, following central sensitization, may carry peripheral pain signals to the CNS?
   A. A-delta
   B. A-beta
   C. C fibers
   D. A-gamma
   E. Schwann cells

6. What electrical study or imaging tool can be used to verify the presence of ongoing spontaneous pain in a patient?
   A. Electroencephalogram (EEG)
   B. Positron emission tomography (PET)
   C. Functional MRI (fMRI)
   D. Magnetoencephalography (MEG)
   E. None of the above

7. A 32-year-old female underwent cesarean section 1 year prior to presenting to your office. She has a well-healed, low transverse scar. She now presents to the pain clinic with severe pain at the far right end of the scar. She describes the pain as intermittent sharp, burning, shooting pain, exacerbated by touch. On examination, you detect a knot at the right distal portion of the incision, and upon light touch, she jumps off the table and curses at you. What is the **MOST LIKELY** way you would describe her pain
   A. Abnormal/Hyperalgesia
   B. Abnormal/Allodynia
   C. Neuropathic pain
   D. Inflammatory pain
   E. Visceral pain

8. It is determined that the aforementioned patient has a neuroma. What **INCORRECTLY** describes the pain that she is experiencing?
   A. Neuromas generate spontaneous ectopic activity that directly contributes to the perception of spontaneous pain.
   B. Neuromas are sensitive to temperature, mechanical, and chemical stimuli.
   C. C-type nerve fibers are involved in spontaneous ectopic activity.
   D. A-type nerve fibers are involved in spontaneous ectopic activity.
   E. Noradrenergic sensitization results in separation of sympathetic and sensory neuronal activity.

9. Which of the following best describes the mechanisms involved in sensitization?
   A. There is decreased release of excitatory neurotransmitters such as glutamate and substance P.
   B. Opioid receptors are down-regulated with neuropathic pain.
   C. Opioid receptors are down-regulated with inflammatory pain.
   D. Potassium chloride (KCl) transporter down-regulation increases the effects of GABA release.
   E. Release of substance P and other peptides closes the N-methyl-D-aspartate (NMDA) glutamate-gated channel.

10. The dimension of pain thought to include interaction with previous experience and involve the prefrontal cortex is termed:
    A. Sensory-discriminative
    B. Cognitive-evaluative
    C. Affective-motivational
    D. Behavioral-cortical
    E. Emotional-receptive

11. Which of the following is true of placebo analgesia?
    A. It cannot be blocked by naloxone.
    B. The endogenous opioid system is involved.
    C. The somatosensory cortex is involved.
    D. There is no correspondence between placebo analgesia and reward.
    E. All of the above

12. Which of the following is **TRUE** regarding bone cancer pain?
    A. Substance P and other neuropeptides, such as CGRP, are unregulated.
    B. Up-regulation of galanin and neuropeptide Y occurs.
    C. Neuropathic pain and bone cancer pain have similar changes with regard to substance P and CGRP.
    D. The greatest change observed in the spinal cord in response to metastatic bone cancer pain is activation of astrocytes.
    E. All of the above

13. You are performing a neurologic sensory exam. The patient shows normal sensation to light touch in the distributions of the radial and median nerves and increased sensitivity to pinprick. What most accurately describes this phenomenon?
    A. Allodynia
    B. Hypesthesia
    C. Paresthesia
    D. Hyperalgesia
    E. Secondary sensitization

14. Chronic pain conditions are consistently associated with decreased activity in which brain structure(s)?
    A. Prefrontal cortex
    B. Thalamus
    C. Reticular activating system
    D. Pons
    E. All of the above

15. Based on brain-imaging studies, which of the following is implicated as a cause for the autonomic symptoms experienced in cluster headaches?
    A. Activation of the first (ophthalmic) division of the trigeminal nerve
    B. Activation of cranial parasympathetic outflow from the seventh cranial nerve
    C. Cortical spreading depression
    D. Activation of the trigeminovascular system
    E. Hyperemia in the occipital cortex

ANSWERS

1. **D.** The transient receptor potential cation channel subfamily V member 1 (TRPV1) receptor, also known as the capsaicin or vanilloid 1 receptor, responds to stimuli including heat, acidity, and hot pepper capsaicin. These stimuli can enhance each other.

2. **D.** Glutamate is the dominant excitatory nociceptor neurotransmitter.

3. **B.** Intracranial recordings show that the earliest pain-induced signals originate near the secondary somatosensory (SII) cortex, implicating SII and adjacent insula regions as the primary brain areas for receiving nociceptive input.

4. **C.** Secondary sensitization leads to enhanced neural transmission distant from the site of injury, thought to result from reorganized spinal cord nociceptive circuitry. Primary sensitization, in contrast, leads to increased transmission near the site of injury.

5. **B.** A-delta and C fibers are the primary nociceptors in healthy organisms. A-beta afferents are large, non-nociceptive, heavily myelinated touch receptors. However, following central sensitization, input from these touch receptors can result in the sensation of pain.

6. **E.** Currently, there is no objective measure of brain activity that can conclusively determine whether an individual is in pain. However, fMRI and PET are able to provide valuable information regarding the pathologic processing of nociception and pain perception.

7. **B.** Although the pain may be described as inflammatory and/or neuropathic, the patient is clearly experiencing an abnormal response to mechanical light touch. This would be described as tactile allodynia, an experience where a typically innocuous sensation such as light touch becomes painful.

8. **E.** Neuromas are sensitive to multiple sensations and generate spontaneous ectopic activity from both A and C fibers. Noradrenergic sensitization can result in *coupling* of sympathetic and sensory inputs.

9. **B.** In sensitization, opioid receptors are down-regulated with neuropathic pain, though (C) *up-regulated* with inflammatory pain; (A) there is an *increased* release of excitatory neurotransmitters; (D) KCl receptor down-regulation *decreases* the effects of GABA release; (E) these peptides *open* the NMDA channel, leading to increased sensitization.

10. **B.** Traditionally, pain perception consists of the following dimensions: sensory-discriminative, cognitive-evaluative, and affective-motivational. The cognitive-evaluative dimension includes previous experiences and cognitive influences on perception of pain intensity and, traditionally, the prefrontal cortex is thought to be involved in this dimension. Note: Neuroimaging studies have assessed paradigms that do not easily fit into these three traditional dimensions and tend to discuss cortical areas and brain regions involved in specific functions instead.

11. **B.** The placebo response involves the endogenous opioid system and *can* be blocked by naloxone. Studies have shown a correspondence between placebo analgesia and reward pathways. The periaqueductal gray (PAG) and amygdala are involved, as well as the prefrontal/rostral anterior cingulate cortex (ACC).

12. **D.** A unique set of neurochemical changes occur at the level of the spinal cord and dorsal root ganglion for each type of pain: inflammatory, neuropathic, or cancer pain. The greatest change in metastatic bone cancer pain is activation of astrocytes at the spinal cord.

13. **D.** Hyperalgesia describes the abnormally increased response to pain for a stimulus that would typically cause pain, but not to the extent observed. (A) Allodynia describes a painful response to a normally non-noxious stimulus such as light touch. (B) Hypesthesia describes diminished sensation. (C) Paresthesia describes abnormal sensation. (E) Secondary sensitization describes enhanced sensation at sites distant from the site of injury.

14. **B.** Clinical brain imaging studies show reduced activity in and transmission through the *thalamus* for chronic clinical pain (as opposed to experimentally induced acute pain). There is, however, increased activity in the *prefrontal cortex* in chronic pain. These changes support the idea that chronic pain conditions are associated with increased involvement of brain regions for *cognition* and *emotion*. Meanwhile, the *sensory* and *nociceptive* regions of the brain (thalamus) show decreased activity. There is also a reduction in neocortical gray matter.

15. **B.** Activation of cranial parasympathetic outflow from cranial nerve VII is thought to result in the autonomic symptoms in cluster headaches. (A) Activation of V1 is thought to mediate the excruciating unilateral pain in cluster headaches. Answer choices C–E apply to migraine headaches.

An Introduction to Pharmacogenetics in Pain Management: Knowledge of How Pharmacogenomics May Affect Clinical Care

QUESTIONS

1. Polymorphism of an enzyme cofactor involved in tetrahydrobiopterin (BH4) synthesis in primary sensory neurons of the dorsal root ganglion following nerve injury may result in which of the following?
   A. Increased encoding of neuropathic pain stimuli
   B. Reduced sensitivity to painful stimuli
   C. Conversion from acute to chronic neuropathic pain
   D. Reduced response to analgesic medications
   E. Prolonged wound healing

2. Which of the following phenotypes is consistent with either multiple copies of a functional allele or an allele with increased gene transcription?
   A. Nonmetabolizer
   B. Poor metabolizer
   C. Intermediate metabolizer
   D. Extensive metabolizer
   E. Ultra-rapid metabolizer

3. A patient with known mutation in the CYP450 enzyme requires analgesic medication. Which of the following are **NOT** metabolized through this system at standard prescribed doses?
   A. Hydromorphone
   B. Tramadol
   C. Codeine
   D. Oxycodone
   E. Hydrocodone

4. Codeine and hydrocodone are prodrugs metabolized by which enzyme to its analgesic active form?
   A. CYP1A2
   B. CYP2D6
   C. CYP2C9
   D. CYP2C19
   E. CYP3A4

5. Which of the following is the name for a field of medicine that includes a patient's genetic background and uses the information to predict how a patient will respond in terms of efficacy and side effects when given a medication?
   A. Pharmacognosy
   B. Pharmacokinetics
   C. Pharmacogenomics
   D. Genesiology
   E. Pharmacodynamics

ANSWERS

1. **B.** Patients with reduced pain sensitivity are thought to have a polymorphism (a genetic variant) in GTP cyclohydrolase, which is the rate-limiting enzyme involved in tetrahydrobiopterin (BH4) synthesis. BH4 has been shown to be involved in regulation of inflammatory and neuropathic pain. It is estimated that this polymorphism is associated with increased pain tolerance and is present in 15% of the population. Similarly, reduced pain tolerance has been linked to polymorphisms in other genes. Different responses to analgesics among patients can also be attributed to genetic variance.

2. **E.** Classification of phenotypes for enzymes includes the following:
   - Poor metabolizers: Two nonfunctional enzyme alleles.
   - Intermediate metabolizers: At least one reduced functional allele.
   - Extensive metabolizers: At least one functional allele.
   - Ultra-rapid metabolizers: Multiple copies of a functional allele or an allele with a promoter mutation that confers increased transcription of that gene.

Phenotype variations can be responsible for the vast difference in clinical effect as well as side effects between two patients taking the same weight-based dosage of medication.

3. **A.** Although 40%–50% of medications are metabolized in the liver through the CYP450 family of enzymes, three common opioids are not, including hydromorphone, morphine, and oxymorphone.

4. **B.** CYP2D6 is the enzyme needed to convert codeine and hydrocodone to the active analgesic drugs morphine and hydromorphone respectively.

5. **C.** By preemptively identifying patients at risk of adverse side effects or poor efficacy from medication, the field of pharmacogenomics may improve health care outcomes and efficiency, including higher success rate after medication administration, lower incidence of side effects, and reduction of cost. As a relatively new field, it shows promise in terms of tailoring medication regimens to each patient.

12 Psychosocial Aspects of Chronic Pain

QUESTIONS

1. Chronic pain is best understood using which of the following models?
   A. Biomedical
   B. Biopsychosocial
   C. Psychogenic
   D. Secondary-gain
   E. Both A and C

2. In regard to psychological factors that play an important role in the experience of pain, which of the following is an affective factor rather than a cognitive factor?
   A. Anger
   B. Catastrophic thinking
   C. Beliefs about pain
   D. Self-efficacy
   E. Coping

3. All of the following are examples of passive coping strategies **EXCEPT:**
   A. Inactivity
   B. Distraction
   C. Medications
   D. Alcohol
   E. Avoidance

4. According to the operant conditioning principles of reinforcement, the following response to a specific behavior will likely decrease the probability of the behavior recurring:
   A. Neglect
   B. Negative reinforcement
   C. Positive reinforcement
   D. Both A and B
   E. All of the above

5. What is an exaggerated negative orientation toward actual or anticipated pain experiences?
   A. Self-efficacy
   B. Fear avoidance
   C. Pain catastrophizing
   D. Anxiety
   E. Negative reinforcement

6. Your patient had significant pain following his physical therapy sessions and now every time he drives by the facility, he becomes tense and his back pain increases in severity. This is considered:
   A. Classical conditioning
   B. Operant conditioning
   C. Negative reinforcement
   D. Punishment
   E. Fear avoidance

7. According to one study, the target of a patient's anger was most commonly acknowledged to be the:
   A. Health care worker
   B. Attorney
   C. Insurance company
   D. Patient themselves
   E. Significant other

ANSWERS

1. **B.** In chronic pain, there may or may not be an identifiable pathologic process or organic cause. Pain can also take a significant emotional toll on the patient, leading to feelings of demoralization, helplessness, hopelessness, depression, and anxiety, to name a few. Since people rarely live in complete isolation, there is a larger social context that impacts and influences a person's chronic pain. Given the multidimensional nature of chronic pain, a biopsychosocial approach is best used to understand this condition. This model focuses on the illness as a whole, which is the result of a complex interaction of biologic, psychological, and social variables. Both the patient's perception of his/her pain and their response to the illness and treatments can be understood more completely by using this model.

2. **A.** Affective factors are emotions and, in chronic pain, they are mainly negative emotions such as depression, anxiety, and even anger. The other factors listed are cognitive factors, which are involved in how someone thinks, perceives, and reasons. Catastrophic thinking is defined as an exaggerated negative orientation toward actual or anticipated pain experiences. It can also be described as a set of maladaptive beliefs. Beliefs about

the meaning of pain influence a person's expectations about pain and can be either positive or negative. Self-efficacy is a personal conviction that one can successfully execute a course of action to produce a desired outcome. This is a positive factor in chronic pain patients that can affect physical and psychological functioning. The concept of coping is basically self-regulation of pain by using purposeful and intentional acts to help deal with, adjust, reduce, or minimize the pain.

3. **B.** Coping is self-regulation of pain by using purposeful and intentional acts to help deal with, adjust, reduce, or minimize the pain. It can be divided into overt and covert strategies or passive and active strategies. Passive coping strategies involve depending on others for help and restriction of activities and are related to greater pain and depression. These include inactivity, avoidance, medications, alcohol, and drugs. Patients utilizing only passive strategies tend to absolve themselves of personal responsibility for managing their pain. Active strategies, on the other hand, have been associated with adaptive functioning and improvement in pain. These include efforts to function despite pain, distracting oneself from pain, relaxation techniques, and reassuring oneself that the pain will diminish.

4. **A.** The operant principles of reinforcement include positive reinforcement, negative reinforcement, punishment, and neglect. Positive and negative reinforcement both increase the likelihood of a behavior recurring (reinforces), but through different consequences—rewarding the behavior or preventing/withdrawing aversive results respectively. Neglect prevents or withdraws positive results, making a behavior less likely to recur. Punishment, although not an option in the question, also decreases the probability of a behavior recurring but by punishing the behavior.

5. **C.** Pain catastrophizing is defined as an *exaggerated* negative orientation toward actual or anticipated pain experiences. Example: "It's terrible, and I think it's never going to get any better." Fear avoidance, although seemingly similar, is a conditioned response where certain activities which have caused pain in the past are avoided because of the anticipation that they will cause pain.

6. **A.** This is an example of classical conditioning. By experiencing pain following repeated physical therapy sessions, the patient became "conditioned" and experienced a negative emotional response toward the facility, which they associated with the activity. The negative emotional response led to tensing of muscles, which increased their pain, ultimately strengthening the association. This may eventually lead to fear avoidance, where the patient avoids physical therapy (or driving by the facility) because of the anticipation of pain. Negative reinforcement and punishment are both principles of operant conditioning, which focuses on modifying the frequency of a given behavior through the use of consequences, either rewarding or aversive.

7. **D.** There have been studies that show anger to be a fairly common emotion in patients with chronic pain, and it is strongly associated with pain intensity, perceived interference, and pain behaviors. Okifuji and colleagues found that the target of anger was most commonly acknowledged as oneself (70% of patients). Other targets include health care providers (60%), significant others (39%), insurance companies (30%), employers (26%), and attorneys (20%). (Okifuji A, Turk DC, Curran SL. Anger in chronic pain: investigations of anger targets and intensity. *J Psychosom Res.* 1999;47(1):1-12.)

History and Physical Examination of the Pain Patient

13

QUESTIONS

1. A 33-year-old man presents for his yearly physical. On physical examination, upon stroking the lateral aspect of the bottom of his foot, you see his great toe extend. This may be a sign of:
   A. Lower motor neuron dysfunction
   B. A sensory deficit in the foot
   C. Autonomic dysfunction
   D. Upper motor neuron dysfunction
   E. Normal finding in males

2. What is the primary benefit of the physician bringing the patient to the room?
   A. Increases patient satisfaction by perceived reduced wait times
   B. Allows identification of potential inconsistencies on examination
   C. Reduces the amount of time needed for documentation
   D. Improves staff morale
   E. Increases work-flow throughput

3. Hoffman's sign:
   A. Can be seen in healthy individuals
   B. Always represents pathology
   C. Can be affected by SSRI use
   D. Is elucidated by squeezing the dorsal aspect of the third distal phalanx
   E. A and C

4. More than three out of five of Waddell's signs:
   A. Indicates the patient is malingering
   B. Necessitates prompt referral to psychological services
   C. Is grounds for dismissal from the clinic

   D. May be seen with true organic pathology
   E. Definitively differentiates between organic and nonorganic pathology

5. Lumbar discogenic pain:
   A. Maybe exacerbated by the Valsalva maneuver
   B. Is predominantly axial
   C. Is reproduced with straight leg raise testing
   D. Can be provoked with Spurling's maneuver
   E. A and B

6. Motor strength testing:
   A. Is purely subjective
   B. Tests A-δ motor fiber function
   C. May be verified with a Hoover test for effort
   D. Is rated 4/5 when giveaway weakness is noted
   E. Requires placing muscles at a mechanical disadvantage

7. Asking a patient to track a moving object in the eight directions of cardinal gaze tests the functions of cranial nerves:
   A. I, II, III
   B. II, V, VIII
   C. III, IV, VI
   D. III, V, VIII
   E. IV, V, VI

8. A 58-year-old male presents for evaluation of peripheral neuropathy. He has a history of significant alcohol abuse. Chronic alcoholism may also result in the inability to:
   A. Protrude the tongue
   B. Oppose the thumb

C. Sequentially supinate and pronate the hand
D. Shrug the shoulders
E. Flex the hip

9. Which of the following cranial nerves innervates the muscles of mastication?
A. CN IV
B. CN V
C. CN VI
D. CN VII
E. CN VIII

10. A 78-year-old patient presents with neck pain radiating to the left upper extremity. MRI of the cervical spine shows C4–5 subarticular disk herniation contacting the exiting C5 nerve root. C5 radiculopathy will result in:
A. Shoulder external rotation weakness, no reflex changes, decreased sensation in the lateral aspect of the arm
B. Forearm flexion and supination weakness, absent biceps reflex, decreased sensation in the lateral aspect of the forearm
C. Shoulder abduction, extension and flexion weakness, absent biceps reflex, decreased sensation in the lateral aspect of the forearm
D. Forearm extension weakness, absent triceps reflex, decreased sensation in the medial aspect of the arm
E. Forearm flexion in the mid-prone position, absent brachioradialis reflex, decreased sensation in the medial aspect of the forearm

11. A 23-year-old professional football player presents to the pain clinic for evaluation of knee pain that started after he was hit on the side of the knee during a tackle. A positive anterior drawer sign indicates damage to which of the following structures?
A. Medial meniscus
B. Posterior cruciate ligament
C. Patellar tendon
D. Anterior cruciate ligament
E. Medial collateral ligament

12. A 54-year-old female presents with neck pain radiating to the left shoulder. Which of the following is most specific for C5–6 root compression?
A. Left neck pain with simultaneous right lateral flexion and extension of the neck
B. Pain with the abduction of the left arm
C. Pain relief by resting the forearm on the head on the left side
D. Pain with the abduction of the right arm
E. Pain relief by resting the forearm on the head on the right side

13. A 17-year-old baseball player presents with left shoulder pain that is worse on abduction and elevation. These examination findings are consistent with:
A. Subdeltoid bursitis
B. Bicipital tendonitis
C. Rotator cuff tear
D. Impingement syndrome
E. Labral tear

14. A 54-year-old male presents with left foot pain. Physical examination reveals Morton's neuroma. Where is the **MOST** common location of pain in Morton's neuroma?
A. First and second toes
B. Second and third toes
C. Third and fourth toes
D. Fourth and fifth toes
E. Not in the foot

15. Which nerve is entrapped in tarsal tunnel syndrome?
A. Posterior tibial
B. Dorsalis pedis
C. Deep peroneal
D. Superficial peroneal
E. Sural

16. When pain is provoked by placing the patient in the prone position with the knee flexed to 90 degrees and downward force placed on the heel, this is best described as a positive:
A. Drawer test
B. Patellar femoral grinding test
C. Apley's compression test
D. FABER test
E. Lasègue's test

17. Normal thoracolumbar spine range of motion consists of:
A. 90 degrees of forward flexion/30 degrees of back extension/60 degrees of lateral rotation
B. 90 degrees of forward flexion/15 degrees of back extension/45 degrees of lateral rotation
C. 80 degrees of forward flexion/30 degrees of back extension/70 degrees of lateral rotation
D. 90 degrees of forward flexion/15 degrees of back extension/60 degrees of lateral rotation
E. None of the above

18. A 62-year-old male presents with S1 radiculopathy. He can perform five-toe raises while standing and lightly holding onto something for balance. You conclude that he has Grade __ gastrocnemius strength.
A. 2
B. 3
C. 4
D. 5
E. None of the above

19. A patient presents with an inability to evert the foot. What nerve root is most likely damaged?
A. L3
B. L4
C. L5
D. S1
E. S2

20. Concerning spinal examination:
A. Lumbar discogenic pain is associated with intolerance of the standing position.
B. In cervical arthropathy, the positional change will improve the range of motion of the cervical spine.
C. Pain with back extension and lateral rotation suggest facet joint arthropathy.

D. The Spurling maneuver is highly sensitive for confirming a diagnosis of cervical radiculopathy.

E. The normal thoracolumbar spine range of motion is 45 degrees in forward flexion.

21. The "corneal blink" reflex is carried out by an afferent and efferent pathway belonging to which of the following nerves respectively?
A. Optic and abducens
B. Trochlear and V2 of the trigeminal
C. Trigeminal and facial
D. Facial and V1 of the trigeminal
E. Scleral branch of the optic and cervical branch of the facial

22. The "gag" reflex is carried out by an afferent and efferent pathway belonging to which of the following nerves respectively?
A. Vagus and glossopharyngeal
B. Chorda timpani (facial) and glossopharyngeal
C. Superior laryngeal branch of the vagus and recurrent pharyngeal of the vagus
D. Glossopharyngeal and vagus
E. The cranial portion of spinal and vagus

23. The following is **TRUE** about the Hoover test:
A. It is used to test the physiologic weakness of the lower extremities.
B. A positive test occurs when the patient exerts a downward force on the heel of the "nonparetic" leg when asked to elevate the paretic leg.
C. A positive test "rules out" psychogenic etiology of the patient's limb weakness.
D. The test is useful to differentiate between proximal muscle weaknesses from ascending paresis.
E. A positive test occurs when the patient fails to exert a downward force on the heel of the "nonparetic" leg when asked to elevate the paretic leg.

24. The following is **FALSE** about coordination and balance testing related to the cerebellum:

A. The vermis controls axial coordination and balance, whereas the hemispheres coordinate the limbs.
B. Vermis integrity can be tested by asking the patient to walk "heel-to-toe" one foot in front of the other.
C. The hemispheric function can be tested with finger-to-nose skills.
D. Heel-to-shin tests can assess the vermian function.
E. Gait and balance are functions of vermis integrity.

25. Which muscle is correctly matched with the appropriate action, nerve root, and nerve?
A. Infraspinatus: shoulder external rotation, C5–6, suprascapular
B. Biceps: forearm flexion/supination, C5–6, radial
C. Brachioradialis: wrist extension, C6–7, radial
D. Flexor carpi ulnaris: wrist flexion and ulnar deviation, C6–7, ulnar
E. Adductor pollicis longus: thumb abduction, C7–8, median

26. Which of the following is true regarding the vestibulocochlear nerve?
A. Nystagmus on eye movement testing may be a sign of vestibular dysfunction.
B. Testing of the nerve includes the Rinne, Weber, and Snellen tests.
C. In patients with sensorineural deafness and normal hearing, bone conduction is better than air conduction.
D. In unilateral sensorineural hearing loss tested with the Weber test, the sound is heard better in the affected ear.
E. It is the cranial nerve IX.

27. Match the deep tendon reflex with the correct nerve root level:
A. Biceps, C5–6
B. Brachioradialis, C7–8
C. Triceps, C5–6
D. Quadriceps femoris, L1–2
E. Gastrocnemius/Achilles, L4–L5

ANSWERS

1. **D.** Babinski's and Hoffman's signs may be present in patients with upper motor neuron dysfunction. The Babinski reflex is normal in children 0–2 years old.

2. **B.** When the examining physician brings the patient back to the room, it allows them to assess mobility and gait. It also allows observation of function outside of the "formal" examination setting, which could potentially present different findings.

3. **E.** Upper motor neuron lesions can cause hyperreflexia, which may be evaluated by Babinski's and Hoffman's testing. In young women and individuals taking selective serotonin reuptake inhibitor antidepressants, a subtly positive Hoffman's may be present and considered normal.

4. **D.** There are five Waddell's signs; the presence of any three of these five signs are suggestive of a nonorganic pain etiology. However, Waddell's signs may not be able to distinguish accurately between organic and nonorganic causes of pain, according to recent findings, because Waddell's signs can also be present even when there is an organic cause of pain. Findings on the examination should be considered in the context of other information obtained from the patient's history and additional diagnostic studies.

5. **E.** Pain provoked by forward flexion is typical of discogenic or vertebral body pain, because flexion causes axial loading. Lumbar discogenic pain is often only in the axial spine, associated with the inability to sit for long periods and increased pain with coughing, sneezing, and Valsalva.

6. **C.** Muscle strength testing depends on patients' understanding and effort. The Hoover test can help detect the psychogenic weakness of the lower extremities.

7. **C.** Cranial nerves III (ophthalmic), IV (trochlear), and VI (abducens) control eye movement and can be tested by asking the patient to track a moving object in the eight positions of cardinal gaze.

8. **C.** Rapid alternating movements (e.g., sequential hand pronation and supination) are adversely affected in patients with cerebellar disease. Chronic alcohol abuse can cause acquired cerebellar degeneration.

9. **B.** The mandibular division of the trigeminal nerve also supplies the muscles of mastication (i.e., temporalis, masseter, medial, and lateral pterygoid muscles).

10. **C.** The C5–6 nerve roots supply: (1) suprascapular nerve (innervates infraspinatus muscle, which helps with shoulder external rotation), (2) axillary nerve (innervates deltoid muscle, which helps with shoulder abduction, extension, and flexion), and (3) musculocutaneous nerve (innervates biceps muscle, which helps with forearm flexion and supination). The biceps tendon reflex is innervated by C5–6, brachioradialis tendon reflex by C6, and triceps tendon reflex by C7–8. C5 supplies the lateral aspect of the arm, and C6 supplies the lateral aspect of the forearm, thumb, and lateral half of the index finger.

11. **D.** Movement of the tibia forward relative to the rest of the leg constitutes a positive anterior drawer sign and suggests a tear of the anterior cruciate ligament.

12. **C.** A positive abduction tension release sign is highly specific for distinguishing shoulder pathology from C5–6 root compression. This test involves having the patient abduct the affected arm and rest the forearm on top of the head. With shoulder pathology, this will cause pain, but with lower cervical root compression, this typically reduces the radicular pain. The Spurling maneuver can also help to distinguish cervical pathology from other types of pain.

13. **D.** Pain on shoulder abduction and elevation is seen with impingement syndrome due to entrapment of soft tissue between the humeral head and the coracoacromial arch. Other conditions, such as bursitis and rotator cuff pathology, can be present at the same time.

14. **C.** Morton's neuroma is characterized by pain between the metatarsal bones, usually between the third and fourth toes, and less commonly between the second and third toes. The pain is reproducible on palpation of the space between the metatarsal heads.

15. **A.** The posterior tibial nerve in tarsal tunnel syndrome is trapped beneath the laciniate ligament, leading to pain and paresthesia in the foot and toes.

16. **C.** Apley's compression or grinding test is used to evaluate for medial and lateral meniscal tears. This is the test described in the question stem.

17. **A.** For the thoracolumbar spine, normal range of motion is 90 degrees of forward flexion, 30 degrees of back extension, 60 degrees of lateral rotation, and 25 degrees of lateral flexion. The normal range of motion of the cervical spine differs.

18. **C.** Muscle strength is commonly assessed with the Medical Research Council scale. Grades 1–3 are relatively objective and less prone to variation. The gastrocnemius muscle presents unique challenges because, in the case of the gastrocnemius, a Grade 3 = able to perform one toe raise with the patient standing and lightly holding onto something for balance (requires more patient participation). Grade 4 = able to perform five toe raises and Grade 5 = able to perform ten toe raises.

19. **C.** Foot eversion involves the peroneus longus, supplied by the superficial peroneal nerve, which has its source from the L5 nerve root.

20. **C.** Pain from back extension and lateral rotation is suggestive of facet arthropathy (results in zygapophyseal joint loading). The Spurling maneuver is highly *specific* for confirming the diagnosis of cervical radiculopathy. Lumbar discogenic pain is often restricted to the axial spine and is associated with intolerance of the *sitting* position and pain provoked by coughing, sneezing, and Valsalva maneuver.

21. **C.** The trigeminal nerve provides the afferent (ascending, sensory) limb, and facial nerve provides efferent (descending, motor) limb of the corneal blink reflex.

22. **D.** Cranial nerve IX, the glossopharyngeal nerve, provides the afferent limb of the gag reflex (taste in posterior third of tongue and sensation in pharynx). Cranial nerve X, the vagus nerve, innervates the efferent limb of the gag reflex (pharyngeal and laryngeal muscles).

23. **E.** The Hoover test helps to evaluate the psychogenic weakness of the lower extremities. A positive test occurs when the patient fails to exert a downward force on the heel of the "nonparetic" leg when asked to elevate the paretic leg.

24. **D.** Cerebellar function can be divided into midline/ vermal and hemispheric functions. The vermis controls axial coordination and balance (gait and standing balance); the hemispheres coordinate the limbs (finger-to-nose and heel-to-shin tests).

25. **A.**

Upper Extremity Muscles: Innervation and Action

Muscle	Action	Nerve Root	Nerve
Infraspinatus	Shoulder external rotation	C5–6	Suprascapular
Deltoid	Shoulder abduction, extension, and flexion	C5–6	Axillary
Biceps	Forearm flexion and supination	C5–6	Musculocutaneous
Triceps	Forearm extension	C7–8	Radial
Brachioradialis	Forearm flexion in the mid-prone position	C6	Radial
Extensor carpi radialis longus and brevis	Wrist extension	C6–7	Radial
Flexor carpi ulnaris	Wrist flexion with ulnar deviation	C8–T1	Ulnar
Flexor digitorum profundus	Flexion at the distal interphalangeal joints	C7–8	Anterior interosseus branch of the median nerve
Abductor pollicis brevis	Abduction of the thumb	C8	Median
Adductor pollicis longus	Abduction of the thumb	C8–T1	Ulnar

26. **A.** Nystagmus noted that eye movement testing might be a sign of vestibular dysfunction (cranial nerve VIII, vestibulocochlear nerve, mediates hearing, and balance).

27. **A.**

Nerve Root Innervation of the Deep Tendon Reflexes

Muscle Tendon	Nerve Root Level
Biceps	C5–6
Brachioradialis	C6
Triceps	C7–8
Quadriceps femoris	L3–4
Gastrocnemius/Achilles tendon	S1–2

14 Electromyography and Evoked Potentials

QUESTIONS

1. What comprises a motor unit?
   A. A group of muscle fibers innervated by a single anterior horn cell
   B. A single muscle fiber innervated by an axonal branch
   C. A group of muscle fibers that make up a single muscle
   D. A group of muscle fibers innervated by a single nerve root
   E. A group of muscle fibers innervated by a single peripheral nerve

2. Which of the following is most likely an absolute contraindication to needle electromyography (EMG)?
   A. Human immunodeficiency virus
   B. Cardiac pacemaker
   C. Pregnancy
   D. Placing a needle through an infected site
   E. Severe thrombocytopenia

3. What is the most common complication of needle electrode examination?
   A. Infection
   B. Bleeding
   C. Bruising
   D. Weakness
   E. Soreness

4. Which of the following disorders would most likely be normal on nerve conduction studies (NCS)/EMG testing?
   A. Peripheral neuropathy
   B. Myopathy
   C. Radiculopathy
   D. Multiple sclerosis
   E. Amyotrophic lateral sclerosis

5. All of the following will affect nerve conduction velocity **EXCEPT:**
   A. Temperature of the limb
   B. Patient's height
   C. Myelination
   D. Patient's BMI
   E. Patient's age

6. What is the motor conduction velocity of a nerve if the distance between the two stimulus points is 10 cm, the proximal motor latency is 5 ms, and the distal motor latency is 3 ms?
   A. 20 cm/s
   B. 20 m/s
   C. 50 m/s
   D. 80 m/s
   E. Cannot calculate with the given information

7. Which of the following conditions is most likely to have EMG findings that are normal?
   A. HIV-associated distal sensorimotor polyneuropathy
   B. Polymyalgia rheumatica
   C. Amyotrophic lateral sclerosis (ALS)
   D. Radiculopathy
   E. Carpal tunnel syndrome

8. EMG and nerve conduction studies provide all of the following diagnoses **EXCEPT:**
   A. Demyelinating neuropathy
   B. Axonal neuropathy
   C. Primary muscular neuropathy
   D. Neuropathy caused by uncontrolled diabetes
   E. Total denervation injury

9. What is the main reason to perform an H-reflex study?
   A. Evaluate for an L4 radiculopathy
   B. Evaluate for an L5 radiculopathy
   C. Evaluate for an S1 radiculopathy
   D. Evaluate for a C8 radiculopathy
   E. None of the above

10. What is the most severe form of nerve injury and consists of severe disruption or transection of the nerve?
    A. Neurotmesis
    B. Axonotmesis
    C. Neuropraxia
    D. Wallerian degeneration
    E. Cryptogenic neuropathy

11. What is the most sensitive diagnostic test for distal small-fiber neuropathy?
    A. Electromyography
    B. Quantitative sudomotor axon reflex test
    C. Somatosensory evoked potentials
    D. Nerve conduction studies
    E. Motor evoked potentials

12. Which of the findings on a needle examination would be typical of an axonal neuropathy?
    A. 2–3-ms burst of electrical activity of 50–250 mV on initial insertion of the needle into the muscle
    B. A "full" interference pattern on maximum voluntary effort
    C. Presence of an F-wave
    D. Positive sharp waves
    E. Polyphasic potentials with reduced amplitude

13. A patient presents to your clinic with right arm pain and weakness. Her recent EMG/NCS report shows normal sensory and motor nerve conduction studies. However, on needle examination, she has active denervation noted in the cervical paraspinals, right flexor carpi radialis, and right brachioradialis. EMG of the triceps brachii and deltoid were normal. What is the likely source of her pain?
    A. Right C5 radiculopathy
    B. Right C6 radiculopathy
    C. Right C8 radiculopathy
    D. Right median neuropathy
    E. Right radial neuropathy

14. Which of the following is the "gold standard" for the electrodiagnostic evaluation of radiculopathies?
    A. Somatosensory evoked potentials
    B. Motor evoked potentials
    C. Event-related potentials
    D. Hoffman's reflex
    E. Electromyography

15. What is the most common visual evoked potential abnormality seen with multiple sclerosis?
    A. Prolonged N75 latency
    B. Prolonged N145 latency
    C. Prolonged P100 latency
    D. Decreased P100 amplitude
    E. Decreased N75 amplitude

16. Which of the following statements is **FALSE** concerning brainstem auditory evoked potentials (BAEPs)?
    A. Abnormal BAEPs are demonstrated in Friedreich's ataxia.
    B. Testing is limited with marked hearing loss.
    C. Abnormal BAEPs are demonstrated in patients with multiple sclerosis.
    D. They are extremely useful in the diagnosis of acoustic neuromas.
    E. Testing is limited in comatose patients or those under general anesthesia.

17. In regard to somatosensory evoked potentials (SEPs), the following is **TRUE:**
    A. Recording of the SEPs response depends on stimulation of large, fast-conducting sensory fibers in the peripheral nerve.
    B. The nerve conduction pathway spares the primary sensory cortex.
    C. There is no accepted correlation between SEPs and disorders affecting joint and position sense.
    D. SEPs cannot be accurately obtained by stimulation of cranial nerves.
    E. SEPs are not useful in patients with peripheral neuropathy.

18. In the somatosensory evoked potential pathway, a stimulus is propagated from the peripheral nerve to the brain via which of the following routes?
    A. Dorsal root ganglion (DRG), contralateral dorsal column, medial lemniscus, thalamus, cortex
    B. DRG, ipsilateral dorsal column, thalamus, medial lemniscus, cortex
    C. DRG, medial lemniscus, contralateral dorsal column, thalamus, cortex
    D. DRG, ipsilateral dorsal column, medial lemniscus, thalamus, cortex
    E. DRG, contralateral dorsal column, thalamus, medial lemniscus, cortex

19. Which of the following SEP responses is thought to reflect activity in the nerve roots of the cauda equina?
    A. L3S
    B. T11S
    C. P37
    D. N45
    E. None of the above

20. In regard to motor evoked potentials (MEPs), the following is **TRUE:**
    A. Electrical stimulation is more common than magnetic stimulation because electrical is more accurate than magnetic.
    B. The clinical utility of MEPs is in the diagnosis of disorders that affect the central or peripheral motor pathways.
    C. The most accepted way of measuring MEPs is by needle insertion.
    D. MEPs are generally not useful in evaluation of parenchymal brain injury, such as in the case of a cerebrovascular accident.
    E. All of the above

ANSWERS

1. **A.** A motor unit is a group of muscle fibers innervated by a single anterior horn cell. All of the motor units within a muscle are considered a motor pool. The junction between a single muscle fiber and a branch of a motor neuron is the neuromuscular junction.

2. **D.** Many sources report no absolute contraindications to EMG; however, the most likely absolute contraindication to needle EMG is placing a needle through an infected site. Relative contraindications include severe thrombocytopenia and lymphedema.

Cardiac devices such as pacemakers and implanted cardiac defibrillators are relative contraindications for stimulation during NCS. Pregnancy and HIV are not contraindications.

3. **E.** Complications from needle electrode examination are rare, but the most common is transient muscle soreness. Other potential complications include infection, bleeding/bruising, nerve injury, and pneumothorax.

4. **D.** Findings on EMG are almost always normal in diseases of the central nervous system, such as multiple sclerosis. Nerve conduction studies are often normal in radiculopathy, and diagnosis is therefore established using needle EMG. NCS/EMG can be used to help diagnose a number of conditions including peripheral neuropathy, myopathy, and amyotrophic lateral sclerosis.

5. **D.** Of the factors listed, temperature of the limb, patient's height, myelination, and a patient's age will affect nerve conduction velocity. The patient's BMI does *not* have an effect on nerve conduction velocity. Nerve conduction velocity is increased with increased limb temperature, decreased height, and with myelinated fibers. Velocity is decreased in infants and older adults. Although not an option in this question, nerve conduction velocity is also affected by the diameter of the fiber—small fibers are slower than large fibers.

6. **C.** Conduction velocity is based on the difference in *latencies* between the two points of stimulation and the *distance* between the two points of stimulation. It is calculated by the following formula:
MCV (m/s) = DMM/(PML – DML)
DMM – distance between two stimulus points in millimeters
PML – proximal motor latency in milliseconds
DML – distal motor latency in milliseconds
MCV – motor conduction velocity in m/second
Therefore:
MCV = 100 mm/(5 ms – 3 ms) = 50 mm/ms = 50 m/s

7. **B.** Although polymyalgia rheumatica is an important cause of muscle pain and weakness, it is not a true myopathy. Strength is maintained, and inflammation is at the level of the synovium and bursa. EMG findings are also normal in patients with this condition. All the other conditions will most likely have abnormal findings on EMG.

8. **D.** EMG and NCS are useful for localizing sites of neuromuscular disorders and providing information about the nature of the process, whether primarily demyelinating, axonal, primary muscular, or radicular. Unfortunately, it cannot provide the cause of the process (diabetes, tumor, Guillain-Barré syndrome).

9. **C.** The H-reflex, or H-reflex latency, is carried mostly in the S1 nerve root distribution; therefore, the main reason for the study is to evaluate for a S1 radiculopathy. The stimulation impulse travels up the sensory fibers of the posterior tibial nerve,

synapses with the alpha motor neuron, and then returns down the motor fibers of the calf muscle. It may be redundant when a depressed ankle reflex has already been noted on physical examination. Also, the opposite leg must be studied to show a normal H-reflex as a contrast because bilateral absent H-reflex may be caused by peripheral neuropathy. Other pitfalls include the lack of a good H-reflex in many older patients and the inability to tell when the injury occurred if needle EMG is normal.

10. **A.** Nerve injury includes, from mildest to most severe, neuropraxia, axonotmesis, and neurotmesis. Neurotmesis is a severe disruption or transection of the nerve. In this type of injury, neuromas may form, which may be painful, and surgical reanastomosis may be required. Neuropraxia is a loss of conduction without associated changes in axonal structure. Axonotmesis is nerve injury where the axon is disrupted in its myelin sheath. It is also the type of nerve injury associated with Wallerian degeneration.

11. **B.** Quantitative sudomotor axon reflex test (QSART) is the most sensitive diagnostic test for distal small-fiber neuropathy. It is a quantitative thermoregulatory sweat test that is used to detect postganglionic sudomotor failure in neuropathies and preganglionic neuropathies with presumed trans-synaptic degeneration.

12. **D.** A 2–3 ms burst of electrical activity of 50–250 mV in amplitude on insertion of the needle into the muscle is normal insertional activity on needle examination. A "full" interference pattern on maximum voluntary effort is the interference pattern in normal muscle. The F-wave is a small, late muscle response that occurs from backfiring of anterior horn cells. It is used for suspected early Guillain-Barré syndrome. Potentials that are reduced in amplitude and polyphasic are seen in myopathies. Positive sharp waves are spontaneous activity seen in denervated muscle from axonal injury.

13. **B.** First, motor and sensory nerve conduction studies are rarely useful in radiculopathies because the lesion is proximal to the dorsal root ganglion. This is why needle examination is needed when evaluating a patient for radiculopathy. This patient has active denervation in the cervical paraspinals; therefore, we know this probably involves a nerve root instead of a peripheral nerve. There is also active denervation in the right flexor carpi radialis (C6, C7, C8) and right brachioradialis (C6, C7). However, EMG of the triceps brachii (C7, C8) and deltoid (C5, C6) were normal, which makes a C5 and C8 radiculopathy less likely.

14. **E.** Electromyography is the gold standard for the electrodiagnostic evaluation of radiculopathies. Somatosensory evoked potentials have been used through "segmentally specific" techniques and spinal SEPs rather than cortical SEPs, but they are controversial. They seem to be most useful for radiculopathies where sensory symptoms predominate.

15. **C.** Visual evoked potentials evaluate pathology affecting the visual pathways and are used primarily for the diagnosis of multiple sclerosis. The VEP response consists of three peaks—N75, P100, and N145 (N for negative, P for positive, and the number indicating latency in milliseconds). N75 and N145 are of less clinical relevance. The VEP abnormality most commonly seen with multiple sclerosis is prolongation of P100 latency.

16. **E.** Brainstem auditory evoked potentials assess the auditory pathway from the middle ear structures through the eighth cranial nerve and brainstem and into the auditory cortex. They are extremely useful for the diagnosis of acoustic neuromas and can also be used to help diagnose multiple sclerosis and Friedreich's ataxia. The status of a patient does not usually affect the ability to obtain a BAEP response, including patients under general anesthesia and those who are comatose. Marked hearing loss can limit testing by degradation of the response.

17. **A.** Recording of the SEPs response depends on stimulation of large, fast-conducting sensory fibers in the peripheral nerve, and the pathway goes from the peripheral nerve to the primary sensory cortex. In peripheral nerve disease, cortical SEPs can be recorded when sensory nerve responses are not recordable by other techniques because of central nervous system amplification. Conduction velocity can be calculated by stimulating two sites along the peripheral nerve and subtracting the cortical SEPs latencies. SEPs can also be used to identify trigeminal nerve lesions in multiple sclerosis and parasellar and cerebellopontine angle tumors affecting the trigeminal nerve. SEPs can be correlated with proprioceptive disorders, but are usually normal when only pain and temperature sensation are affected.

18. **D.** The somatosensory evoked potential pathway starts with stimulation of large, fast-conducting sensory fibers in the peripheral nerve. The impulse then enters the spinal cord through the dorsal root ganglion and ascends in the ipsilateral dorsal columns. It then crosses to the contralateral side at the medial lemniscus and continues to the contralateral ventroposterolateral nucleus. It then proceeds to the primary sensory cortex.

19. **A.** When the tibial nerve is stimulated at the ankle during somatosensory evoked potentials testing, four peaks are expected: L3S (negative with 19 ms latency), T11S (negative with 21 ms latency), P37 (positive with 37 ms latency), and N45 (negative with 45 ms latency). The L3S peak is thought to reflect activity in the nerve roots of the cauda equina (T11 response from the dorsal fibers of the spinal cord, P37 and N45 from thalamocortical activity).

20. **B.** Motor-evoked potentials are an extension of conventional NCS by allowing assessment of motor pathways in peripheral neuronal structures and central motor conduction pathways. Stimulation is applied centrally and recorded peripherally. Electrical or magnetic stimulation can be used, but magnetic stimulation is preferred because it is relatively painless. Because it assesses the central motor conduction pathways, it can be used to evaluate CNS pathology such as multiple sclerosis, Parkinson's disease, cerebrovascular accident, myelopathy in the cervical and lumbar spine, plexus lesions, and motor neuron disorders.

15 Radiologic Assessment of the Patient With Spine Pain

QUESTIONS

1. In the primary care setting, which of the following is the most common systemic pathologic process causing low back pain?
   A. Metastatic neoplasm
   B. Osteoporotic compression fracture
   C. Discitis
   D. Inflammatory spondyloarthropathy
   E. Epidural abscess

2. Which of the following is true about imaging of *asymptomatic* patients?
   A. Up to 95% of patients over the age of 50 years have age-related disk changes on lumbar X-ray examination (disk space narrowing, anterior osteophytes, vacuum phenomena).
   B. Approximately 60% of patients older than 60 years undergoing lumbar magnetic resonance imaging (MRI) have abnormalities that would be considered significant in an appropriate clinical setting.
   C. In young adults aged 20–22 years, lumbar MRI reveals grade 3 or higher Pfirrmann disk degeneration in approximately half of individuals.
   D. In healthy adults with a mean age of 40 years, T2 signal loss and disk herniations are most common at the L4 and L5 segmental levels (25%–35% of disks) with a high prevalence of asymptomatic high intensity zones (24% at L4 and L5).
   E. All of the above

3. Position and loading play an important role in spinal anatomy and affect imaging sensitivity. All of the following are true **EXCEPT:**
   A. Lumbar extension reduces cross-sectional area of the central canal.
   B. Lumbar flexion decreases neuroforaminal cross-sectional area.
   C. Cervical extension reduces cross-sectional area of the central canal.
   D. Cervical flexion reduces cross-sectional area of the central canal, but less so than extension.
   E. Cervical flexion increases neuroforaminal cross-sectional area.

4. Radiation exposure from spinal imaging is a significant health concern. Which of the following statements is **FALSE?**
   A. A conventional chest X-ray provides 1/30 (0.1 mSv) of the annual natural background radiation exposure in North America (3 mSv).
   B. A three-view lumbar spine X-ray is equivalent in radiation exposure to five chest X-rays.
   C. A cervical x-ray is equivalent in radiation exposure to two chest X-rays.
   D. A lumbar computed tomography (CT) scan provides 6 mSv of exposure, a value equivalent to 60 chest X-rays.
   E. A technetium bone scan has a radiation dose of 6.3 mSv or 63 chest X-rays.

5. Which of the following is the strongest red flag predictor of a neoplastic process underlying a patient's spine pain?
   A. Unexplained weight loss
   B. Age > 70 years
   C. History of cancer
   D. Immunosuppression
   E. Progressive neurologic deficit

6. What type of Modic change is seen at the top of the L5 vertebral body in Fig. 15.1?
   A. Type I
   B. Type II
   C. Type III
   D. None of the above
   E. Both A and B

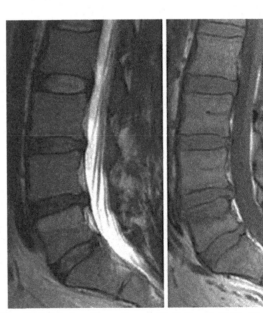

Fig. 15.1 Reprinted from Benzon H, Rathmell JP, Wu CL, et al. *Practical Management of Pain.* 5th ed. Philadelphia, PA: Elsevier Mosby; 2014:200.

7. Which of the following statements is most accurate regarding imaging correlates of discogenic pain as predicted by positive diskography?
   A. Loss of nuclear disk signal is thought to be most predictive.
   B. Severity of disk height loss is not predictive of discogenic pain.
   C. High-intensity zones (HIZ) are always indicative of painful disks.
   D. Modic marrow endplate changes are less significant when they involve >25% of the vertebral body.
   E. Only Modic I changes have correlated with positive diskography.

8. Which of the following is true regarding imaging of zygapophyseal joints and facet joint pain?
   A. Morphologic facet changes such as subchondral sclerosis, erosions, cysts, osteophytes, or joint space narrowing are nonspecific age-related changes.
   B. There is no association between MRI findings of structural facet arthrosis and pain relief with dual medial branch blocks.
   C. T2 hyperintensity within and around the facet joint including the adjacent pedicle and multifidus muscle has been associated with axial pain of facet origin.
   D. Gadolinium enhancement of the facet joint is suggestive of facet synovitis and possibly pain of facet origin.
   E. All of the above

9. Which of the following is **FALSE** regarding imaging of the sacroiliac (SI) joint and SI joint pain?
   A. The inferior and anterosuperior aspects of the radiographically visualized joint are synovial.
   B. Although the surface area of the joint is large, its synovial space volume is small ranging from 1–2.5 cc.
   C. Radiographic narrowing of the SI joint, subchondral sclerosis, osteophyte formation, and vacuum phenomena within the joint indicate that the patient has SI joint pain.
   D. Technetium bone scans are more specific than radiography for identifying patients with SI joint pain as referenced by intraarticular injections.
   E. MRI evidence of active SI joint inflammation with gadolinium enhancement has been correlated with disease activity in sacroiliitis secondary to spondyloarthropathy.

10. A 75-year-old patient presents with focal midline lumbar pain and intermittent bilateral leg pain, worse with extension and ambulation. Imaging with MRI (Fig. 15.2) reveals a posterior midline epidural cyst with neural compression. There is apposition of the L4 and L5 spinous processes. The most likely etiology is:
    A. Bertolotti's syndrome
    B. Baastrup's disease
    C. Zygapophyseal joint arthropathy
    D. Epidural metastasis
    E. Epidural abscess

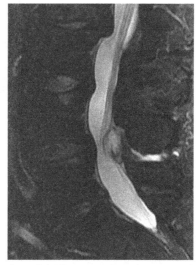

Fig. 15.2 Reprinted from Benzon H, Rathmell JP, Wu CL, et al. *Practical Management of Pain.* 5th ed. Philadelphia, PA: Elsevier Mosby; 2014:210.

11. Pain in Bertolotti's syndrome may emanate from which structure?
    A. Transitional segment neoarticulation
    B. Contralateral facet joint at the level of an asymmetric neoarticulation
    C. Discogenic pain from the disk above the transitional segment
    D. Radicular pain from herniation in the superior adjacent segment disk
    E. All of the above

12. A patient presents with radiculopathy and an MRI image is obtained (Fig. 15.3). Using the appropriate nomenclature, describe the L5–S1 herniation and the anticipated level of radiculopathy.
    A. Focal protrusion, left L5 radiculopathy
    B. Focal protrusion, left S1 radiculopathy
    C. Extrusion, left L5 radiculopathy
    D. Extrusion, left S1 radiculopathy
    E. Sequestration, left L5 radiculopathy

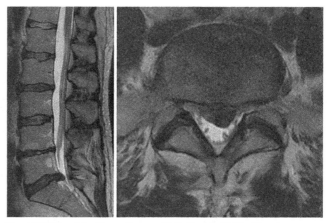

Fig. 15.3 Reprinted from Benzon H, Rathmell JP, Wu CL, et al. *Practical Management of Pain.* 5th ed. Philadelphia, PA: Elsevier Mosby; 2014:216.

13. What is the best imaging modality for distinguishing postoperative epidural scarring from recurrent disk herniation?
    A. CT myelography
    B. MRI without contrast
    C. MRI with contrast
    D. Bone scan
    E. SPECT/CT

14. Which of the following is **FALSE** regarding cervical radicular pain and disk herniations?
    A. The C5 and C6 nerve roots are most commonly affected.
    B. Cervical radicular pain is typically caused by a multifactorial etiology including uncovertebral and facet joint hypertrophy, loss of disk height, and, less commonly, disk herniation.
    C. The vector of cervical disk herniation is typically posterolateral.
    D. Since cervical nerves exit low in the foramen, a herniation will likely affect the exiting nerve rather than the traversing nerve.
    E. Since most cervical radiculopathy etiologies are at least in part bony, complete resolution of pain is less likely than in the lumbar region where a purely disk etiology is more common.

15. What is the dominant structural cause of this patient's lumbar spinal stenosis (Fig. 15.4)?
    A. Disk bulge

B. Facet hypertrophy
C. Ligamentum flavum hypertrophy
D. Short pedicles
E. Spondylolisthesis

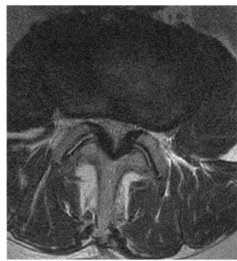

Fig. 15.4 Reprinted from Benzon H, Rathmell JP, Wu CL, et al. *Practical Management of Pain.* 5th ed. Philadelphia, PA: Elsevier Mosby; 2014:225.

ANSWERS

1. **B.** Osteoporotic compression fractures are the most common systemic pathologic process underlying low back pain in the primary care setting (4% of patients). Only 0.7% suffer from undiagnosed metastatic neoplasm. Spine infection (diskitis, epidural abscess) is present in only 0.01% of patients. Inflammatory spondyloarthropathies, such as ankylosing spondylitis, account for 0.3% of presentations.

2. **E.** The evidence is robust that a significant percentage of *asymptomatic* patients present with age-related changes on imaging that are nonspecific for pain. As such, correlation of imaging findings with pain presentation is essential.

3. **B.** Lumbar flexion increases both neuroforaminal and central cross-sectional area. In the cervical spine, however, flexion somewhat reduces central canal area relative to the neutral position, but increases neuroforaminal area.

4. **B.** A typical lumbar spine series (1.5 mSv) has radiation exposure of 15 chest X-rays (0.1 mSv).

5. **C.** History of cancer is the strongest predictor of a neoplastic process as the underlying cause of new onset spine pain.

6. **A.** Type I Modic change exhibits hypointense (dark) signal on T1 and hyperintense (bright) signal on T2 MRI and may enhance with gadolinium. It is indicative of vascularized granulation tissue.

7. **A.** The rank correlation of MRI findings with a positive diskogram was as follows: signal abnormality > disk height > disk contour > HIZ > end plate change. Disk signal change alone was as accurate as other individual parameters or combinations.

8. **E.** Facet morphologic changes are nonspecific for pain and occur universally with age. Signs of edema, hyperemia, and accelerated metabolic activity suggestive of active inflammation, best detected by bone scan or SPECT/CT as well as T2 signal, may be most predictive of facet-mediated pain.

9. **C.** Like the facet joint, age-related morphologic changes of the SI joint are common above the age of 40 years and not predictive of SI joint pain.

10. **B.** This is an interesting presentation of Baastrup's disease, whereby the L4 and L5 spinous processes are in midline contact, resulting in formation of a pseudobursa that extends anteriorly through a midline cleft in the ligamentum flavum and presents

as a midline posterior epidural cyst with claudication symptoms caused by spinal stenosis.

11. **E.** Bertolotti's syndrome involves transitional lumbosacral segment–related pain, which may arise from multiple pain generators, as listed in the question stem.

12. **D.** This L5–S1 disk herniation is an extrusion by sagittal imaging; its paracentral and subarticular location will impact the traversing/descending left S1 nerve root, resulting in the left S1 radiculopathy described.

13. **C.** MRI with gadolinium enhancement is very accurate in distinguishing recurrent disk herniation from epidural fibrosis. Epidural fibrosis enhances rapidly and uniformly following gadolinium administration; disk material does not enhance for the first 20–30 minutes. Early postgadolinium images in the postoperative patient will show recurrent disk herniation as a nonenhancing zone; enhancing epidural fibrosis may surround this.

14. **A.** The most commonly affected cervical nerve roots from disk herniation are the C6 and C7 nerve roots. These herniations typically take place at the C5–6 and C6–7 levels, respectively.

15. **C.** The ligamentum flavum (dark) is the dominant structure causing this patient's lumbar spinal stenosis. While the facet joint does demonstrate hypertrophy, it is not the primary cause of this patient's spinal narrowing. Short pedicles and spondylolisthesis cannot be identified from this axial MRI slice. The disk shows no posterior herniation or bulge.

16 Psychological and Behavioral Assessment

QUESTIONS

1. Which of the following domains is assessed by the Patient Outcome Questionnaire?
   A. Physical functioning
   B. Pain beliefs and coping
   C. Quality of care
   D. Personality
   E. Emotional functioning

2. According to the Initiative on Methods, Measurement, and Pain Assessment in Clinical Trials (IMMPACT) committee's review, which pain intensity scale is recommended for chronic pain clinical trials in adults?
   A. Numerical Rating Scale (NRS)
   B. Verbal Rating Scale (VRS)
   C. Visual Analog Scale (VAS)
   D. FACES Pain Scale
   E. Color Analog Scale (CAS)

3. Psychological and behavioral assessment can be used for all of the following goals **EXCEPT:**
   A. Provide multidimensional information regarding the patient's pain
   B. Determine whether the patient is malingering
   C. Determine whether the patient requires adjunctive psychological treatment
   D. Determine the patient's baseline pain complaint and functioning
   E. Provide information about a patient's suitability for invasive procedures

4. One of your patients with chronic pain is given an assessment that classified him as "interpersonally distressed." Which assessment was he mostly likely given?
   A. Minnesota Multiphasic Personality Inventory
   B. Survey of Pain Attitudes

C. Patient Outcome Questionnaire
D. McGill Pain Questionnaire
E. West Haven-Yale Multidimensional Pain Inventory

5. During biofeedback treatments, which of the following assessments is most commonly used?
   A. Psychophysical measures
   B. Questionnaires and inventories
   C. Behavioral observations
   D. Diaries
   E. Reports from family and significant others

6. The IMMPACT group encouraged the use of measures that were developed and normed for a specific population (e.g., osteoarthritis). Which of the following is a disease-specific measure?
   A. Pain Catastrophizing Scale
   B. Pain Disability Index
   C. Beck Depression Inventory
   D. Oswestry Disability Questionnaire
   E. McGill Pain Questionnaire

7. Which inventory primarily measures physical function?
   A. West Haven-Yale Multidimensional Pain Inventory
   B. Beck Depression Inventory
   C. Brief Pain Inventory
   D. Patient Outcome Questionnaire
   E. Patient-Reported Outcomes Measurement Information System

ANSWERS

1. **C.** The Patient Outcome Questionnaire (POQ) was produced by the American Pain Society to assess the quality of patient care, specifically the patient's perceived quality of pain treatment. The questionnaire consists of 12 items that assess pain severity; the impact of pain on affect, sleep, and activity; side effects; satisfaction with information provided about the pain treatment; shared decision making; and use of nonpharmacologic strategies.

2. **A.** All of the choices are valid measures of pain intensity; however, the IMMPACT group recommended the 11-point numerical rating scale (NRS) to assess pain intensity for chronic pain clinical trials. The main reason was that respondents may prefer VRS and NRS over the VAS. Also, the VAS instruments are more likely to result in missing or incomplete data, and respondents with limited vocabulary or command of English may

have difficulty with the VRS. They recommended the verbal rating scale as an adjunct. The FACES Pain Scale and CAS are primarily used for measuring pain in children.

3. **B.** Psychological and behavioral assessment of pain can be used for the following:
   - Provide information about a patient's pain experiences, treatment history, emotional and physical functioning, and belief about pain
   - Identify a patient's strengths and weaknesses, and the factors that contribute to the development and maintenance of problems in physical, social, and emotional functioning
   - Identify comorbid psychiatric or behavioral conditions that may interfere with pain coping and overall adjustment
   - Determine whether the patient is psychologically appropriate and likely to benefit from surgical or invasive procedures if medically indicated
   - Determine the patient's pain complaint and functioning at baseline

   It is not designed to differentiate between organic and psychogenic pain.

4. **E.** The West Haven-Yale Multidimensional Pain Inventory was designed to measure the psychosocial and behavioral aspects of chronic pain. It is a 52-item, self-report instrument using 7-point Likert scales. It classifies patients with persistent pain into one of three profiles: dysfunctional, interpersonally distressed, or adaptive copers.

5. **A.** Of the assessment strategies listed, psychophysical measures are most commonly used during biofeedback treatments. Psychophysical measures demonstrate that psychological factors can influence biologic reactions, including pain symptoms. When patients are aware of this, behavioral strategies are more successful and patients are more likely to participate in these strategies. Biofeedback uses these measures to teach patients how to modify bodily reactions voluntarily by providing feedback of physiologic processes. Psychophysical measures include surface EMG, blood flow, peripheral skin temperature, and heart rate variability.

6. **D.** The Oswestry Disability Questionnaire assesses a patient's ability to engage in everyday activities and the manner in which pain interferes in functioning. It is disease specific, focusing specifically on chronic lower back pain. None of the other options is disease-specific. The Pain Catastrophizing Scale measures pain-related catastrophic thoughts. The Beck Depression Inventory measures depression, as the name implies, in adolescents and adults. The McGill Pain Questionnaire measures pain intensity, but also pain quality, location, and exacerbating and ameliorating factors.

7. **C.** Originally developed to measure pain intensity and interference, the Brief Pain Inventory is now widely used for non-cancer–related pain. It has demonstrated validity and reliability and was recommended by IMMPACT for use as a measure of physical functioning in pain clinical trials. The West Haven-Yale Multidimensional Pain Inventory and the Patient-Reported Outcomes Measurement Information System both measure psychosocial impact. The Beck Depression Inventory measures emotional function (depression). The Patient Outcome Questionnaire is a quality measure.

17 Disability Assessment

QUESTIONS

1. A patient had a left above-the-knee amputation because of traumatic injury while operating a forklift at his warehouse job. As a result of his accident, he has lost his job and has no financial support to fall back on. Which of the following elements of the Institute of Medicine (IOM) model of disability is this a function?
   A. Medical impairment
   B. Quality of life
   C. Work disability
   D. Functional limitations
   E. All of the above

2. The International Classification of Functioning, Disabilities, and Health (ICF) differs from the International Classification of Impairments, Disabilities, and Handicaps (ICDIH) in that:
   A. It is rooted in the medical model of disease.
   B. It is based upon a linear relationship between the individual and their health condition.
   C. Environmental and personal modifiers affect outcomes.
   D. It is the least accepted model of disablement in the United States.
   E. None of the above

3. A patient presents to your clinic after fracturing their L5 vertebra in a work-related accident. When, under Workers' Compensation (WC) law, is the deadline they have to report their injury to their employer, lest they forfeit benefits?
   A. 3 business days
   B. 2 weeks
   C. 30 days
   D. 3 months
   E. 1 year

4. Maximum medical improvement (MMI) is the point at which a condition (impairment) has stabilized and is unlikely to change (improve or worsen) substantially in what period of time?
   A. 6 months
   B. 12 months
   C. 24 months
   D. 10 years
   E. Indefinite

5. The opinions set forth in the Independent Medical Evaluation (IME) report are expected to be expressed in terms of medical probability versus medical possibility. Which of the following is accurate?
   A. Medical possibility: Something could occur as a result of a particular cause with a probability of greater than 50%.
   B. Medical probability: Something is more likely to occur than not with a probability of greater than 50%.
   C. Medical probability: Something is equally likely to occur than not.
   D. The two terms are interchangeable.
   E. Medical possibility: Something occurs as a cause of an event with high certainty.

6. Which of the following is **NOT** a component of the ICF classification system?
   A. Body functions and body structure
   B. Activity limitations
   C. Participation
   D. Quality of life measures
   E. Impairments

7. A 36-year-old man is working at a fast-food restaurant when he lifts a 50-lb bag of frozen fries and falls over in pain, pointing to his back. The worker has a history of low back problems. He does not return to work for 1 month, but after some physical therapy and medications, his back pain is resolved and he is fully functional. Which of the following terms does this situation define?
   A. Aggravation
   B. Exacerbation
   C. Impairment
   D. Disability
   E. Agitation

8. The World Health Organization's International Classification defines _____ as: "any loss or abnormality of psychological, physiological or anatomical structure or function resulting from a pathology."
   A. Pathology
   B. Impairment
   C. Disability
   D. Handicap
   E. Limitation

9. When measuring disability for compensation purposes, which of the following terms has the highest value and most weight?
   A. Medical impairment
   B. Work impairment
   C. Non-work impairment
   D. Quality of life impairment
   E. Psychiatric impairment

10. The inability to stand because of a spinal cord injury is best described as:
    A. Pathology
    B. Impairment
    C. Disability
    D. Handicap
    E. Psychogenic

11. Which of the following is true regarding the Workers' Compensation system?
    A. Injury must be reported to the employer within 90 days of injury.
    B. A causality determination related to work does not have to be made.
    C. The Social Security Administration adjudicates.
    D. Benefits may be forfeited if refusing to return to work when cleared.
    E. The work injury is typically the fault of the employer

12. Which of the following is **NOT** a component of the biopsychosocial model of disability?

A. The psychological component
B. The economic component
C. The social component
D. The medical component
E. The personal component

13. Which of the following is true about Social Security Administration (SSA)?
    A. Social Security Disability Insurance (SSDI) extends coverage to disabled workers who would have worked in a qualified job for 5 of the 10 preceding years and who are younger than 65 years of age.
    B. SSDI is funded through Federal Insurance Contribution Act (FICA) payroll taxes.
    C. Supplemental Security Income (SSI) provides income for medically indigent persons who suffer from blindness, disability, or are more than 65 years of age.
    D. SSI does not require a work history to be eligible.
    E. All of the above

14. Which organization is recognized nationally and globally as the preferred reference for medical impairment ratings?
    A. The International Association of Impairment Ratings
    B. The Veterans Benefits Administration
    C. The Social Security Administration
    D. The ICF of the World Health Organization
    E. The American Medical Association

ANSWERS

1. **C.** The IOM developed a generalized model to demonstrate common features to all disability models. This model consists of five domains. Medical impairment is the first domain and can be measured objectively. Functional limitation is the second domain and is measured in terms of basic and advanced activities of daily living. Work disability is the third domain and can be attributed to financial losses resulting from work impairment. Non-work disability is the fourth domain and describes losses in terms of social aspects, hobbies, and recreational pursuits. Quality of life is the fifth domain and pertains to diminished life satisfaction.

2. **C.** The ICF portrays a more nonlinear, interactive association between an individual with a health condition and takes into consideration factors of personal and environmental nature, as opposed to the ICIDH system, which is more linear, with a unidirectional and causal relationship that is rooted in the medical model of disease.

3. **C.** A causality determination must be made that the injury or illness arose out of the course of employment and occurred while the employee was at work and actively participating in work activities. Injury or illness

must be reported to the employer within 30 days of the inciting event and a claim filed within 1 year for disability and 2 years for death.

4. **B.** MMI is the point at which a condition has stabilized and is unlikely to change (improve or worsen) substantially in the next 12 months, with or without treatment. It does not preclude any further deterioration of a condition beyond this time period and does not preclude allowances for ongoing follow-up or maintenance care.

5. **B.** Medical *possibility* refers to when something *could* occur as a result of a particular cause with a probability of 50% or less. Medical *probability* refers to when something is *more likely to occur* than not with a probability exceeding 50%.

6. **D.** The World Health Organization's ICF classification system falls short in its adequate attention given to measures of quality of life.

7. **B.** Exacerbation is a circumstance that *temporarily* worsens a preexisting condition. Aggravation is a circumstance or event that *permanently* worsens a preexisting condition. Impairment is a significant

deviation, loss, or loss of use of any body structure or function in an individual with a health condition. Disability is any restriction to perform an activity within the range considered normal.

8. **B.** Impairment is "any loss or abnormality of a psychological, physiological or anatomical structure or function resulting from a pathology." Pathology is a disease or trauma acting at a tissue, anatomic, or physiologic level potentially to alter the structure and functioning of an organ. Disability is any restriction or lack of ability to perform an activity in the manner or within the range considered normal. Handicap is a disadvantage for an individual that limits fulfillment of a role that is normal for that individual.

9. **A.** Medical impairment, the first domain of the IOM, carries the most weight because it is anatomically and physiologically based and therefore more suitable to objective measurement.

10. **C.** Disability is commonly conceptualized in terms of limitations in activities within one's personal sphere, including mobility and self-care. It is the functional consequences of or abilities lost from an injury.

11. **D.** Injury must be reported to the employer within 30 days. Workers' Compensation is a no-fault system where the employee foregoes the right to sue the employer in exchange for coverage when requirements are met. Benefits may be forfeited in cases of substance abuse or intoxication at time of injury, refusal to comply with safety rules and equipment, being incarcerated, or refusing to return back to work after being medically cleared.

12. **B.** The biopsychosocial model of disability is the accepted and preferred conceptual model for disablement. It recognizes contributions of medical, social, personal, and psychological determinants of disability.

13. **E.** SSA offers two separate disability programs, SSDI and SSI. SSDI is funded through payroll tax at a federal level and SSI is funded through a federal and state partnership with funds derived from both federal and state income tax. SSI does not require a work history to be eligible.

14. **E.** The AMA has produced ratings manuals to assist physicians in rating impairment. Original ratings articles were published in 1971 and have been periodically updated and revised. The AMA Guidelines to the Evaluation of Permanent Impairment is recognized nationally and globally and is the preferred reference for medical impairment ratings. It is recognized in most of Canada, the Netherlands, Australia, New Zealand, Hong Kong, and Korea.

PART 4

CLINICAL CONDITIONS

Postoperative Pain and Other Acute Pain Syndromes

18

QUESTIONS

1. Preventive analgesia is best described as:
   A. Preventing central sensitization
   B. Preventing painful insult
   C. Preventing the inflammatory reaction after an insult
   D. Preventing the need for multimodal analgesia
   E. None of the above

2. All of the following are true regarding ketamine **EXCEPT:**
   A. It is an NMDA (N-methyl-D-aspartate) receptor antagonist.
   B. It is recommended for neuraxial anesthesia.
   C. It is beneficial in low doses.
   D. It is helpful in the management of opioid-induced hyperalgesia.
   E. It can attenuate central sensitization.

3. Each of the following is an example of multimodal analgesia **EXCEPT:**
   A. Intravenous (IV) acetaminophen with oral (PO) ibuprofen
   B. Paravertebral block with IV fentanyl
   C. IV ketorolac with PO ibuprofen
   D. PO acetaminophen with IV patient-controlled analgesia (PCA) morphine
   E. Preoperative PO gabapentin with intraoperative lidocaine skin infiltration

4. All of the following are advantages of IV PCA morphine over traditional "as-needed" (PRN) analgesic regimens **EXCEPT:**
   A. Addresses interpatient and intrapatient variability in analgesic needs
   B. Provides superior analgesia

   C. Decreased respiratory depression
   D. Fewer pulmonary complications
   E. Improved patient satisfaction

5. Which of the following statements about neuraxial spread of opioid is correct?
   A. Sufentanil spreads more rostral than morphine.
   B. Fentanyl spreads more rostral than morphine.
   C. Fentanyl spreads more rostral than hydromorphone.
   D. Morphine spreads more rostral than sufentanil.
   E. None of the above

6. Which of the following statements regarding acetaminophen is true?
   A. It is available in oral, rectal, intramuscular (IM) depot, and IV formulations.
   B. Its mechanism of action is more peripheral than central.
   C. When compared with PO route, IV acetaminophen provides faster onset of pain relief, but the time to maximal pain relief is the same.
   D. Coadministration with opioids appears to provide opioid-sparing analgesia but may not reduce opioid-related side effects.
   E. It is associated with renal toxicity.

7. All of the following statements about gabapentin are true **EXCEPT:**
   A. It may decrease postoperative requirement of opioids.
   B. It can cause postoperative dizziness and sedation.
   C. It is structurally similar to γ-aminobutyric acid (GABA).
   D. It works through the GABA receptor.
   E. It works through calcium channel inhibition.

8. All are advantages of continuous epidural analgesia **EXCEPT:**
   A. Decreases pulmonary and cardiovascular complications
   B. Leads to shorter length of hospital stay when compared with IV PCA
   C. Can be used as fixed-rate infusion, patient-controlled boluses, or combinations of both
   D. May decrease opioid side effects
   E. More efficacious analgesia than IV PCA

9. What is the most common side effect of neuraxial opioids?
   A. Nausea and vomiting
   B. Pruritus
   C. Urinary retention
   D. Respiratory depression
   E. Double vision

10. All of the following are true regarding ultrasound-guided regional anesthesia (UGRA) when compared with nerve stimulation **EXCEPT:**
    A. UGRA offers a faster onset of sensory blockade and a greater block success rate.
    B. UGRA is associated with fewer complications.
    C. UGRA achieves faster block performance and requires fewer needle passes.
    D. UGRA causes less block-related discomfort, thus making this technique better received by patients.
    E. All of the above are true.

11. Which of the following is uncommon with interscalene block?
    A. Phrenic nerve block
    B. Ulnar nerve block
    C. Superior trunk block
    D. Middle trunk block
    E. Musculocutaneous nerve block

12. Which site is the most stable for placing a catheter to block the brachial plexus?
    A. Interscalene
    B. Supraclavicular
    C. Infraclavicular
    D. Axillary
    E. Antecubital

13. All of the following nerves are blocked in a lumbar plexus block **EXCEPT:**
    A. Obturator
    B. Sciatic
    C. Saphenous
    D. Lateral femoral cutaneous
    E. Femoral

14. All of the following are advantages of continuous femoral infusion versus IV PCA in patients undergoing total knee replacement **EXCEPT:**
    A. Complete analgesia of lower extremity
    B. Reduction in postoperative bleeding
    C. Lower opioid consumption
    D. Early ambulation
    E. Decrease in the length of hospitalization

15. Which statement about popliteal blocks is true?
    A. The lateral approach is considered superior to posterior approach.
    B. Popliteal fossa block provides effective postoperative analgesia for all foot and ankle procedures.
    C. Blocking the tibial and common peroneal nerves in the popliteal fossa separately at the bifurcation provides a faster onset than does a prebifurcation sciatic block.
    D. Continuous-infusion nerve blocks and single-injection blocks have similar outcomes.
    E. All of the above

16. All of the following statements about intraarticular injections are true **EXCEPT:**
    A. Intraarticular morphine provides benefit mainly for highly inflammatory joint surgery.
    B. Intraarticular neostigmine is usually associated with increased postoperative nausea and vomiting (PONV).
    C. Clonidine is equivalent to morphine in terms of analgesia.
    D. Meperidine has dual opioid and local anesthetic effects.
    E. Regional anesthesia might be superior to intraarticular injection of local anesthetics.

17. Which of the following should be avoided when managing acute pain in opioid-tolerant patients?
    A. Parenteral hydromorphone
    B. Ketorolac
    C. Buprenorphine
    D. Ketamine
    E. Methadone

18. Which of the following is an age-related change in the elderly?
    A. Increased pain perception
    B. Decreased sensitivity to opioids
    C. Postoperative gastrointestinal hyperactivity
    D. Increased incidence of pulmonary complications with use of PCA morphine
    E. Increased safety profile of semisynthetic opioids such as oxymorphone

19. A chronic alcoholic patient fell down the stairs and presented with multiple left rib fractures. You can smell alcohol on his breath. He is cooperative and is in severe pain. Which is the best option for pain management?
    A. Morphine
    B. Acetaminophen
    C. Codeine
    D. Paravertebral or intercostal block
    E. Intravenous patient-controlled analgesia

20. A young man has had a motor vehicle accident causing fractures of both arms and suspected head injury. Which of the following therapies is a good choice for initial management of pain related to examination and fracture manipulation?
    A. Acetaminophen

B. Fentanyl
C. Ketorolac
D. Nitrous oxide
E. Hydromorphone

A. Fentanyl
B. Ibuprofen
C. Ketamine
D. Lidocaine
E. Femoral nerve block

21. Which of the following is **LEAST** beneficial to manage pain in a patient suffering from third-degree burns of the back, chest, and lower extremities?

ANSWERS

1. **A.** Preventive analgesia is a method of preventing or attenuating the central sensitization that results from a painful insult and the inflammatory reaction that develops after the insult. For preventive analgesia to effectively prevent central sensitization and reduce postoperative and chronic pain, intensive multimodal analgesic interventions should be used during the perioperative period.

2. **B.** Ketamine is an N-methyl-D-aspartate (NMDA) receptor antagonist. In low doses (0.25 mg/kg), it may attenuate central sensitization (chronic postsurgical pain) and opioid tolerance without cognitive impairments or psychotomimetic effects. It may attenuate opioid-related side effects, postoperative pain, chronic pain, and opioid-induced hyperalgesia. Reports of epidural and intrathecal ketamine have been published, but neuraxial use of ketamine is discouraged until further safety and neurotoxicity data are available.

3. **C.** Multimodal analgesia involves the administration of two or more analgesic agents by one or more routes that exert their effects via different analgesic mechanisms and ideally act synergistically at different sites in the nervous system, thereby providing superior analgesia with fewer side effects. The concept of a multimodal strategy, including regional analgesia, was introduced to allow early ambulation, promote better rehabilitation, accelerate recovery, and reduce the length of hospital stay. Ketorolac and ibuprofen are both nonsteroidal anti-inflammatory drugs (NSAIDs) belonging to the same class of analgesics; thus, a combination of these is not an example of multimodal analgesia.

4. **C.** IV PCA allows the clinician to compensate for several factors, including the wide interpatient and intrapatient variability in analgesic needs, variability in serum drug levels, and administrative delays, which might result in inadequate postoperative analgesia. When compared with traditional PRN analgesic regimens, the use of IV PCA may be associated with improved patient outcomes, including superior postoperative analgesia, improved patient satisfaction, and possibly decreased risk for pulmonary complications. The incidence of opioid-related side effects, including respiratory depression (0.5%), from IV PCA does not appear to differ

significantly from that of other administration routes (e.g., IV, IM, or subcutaneous).

5. **D.** Hydrophilic opioids (e.g., morphine and hydromorphone) tend to remain within cerebrospinal fluid (CSF) after neuraxial administration and usually produce a delayed but longer duration of analgesia. They also tend to cause a higher incidence of side effects because of CSF spread rostrally, unlike lipophilic opioids (e.g., fentanyl and sufentanil), which tend to provide a faster onset but shorter duration of analgesia as a result of rapid clearance from CSF.

6. **D.** Coadministration of acetaminophen with opioids appears to provide opioid-sparing analgesia but may not reduce opioid-related side effects. Acetaminophen rapidly crosses the blood-brain barrier and inhibits central prostaglandins via the COX pathways. It also triggers the activation of cannabinoid receptors and inhibits nitric oxide pathways. Acetaminophen has weak peripheral anti-inflammatory activity. When compared with oral acetaminophen, IV acetaminophen provides faster onset of pain relief, reduces the duration of meaningful pain, and decreases the time to maximal pain relief. Acetaminophen is available in rectal, oral, and IV formulations. It is often associated with hepatic, not renal toxicity.

7. **D.** Gabapentin is analogous in molecular structure to GABA (γ-aminobutyric acid), but does not act on the GABA receptor. Studies have shown benefit in acute pain management when an oral dose of 1200 mg gabapentin was administered preoperatively. One of these studies also incorporated a limited postoperative dosing course (for 10 days after breast surgery) and reported lower opioid requirements and pain scores with movement. Side effects are sedation, dizziness, and visual disturbance. It may be useful for acute analgesia and chronic antihyperalgesia.

8. **B.** Continuous epidural analgesia may provide a longer duration of analgesia than an individual injection and analgesia superior to that with systemic opioids. Postoperative use of continuous epidural analgesia may be associated with improved patient morbidity by decreasing pulmonary, cardiovascular, and gastrointestinal complications in high-risk patients and after high-risk procedures. Postoperative epidural analgesia may be delivered as a fixed continuous

infusion or as patient-controlled epidural analgesia (PCEA). Based on the principles of PCA, PCEA allows individualization of postoperative analgesic requirements, reduces drug use, improves patient satisfaction, and provides superior analgesia.

9. **C.** Neuraxial opioids are associated with side effects that could affect patients' quality of recovery. Side effects include nausea and vomiting in more than 50% of patients, and pruritus in up to 60%, as opposed to 15%–18% for PCEA with local anesthetic or systemic opioids. Other adverse effects include urinary retention in up to 80% of patients and respiratory depression in 0.2%–1.9%. These side effects are not limited to any specific opioid and it is not clear whether their incidence is dose dependent.

10. **B.** Studies have shown that when compared with nerve stimulation, the use of UGRA for upper or lower extremity blocks and placement of catheters offers a faster onset of sensory blockade and a greater block success rate. UGRA has also been shown to achieve faster block performance, require fewer needle passes, and induce less block-related discomfort, thus making this technique better received by patients. An analysis of neurologic complications in 1000 UGRA procedures for elective orthopedic surgery showed that the rate of postoperative neurologic symptoms was very similar to that previously reported for traditional techniques.

11. **B.** The interscalene approach typically provides a complete block for the superior and middle trunk, but the inferior trunk is often blocked incompletely, thus making this approach unsuitable for forearm and hand procedures. For elbow procedures, the interscalene block is frequently supplemented by other nerve blocks such as the intercostobrachial, medial cutaneous and medial antebrachial cutaneous, and ulnar.

12. **C.** Infraclavicular block approaches the brachial plexus where it is compact at the level of the cords. This block can be used for procedures involving the elbow, forearm, and hand. It is especially useful in patients unable to abduct their shoulder to allow access to the axilla. This approach also results in the most secure catheter insertion site for the brachial plexus.

13. **B.** Lumbar plexus block (LPB) is a reliable way to block the femoral, lateral femoral cutaneous, and obturator nerves with a single injection. Since the saphenous nerve is an extension of the femoral nerve, it is blocked too. The sciatic nerve arises from the sacral plexus (L4–5, S1–3) and is not covered.

14. **A.** A femoral block must often be supplemented with a single-shot or continuous sciatic nerve block for complete analgesia of lower extremity, because it does not cover the sacral plexus. In a study of patients undergoing total knee replacement, continuous femoral infusion patients (vs. IV PCA patients) had a 72% reduction in postoperative bleeding ($P = 0.05$), achieved better performance on continuous passive

motion, had a 90% decrease in serious complications, ambulated sooner (2.5 vs. 3.5 days), and had a 20% decrease in the length of hospitalization (4 vs. 5.5 days).

15. **C.** The popliteal nerve can be blocked from the posterior or lateral approach, although the lateral approach may be superior when there are concerns regarding patient positioning. A popliteal fossa block, when supplemented with a saphenous nerve block, provides effective postoperative analgesia for all foot and ankle procedures. When the UGRA technique is used, blocking the tibial and common peroneal nerves in the popliteal fossa separately at the bifurcation provides a faster onset than does a prebifurcation sciatic block.

16. **B.** Combination drug therapies for intraarticular analgesia have been shown to produce maximum benefit with fewer side effects. Intraarticular morphine provides benefit mainly for highly inflammatory joint surgery. Intraarticular meperidine has a dual opioid and local anesthetic effect. Intraarticular administration of neostigmine (0.5 mg) was shown to provide more pain relief than morphine (2 mg) in patients undergoing knee arthroscopy. Intraarticular neostigmine (0.5 mg) has not been reported to increase PONV. Clonidine (150 µg) was found to be equivalent to morphine (2 mg) and superior to placebo, but the combination of clonidine and morphine provided no additional benefit. Evidence suggests that regional anesthesia might be superior to intraarticular injection of local anesthetics. Continuous perineural analgesia provides better analgesia than intraarticular injection of local anesthetics but requires strong technical skills.

17. **C.** Opioid-tolerant patients could be those who use opioids legitimately for the treatment of chronic pain, those who obtain and use opioid medications illicitly, and those who abuse heroin. Ketorolac is particularly useful because it has been shown to decrease morphine use and morphine-related side effects. NMDA receptor antagonists such as ketamine potentiate the analgesic effects of opioids and may decrease opioid tolerance. Methadone, commonly used in maintenance therapy as an anti-addictive agent for patients with opioid dependency, should be continued. The use of opioid agonists/antagonists such as buprenorphine and nalbuphine should be avoided in opioid-tolerant patients because they may potentiate acute opioid withdrawal reactions.

18. **E.** Studies have indicated that pain perception may decrease with increasing age, in part because of decreased Aδ- and C-fiber function and delays in central sensitization. Older patients have increased sensitivity to and bioavailability of opioids because of a decrease in the number and affinity of tissue receptors and diminished first-pass activity. The use of IV titration of opioids or PCA in the elderly is safe. No difference in the incidence of pulmonary

complications has been observed in the elderly with the use of PCA and systemic injections. Semisynthetic opioid agonists such as oxymorphone are particularly safe to use because they are not metabolized through the cytochrome P-450 system. Hence, they have less risk for drug interaction. The elderly are more prone to the development of postoperative ileus.

19. **D.** Administration of sedative or opioid medications places an intoxicated patient at risk of increased CNS and respiratory depression because of the additive effects with alcohol. Therefore, morphine is not the best choice. In patients with alcoholic cirrhosis and advanced liver disease, altered metabolism and excretion of drugs will change the dosing of hepatically metabolized medications (such as codeine). Neuraxial or regional techniques such as intercostal nerve or paravertebral blocks should be considered as long as coagulopathy has been ruled out.

20. **A.** To minimize the sedating effects of opioids, analgesic treatments should include the use of nonsedating analgesic agents and opioid-reducing strategies whenever possible. IV acetaminophen is a good choice for mild to moderate pain. In patients where head trauma is suspected, infusion of remifentanil, an ultrashort-acting opioid, is safe. It allows rapid neurologic evaluation. NSAIDs such as ibuprofen and ketorolac are best avoided in any patient at risk of intracranial bleeding because of the platelet-inhibiting effects of this drug class. Nitrous oxide is contraindicated if the patient potentially has pneumothorax or bowel obstruction. Isolated peripheral nerve blocks may also be useful in the management of extremity injuries. The use of continuous-infusion peripheral nerve catheters should be considered in patients with more extensive trauma for which the duration of severe pain is expected to be longer than 1–2 days.

21. **E.** Opioids continue to be the primary therapy for the management of background and procedural pain in burn patients. Regional anesthetic techniques are of limited use in patients with extensive burns but could be used in cases of mild, isolated extremity burns.

19

The Prediction and Prevention of Persistent Postsurgical Pain

QUESTIONS

1. Persistent postsurgical pain is seen in:
   A. <1% of patients
   B. 1%–10% of patients
   C. 10%–20% of patients
   D. 20%–30% of patients
   E. >30% of patients

2. An intervention that is initiated before a nociceptive stimulus (e.g., surgical incision) and then continued until the major nociceptive stimulus has abated is called:
   A. Preemptive analgesia
   B. Preventive analgesia
   C. Protective analgesia
   D. Sensitization
   E. Antinociceptive analgesia

3. Which approach for thoracotomy is associated with the highest incidence of persistent chronic pain?
   A. Video-assisted thoracoscopic surgery
   B. Posterolateral
   C. Anterior
   D. Equal for all of the above
   E. Equally high for anterior and posterolateral approach

4. Which surgical procedure has the greatest association with persistent postsurgical pain?
   A. Mastectomy
   B. Thoracotomy
   C. Amputation
   D. Cesarean section
   E. Cholecystectomy

5. All of the following statements about persistent postsurgical pain (PPSP) are true **EXCEPT:**
   A. Outcomes are worse when a procedure is performed in a low-volume institution.

   B. Radiation therapy for women undergoing breast and axillary surgery is associated with decreased probability of chronic pain.
   C. Interpatient variability may predict the evolution of acute pain to chronic pain.
   D. Psychological vulnerability has been found to be a predictor of long-term pain.
   E. B and D

6. What is the best intervention to decrease postoperative pain in breast surgery patients?
   A. Paravertebral block
   B. Perioperative methylprednisolone
   C. Perioperative parecoxib
   D. Perioperative gabapentin
   E. EMLA cream

7. All of the following are predictors of worse outcome following total hip arthroplasty (THA) **EXCEPT:**
   A. Preoperative report of pain in multiple joints
   B. Older age
   C. Female gender
   D. Depression
   E. All of the above are associated with worse outcome.

8. Which of the following should be avoided in thoracic surgery?
   A. Gabapentin
   B. Ketamine in epidural infusions
   C. Remifentanil at high doses
   D. Intercostal sutures
   E. Paravertebral blocks

ANSWERS

1. **E.** Cross-sectional quality-of-life surveys reveal that 40% of the population who underwent surgery in the last 3 years reported persistent pain at the surgical site.

2. **B.** Preventive analgesia is defined as an intervention that is initiated before a nociceptive stimulus (e.g., surgical incision) and continued until the major nociceptive stimulus has abated. The intervention needs to

decrease significantly or eliminate the usual immediate effect of the nociceptive stimulus (e.g., pain, central sensitization).

3. **B.** For thoracotomy, an anterior approach appears to be associated with less acute and chronic pain than the classic posterolateral approach. Additionally, there may be less acute and chronic pain with video-assisted thoracoscopic surgery than with the same operation performed as an open procedure. There are data to support the hypothesis that minimally invasive surgical procedures are associated with less chronic pain than the same operations performed as open procedures.

4. **C.** Procedures such as lower extremity amputation and posterolateral thoracotomy have a high prevalence of chronic pain (>50%), with lower extremity amputation having the highest prevalence. Chronic pain is not as prevalent in other procedures, such as cataract surgery. Additionally, the prevalence of pain may decrease following certain surgeries (hip arthroplasty, lumbar laminectomy for a herniated disk) but increase following other surgeries (thoracotomy, breast surgery).

5. **B.** For a number of major high-risk surgeries, outcome is worse when the procedure is performed in a low-volume institution and a large part of the risk can be attributed to low-volume surgeons. Adjuvant treatments associated with a number of surgical procedures for cancer may also play a role in the development of PPSP. In particular, radiation therapy for women undergoing breast and axillary surgery is associated with an increased probability of chronic pain.

6. **A.** Two randomized controlled studies evaluating the influence of perioperative paravertebral blockade on persistent pain following breast surgery both uncovered a significantly lower prevalence of chronic pain in women who had the block.

7. **C.** Predictors of a worse outcome after THA include a preoperative report of pain in multiple joints, older age, and male gender. One finding that has become obvious recently is that the presence of pain at other sites is a major predictor of persistent pain following THA. Additionally, mental health has an effect, with depression being associated with a higher probability of persistent pain or worse score on the mental health component of the 36-item Short Form Health Survey (SF-36). Depression has been associated with worse outcomes and is a predictor of PPSP.

8. **C.** High-dose remifentanil is associated with increased allodynia and increased pain for up to 6 months.

20 Pediatric Acute Pain Management

QUESTIONS

1. What is an advantage of the FLACC (face, legs, activity, cry, consolability) scale for pain?
   A. It can be used for all ages and for mentally challenged children.
   B. It allows the patient to characterize their pain.
   C. It includes history from the child's parents.
   D. It gives analgesic recommendations based on the pain score.
   E. It aids in identifying the source of the pain.

2. Controlled trials demonstrated safe patient-controlled analgesia (PCA) use above what age?
   A. 15 years old
   B. 12 years old
   C. 10 years old
   D. 6 years old
   E. 3 years old

3. Which of the following is appropriate to administer first-line for mild procedural pain in infants less than 6 months old?
   A. Hydromorphone
   B. Sucrose
   C. Acetaminophen
   D. Codeine
   E. Morphine

4. Which of the following is a concern when administering opioids to neonates and infants?
   A. Neonates and infants are more prone to nausea and vomiting from opioids.
   B. Opioids do not provide analgesia for moderate to severe pain in neonates and infants.
   C. Neonates and infants are more prone to opioid-induced respiratory depression.
   D. Opioids increase risk of bleeding resulting from platelet dysfunction in neonates and infants.
   E. Opioids are associated with dose-dependent hepatotoxicity in neonates and infants.

5. Which of the following is the best choice for long-lasting analgesia in children undergoing major foot and ankle surgery?
   A. Continuous sciatic nerve catheter
   B. Epidural anesthesia
   C. Spinal anesthesia
   D. Caudal anesthesia
   E. Single-shot femoral nerve block

ANSWERS

1. **A.** The FLACC scale ranges from zero to ten points and is solely based on clinician observation of behavior. It does not require the patient or the patient's parents to answer questions. This lack of self-reporting is beneficial because the scale can be used for all age ranges and for mentally challenged children. Scoring is based on five parameters, including face, legs, activity, cry, and consolability, with points ranging from zero (no signs of distress) to two (maximum signs of distress) for each parameter.

2. **D.** Trials have demonstrated effective PCA analgesia in patients aged 6 years and older. Unlike PCA use in adult patients, use of PCA in pediatric patients can be extended to include the initiation of a dose by the patient's nurse or parent. Although this can be somewhat controversial, it is commonplace for individuals other than the patient to administer doses cautiously from a PCA in pediatric pain management.

3. **B.** Sucrose is thought to stimulate the ventral striatum and cingulate gyrus in a similar manner to opioids and can have analgesic benefits; it is appropriate for first-line treatment of mild procedural pain for infants less than 6 months old.

4. **C.** As with adults, a multimodal approach to pain management is desirable when caring for pediatric patients. Although they are effective analgesics, opioid doses should be minimized, especially in patients less than 6 months old because of lower rate of clearance. Neonates and infants have immature respiratory reflexes to airway obstruction and hypoxemia and are therefore more prone to respiratory depression after opioid administration. Hepatotoxicity is associated with acetaminophen administration and can vary because of hepatic immaturity as well as the dose of acetaminophen that is given. Increased risk of bleeding/platelet

dysfunction is associated with NSAIDs and it does not seem to be more pronounced in the pediatric population.

5. **A.** Placement of a continuous nerve catheter is advantageous over a single-shot block when long-lasting analgesia is desired. In addition, continuous nerve catheters have been associated with fewer adverse events when compared with epidural anesthesia in the pediatric population. The placement of a sciatic continuous nerve catheter in a patient undergoing foot or ankle surgery would allow the patient to participate in physical therapy postoperatively. If surgery is more proximal (femur or knee), a femoral nerve catheter would be more appropriate.

21 Low Back Pain

1. A 50-year-old is complaining about pain in an inner thigh area. Which of the following nerve roots is likely impinged?
   A. The L5 nerve root
   B. The L4 nerve root
   C. The S1 nerve root
   D. The L2 and L3 nerve roots
   E. The T12 nerve root

2. An 18-year-old female presents to the emergency department with pain of the lower back for 3 days. She denies any recent trauma. She is in severe distress and cannot find relief with any position or analgesics. She denies bladder or bowel changes. On further questioning, she does admit to regular IV drug use. She has a fever of 100.3°F and is extremely tender on palpation over the mid-lumbar spine. Lower extremity examination is unremarkable, but there is noticeable guarding due to back pain. Which of the following is a red flag in this patient?
   A. History of IV drug use
   B. Age < 20 years
   C. Acute symptoms of < 3 months
   D. Unrelenting pain
   E. All of the above

3. Which of the following about EMG/NCS is **FALSE?**
   A. It is the gold standard for evaluating lower back pain.
   B. It is useful in differentiating between lumbar radiculopathy and peripheral neuropathy.
   C. It correlates poorly with the anatomic level of radicular symptoms.
   D. Combined EMG and NCS have a high specificity.
   E. All of the above are true statements.

4. Which of the following describes a disk extrusion?
   A. The neck of the displaced disk is narrower than the widest diameter of the displaced disk in any plane.
   B. A lack of continuity exists between the displaced disk material and the parent disk.
   C. The neck of the displaced disk is larger than the diameter of the displaced disk in any plane.
   D. The neck of the displaced disk is equal to the diameter of the displaced disk in any plane.
   E. None of the above

5. Which physical examination finding, if positive, is most specific for lower lumbar nerve root irritation?
   A. Straight leg raise
   B. Crossed straight leg raise
   C. Tripod test
   D. Femoral stretch
   E. Patrick's test

6. Nonoperative treatment of lumbar spinal stenosis includes all of the following **EXCEPT:**
   A. Modification of activity
   B. Bracing
   C. Epidural steroid injection (ESI)
   D. Lumbar medial branch block (LMBB)
   E. Calcitonin therapy

7. Which of the following is true regarding herniated disks?
   A. The natural course is enlarging of the herniation.
   B. Small disk herniations tend to recede more often than large herniations.
   C. L5/S1 is the most commonly herniated level.
   D. Avoidance of strict bed rest leads to more rapid recovery.
   E. There must be neural compression to lead to radicular features.

8. A positive straight leg raise test:
   A. Is often absent in lumbar spinal stenosis
   B. Indicates discogenic pain
   C. Is often exaggerated by ankle plantar flexion
   D. Can be observed with compression of the L2 nerve rootlet
   E. Is useful for facet syndrome diagnosis

9. Which of the following is **FALSE** regarding cauda equina syndrome (CES)?
   A. The most frequent cause is massive midline disk herniation or smaller disk herniation in a previously stenotic spine.
   B. It can be conservatively treated with physical therapy and NSAIDs.
   C. Symptoms involve pain, often worse in one leg than the other, and weakness.
   D. Signs involve saddle anesthesia, diminished sphincter tone, and bladder retention.
   E. The gold standard diagnostic test is MRI.

10. Which of the following serious conditions regarding back pain in patients younger than 20 years old is true?
    A. More likely to be related to infection
    B. More likely to be related to neoplasm
    C. More likely to be related to congenital anomalies
    D. More likely to related to an extraspinal process
    E. More likely to be related to pathologic fracture

11. Predictors of favorable outcomes with regard to conservative therapy for treatment of herniated disk include:
    A. Minimal response to ESI
    B. Positive crossed straight leg raise test
    C. Absence of Workers' Compensation claim
    D. Leg pain on extension of spine
    E. Patients with 2 years of high school education who join the workforce early

12. Which of the following features of the intervertebral disk (IVD) is correct?
    A. The scavenger cells of the IVD signal a cascade of inflammatory cells during mechanical injury.
    B. The annulus fibrosis is more fibrous with a lower collagen content.
    C. A healthy IVD is richly supplied with blood and can readily repair internal damages.
    D. There are mechanoreceptors throughout the annulus fibrosis and nucleus pulposus responsible for intense pain when disk pathology exists.
    E. The matrix of the nucleus pulposus (NP) has a high water content and proteoglycans.

13. Clinical features of lumbar facet syndrome include all of the following **EXCEPT:**
    A. Low back pain
    B. Pain to the groin, hip, posterior aspect of thigh, and below the knee

C. Pain with prolonged sitting or standing and relieved by rest and walking
    D. Normal straight leg raise (SLR) test
    E. All of the above are features.

14. An 86-year-old retired schoolteacher comes to your clinic for a routine follow-up examination. She states that she has gradually experienced more intense lower back pain that worsens with standing and improves with rest. Her family states that she can no longer grocery shop without having to rest and she leans on the cart while walking. She most likely suffers from:
    A. A herniated lumbar disk
    B. A compression fracture of the lumbar spine
    C. Infection of the lumbar spine
    D. Lumbar spinal stenosis
    E. A spinal tumor

15. Which of the following is beneficial in lumbar spinal stenosis (LSS), especially LSS resulting from Paget's disease?
    A. Calcium
    B. Methotrexate
    C. Alendronate
    D. Vitamin D
    E. Calcitonin

16. Under what circumstance would contrast-enhanced MRI be superior to standard MRI for evaluation of low back and radicular pain?
    A. When visualization of the central canal is primary concern
    B. In a postsurgical patient where disk re-herniation is a concern
    C. When evaluating for pathologic fractures
    D. For patients with implantable metallic objects
    E. For obese patients

ANSWERS

1. **D.** Impingement of the L2 and L3 nerve roots can present as pain radiating into the groin. The L5 nerve root typically presents as abnormal sensation along the lateral thigh and calf; the L4 nerve root, along the anterolateral thigh axis and immediately below the knee along the medial leg; the S1 nerve root, along the posterior lateral thigh into the lateral foot.

2. **E.** There are several warning signs to be aware of during an evaluation. Age <20 years can suggest congenital disorders. History of IV drug use, being immunocompromised, or history of HIV can increase risk of osteomyelitis, abscess, or possibly diskitis. These infectious etiologies typically present as acute, unrelenting pain associated with fevers. Cauda equina compression, another condition warranting more urgent evaluation and treatment, typically presents with incontinence, saddle anesthesia, and lower extremity symptoms.

3. **A.** MRI is considered the gold standard for evaluation of lower back pain and radicular symptoms. Computed tomography can be useful for evaluation of bony pathology and can be comparable to MRI for evaluation of spinal canal lesions when combined with myelography. EMG/NCS can be useful in differentiating between lumbar radicular symptoms and those from peripheral neuropathy and have a high specificity when combined, but correlate poorly with the anatomic level of radicular symptom.

4. **A.** A disk extrusion is characterized by the neck of the displaced disk being narrower than the widest diameter of the displaced disk in any plane. A disk protrusion is characterized by the neck of the displaced disk material being wider than the diameter of the displaced disk. A disk sequestration is characterized by lack of continuity between the disk material and the parent disk.

5. **B.** Although straight leg raise is sensitive for nerve root irritation, crossed straight leg raise is the most specific. Tripod testing helps to confirm a positive straight leg raise. A positive femoral stretch is indicative of L2 and L3 nerve root tension.

6. **D.** Nonoperative treatment for lumbar stenosis includes medications such as acetaminophen and NSAIDs. Calcitonin has also been shown to be beneficial especially in cases of Paget's disease. Modification of activity can also be beneficial with avoidance of aggravating factors and strict bed rest. Lumbar binders can reduce load across the lumbar spine and provide some pain relief. Epidural steroid injections have been shown to provide short-term relief and symptomatic control of acute flare-ups related to stenosis. Medial branch blocks are used for facetogenic rather than neurogenic pain symptoms such as spinal stenosis.

7. **D.** Sixty percent of patients will experience resolution of symptoms with resolution of radiographic findings. Larger disk herniations tend to decrease in size more than smaller ones. The L4/5 level is the most commonly herniated level. Observations suggest that mechanisms other than direct mechanical compression of neural tissue are involved in mediating radicular symptoms. Continuation of activity as tolerated leads to a more rapid recovery.

8. **A.** A positive straight leg raise is often absent in lumbar spinal stenosis with an incidence of only 10%–23%. When positive, it is indicative of nerve irritation, typically at the lower lumbar levels of L4, L5, and S1. It is often exaggerated by ankle dorsiflexion.

9. **B.** Over 70% of CES cases relate a history of prior back pain. Signs and symptoms involve saddle anesthesia, diminished sphincter tone, bladder retention, weakness in the lower extremities, and pain in the legs with one side being worse. Abdominal pain may also be present from bladder distention secondary to urinary retention. The most frequent cause is massive midline disk herniation or smaller disk herniation in an already stenotic spine. CES is a neurosurgical emergency requiring immediate decompression of the spine; conservative therapy will only delay surgical treatment and is not appropriate.

10. **C.** Patients younger than 20 years experiencing lower back pain are more likely to have congenital and developmental anomalies.

11. **C.** Predictors of favorable outcomes include a negative extended SLR test, absence of leg pain with spine extension, absence of stenosis on spine imaging, favorable response to ESIs, recovery of any neurologic deficits within 12 weeks, a motivated physically fit patient with more than 12 years of education, no Workers' Compensation claims, and a normal psychological profile.

12. **E.** The matrix of the NP has a high water content and proteoglycans. The annulus fibrosis is more fibrous with a high collagen content. The IVD is scantily innervated and is the largest avascular structure in the body. Mechanoreceptors of the IVD are located in the outer third of the annulus fibrosis. The IVD lacks any scavenger cells, which may result in the build-up of metabolites over time.

13. **B.** Lumbar facet pain is characterized by low back pain, pain to the groin/hip/posterior thigh but not below the knee, pain with prolonged sitting or standing, negative neurologic symptoms, and a negative SLR. It is often improved with lying down or walking.

14. **D.** Patients with lumbar spinal stenosis often walk with a stooped, forward posture. Pain is worsened with extension and improves with rest. Forward flexion can also help alleviate symptoms of pain. Onset is typically slow with sensorimotor deficits less pronounced. SLR testing is often negative.

15. **E.** Medication therapy for LSS includes acetaminophen, NSAIDs, and calcitonin. Calcitonin is especially used in Paget's disease. There is lack of data for all other choices.

16. **B.** MRI with contrast can help differentiate between postsurgical scar versus disk re-herniation. CT myelography can be comparable to MRI in evaluation of spinal canal pathology. CT without myelography is not as reliable for evaluating spinal pathology, although CT is superior in evaluating most osseous abnormalities. For implantable metallic objects, MRI may contraindicated.

Neurosurgical Approaches to Pain Management

QUESTIONS

1. Which of the following is **FALSE** regarding neuroablative medial thalamotomy?
   A. Three main medial thalamic nuclei are targeted including the centralis lateralis, centrum medianum, and parafascicularis.
   B. This ablative procedure is primarily used to treat cancer pain syndromes.
   C. A wide variety of pain syndromes have been treated with medial thalamotomy, including central and peripheral deafferentation pain, spinal cord injury, and Parkinson's neuropathic pain.
   D. The most frequently targeted nucleus is the parafascicularis.
   E. Historically, the first thalamic nucleus targeted was the ventral caudal (Vc) nucleus, but this was associated with significant deafferentation pain resulting in procedure modification to target the medial thalamus instead.

2. A 68-year-old female presents for intractable cancer pain secondary to widespread metastatic melanoma. She has failed intrathecal therapy secondary to side effects. She is significantly depressed and anxious because of the intractable pain. Which neurosurgical procedure would be a reasonable therapeutic option?
   A. Stereotactic cingulotomy
   B. Medial thalamotomy
   C. Frontal lobotomy
   D. Motor cortex stimulation
   E. Deep brain stimulation

3. Which neurosurgical procedure targets the caudal portion of the spinal trigeminal nucleus for intractable trigeminal anesthesia dolorosa unresponsive to more conservative therapies?
   A. Caudalis dorsal root entry zone (DREZ) procedure
   B. Stereotactic cingulotomy
   C. Medial thalamotomy
   D. Extralemniscal myelotomy
   E. Anterolateral cordotomy

4. Anterolateral cordotomy involves lesioning of which spinal nerve tract to help control intractable pain?
   A. Lateral corticospinal tract
   B. Lateral spinothalamic tract
   C. Anterior spinocerebellar tract
   D. Rubrospinal tract
   E. Anterior corticospinal tract

5. Which of the following is **TRUE** regarding the lateral spinothalamic tract?
   A. It relays descending pain transmission signals.
   B. It carries information about pain and vibration.
   C. It synapses directly onto the sensory cortex.
   D. Lesions of the lateral spinothalamic tract produce an ipsilateral deficit in pain and temperature sensation two to five segments below the level of the cordotomy.
   E. Fibers in the lateral spinothalamic tract have a somatotopic arrangement.

6. Sensory information from all of the following cranial nerves is carried by the trigeminal tract into the trigeminal tract spinal nucleus **EXCEPT:**
   A. CN III
   B. CN V
   C. CN VII
   D. CN IX
   E. CN X

7. A 61-year-old female presents with debilitating visceral pain secondary to uterine cancer, unresponsive to conservative measures. Which ascending neural pathway is thought to carry visceral nociceptive information for this patient's pain?
   A. Lateral corticospinal tract
   B. Extralemniscal pathway
   C. Rubrospinal tract
   D. Anterior corticospinal tract
   E. Spinocerebellar tract

8. Which of the following is **TRUE** regarding the cervical DREZ ablative procedure?
   A. It is intended for patients with deafferentation pain of the lower extremity.
   B. A prerequisite is complete functional use of the targeted limb.
   C. Complete sensory denervation of the targeted limb is expected postprocedurally.
   D. Complete motor denervation of the targeted limb is expected postprocedurally.
   E. Dysesthesias in the targeted limb are not experienced postprocedurally.

9. All of the following are true regarding deep brain stimulation (DBS) for pain control **EXCEPT:**
   A. DBS implantable hardware is not FDA approved for pain control procedures.
   B. The thalamus, periventricular grey matter (PVG), and periaqueductal grey matter (PAG) are the most commonly targeted sites for DBS implants for pain.
   C. It is postulated that the analgesic mechanism of DBS of the PVG and PAG is caused by activation of multiple supraspinal descending pain inhibitory systems.
   D. Thalamic DBS is thought to activate the nucleus raphe magnus of the rostroventral medulla, which activates descending endogenous analgesic systems.
   E. There is robust randomized control trial data supporting the usefulness of DBS stimulation for analgesia.

10. Motor cortex epidural stimulation (MCS) is thought to exert its analgesic benefit by which of the following mechanisms?
    A. Increased blood flow to the ipsilateral cingulate gyrus
    B. Increased blood flow to the ipsilateral thalamus
    C. Increased blood flow to the ipsilateral orbitofrontal cortex
    D. Increased blood flow to the ipsilateral insula and brainstem
    E. All of the above

11. Bulbar poststroke pain from Wallenberg's syndrome has been treated with which of the following advanced neurosurgical techniques?
    A. Motor cortex epidural stimulation
    B. Caudalis DREZ

C. Deep brain stimulation
D. Anterolateral cordotomy
E. Extralemniscal myelotomy

12. Placement of an intracerebral ventricular catheter for the delivery of intraventricular opioids is accomplished by placing a catheter into the:
    A. Lateral ventricle near the foramen of Monro
    B. Foramen of Luschka
    C. Rostrum of the corpus callosum
    D. Internal capsule
    E. Prefrontal cortex

13. Opioid receptors are abundant around which of the following brain structures?
    A. Wall of the third ventricle
    B. Aqueduct
    C. Periventricular gray matter
    D. Periaqueductal gray matter
    E. All of the above

14. A 68-year-old man presents with intractable postthoracotomy chest pain following an esophagectomy for esophageal cancer. A neurosurgeon offered him anterolateral cordotomy to help relieve his chest pain. On examination, he is most sensitive along the right chest wall at T7–9. If the patient were to undergo the procedure, where would the procedure most likely be performed?
    A. Left T3–6
    B. Right T3–6
    C. Left C4–6
    D. Right C4–6
    E. Left T10–12

ANSWERS

1. **D.** The most frequently targeted nucleus in neuroablative medial thalamotomy is the centrum medianum.

2. **A.** Patients with intractable metastatic cancer pain unresponsive to intrathecal therapy with significant emotional factors are reasonable candidates for stereotactic cingulotomy, which is thought to provide analgesia by altering a patient's emotional response to pain.

3. **A.** The Caudalis DREZ procedure involves destroying the caudal portion of the spinal trigeminal nucleus for intractable trigeminal neuralgia or trigeminal postherpetic neuralgia.

4. **B.** The lateral spinothalamic tract is targeted during anterolateral cordotomy lesioning.

5. **E.** The lateral spinothalamic tract is an ascending, somatotopically arranged pain transmission pathway carrying contralateral pain and temperature information to the thalamus.

6. **A.** Sensory information from cranial nerves V, VII, IX, and X is carried in the trigeminal tract into the trigeminal tract spinal nucleus.

7. **B.** Extralemniscal myelotomy targets visceral pain conducting extralemniscal tracts lying deep to the midline dorsal column.

8. **C.** The cervical DREZ destructive procedure is generally intended for patients with brachial plexus avulsion or brachial plexus cancer invasion with lack of functional use of the extremity, since the procedure will cause complete sensory denervation of the limb. Sensory dysesthesia can be experienced postprocedurally.

9. **E.** Data is sparse, supporting the use of DBS for analgesia. All of the other statements are correct.

10. **E.** All answer choices are correct.

11. **A.** Epidural motor cortex stimulation has been utilized to treat neuropathic pain associated with bulbar poststroke pain.

12. **A.** The surgical technique for implanting a chronic intraventricular morphine infusion involves catheter placement into the lateral ventricle near the foramen of Monro.

13. **E.** All answer choices are correct.

14. **A.** Anterolateral cordotomy involves lesioning the anterolateral tract—this produces a contralateral deficit in pain and temperature sensation two to five segments below the level of the cordotomy.

23 Cancer Pain

QUESTIONS

1. Which of the following is true regarding cancer-related neuropathic pain?
   A. It tends to respond best to multimodal drug therapy, including opioids, corticosteroids, and tricyclic antidepressants.
   B. Vinca alkaloids can cause chemotherapy-induced neuropathy.
   C. It can be associated with treatment with bortezomib.
   D. None of the above
   E. All of the above

2. A 58-year-old male presents with lethargy, confusion, frequent urination, and nausea/vomiting. The basic metabolic panel shows serum calcium level to be 18 mg/dL. X-ray examination of the skull shows multiple punched-out lesions, which can be indicative of multiple myeloma. Which of the following is true regarding imaging for osseous lesions?
   A. Greater than 50% decalcification must occur before osseous lesions are visible on X-ray images.
   B. A bone scan is preferred for detecting bone metastases.
   C. With primary bone tumors, thyroid cancer, and multiple myeloma, plain films are considered more sensitive.
   D. All of the above
   E. None of the above

3. When a cancer patient is capable of only limited self-care, confined to bed or chair for more than 50% of waking hours, what is their Eastern Cooperative Oncology Group (ECOG) status?
   A. 1
   B. 2
   C. 3
   D. 4
   E. 5

4. A 58-year-old male with metastatic lung cancer presents with intractable chest and abdominal pain. Restaging scans show the progression of the disease with numerous liver metastases and a right paraxial soft tissue mass eroding into the 10th and 11th ribs. Pain remains uncontrolled on methadone 20 mg q12 hours, gabapentin 1200 mg q8 hours, and hydromorphone PCA. Neuraxial analgesia is being considered. What is the "break-even" point for implementing intrathecal therapy compared with epidural therapy?
   A. 1 month
   B. 3 months
   C. 6 months
   D. 1 year
   E. The two cannot be compared because they are different modes of providing analgesia.

5. When considering intrathecal therapy with an intraspinal catheter and pump for a patient, what should be the life expectancy to justify implantation?
   A. >1 year
   B. >6 months
   C. >3 months
   D. >2 months
   E. Life expectancy is irrelevant.

6. Bone metastasis is cited as the most common cause of cancer pain. Which of the following cancers is most often associated with bone metastases?
   A. Lung
   B. Thyroid
   C. Bladder
   D. Colon
   E. All of the above

7. A randomized trial by Klazen et al. published in 2010 in *The Lancet*, evaluating the use of percutaneous vertebroplasty for the treatment of vertebral compression fractures, demonstrated superior pain relief compared with placebo at which benchmark?
   A. 1 month
   B. 8 weeks
   C. 3 months
   D. 6 months
   E. 12 months

8. Which of the following agents is commonly involved in the production of painful polyneuropathy (sensory and motor involvement)?
   A. Methotrexate
   B. Doxorubicin
   C. Bleomycin
   D. Vincristine
   E. All of the above

9. In the majority of cases, cancer-related pain is caused by:
   A. Invasion of organic structures by the tumor (directly or by metastasis)
   B. Related to cancer treatment (surgery, chemotherapy, radiation therapy)
   C. Chronic pain syndromes
   D. Depression and anxiety
   E. None of the above

10. Plexopathies are the result of tumor growth around nerve plexuses in the upper or lower extremity. Which of the following is true regarding plexopathies?

A. The lower cord of the plexus is most commonly affected in brachial plexopathy.
B. Brachial plexopathy responds better than lumbosacral plexopathy to medications such as opioids and other oral adjuvants.
C. Lumbosacral plexopathy may require earlier escalation to invasive interventions such as intrathecal therapy to control pain.
D. All of the above
E. None of the above

ANSWERS

1. **E.** Chemotherapeutic agents that may lead to nerve injury and neuropathic pain include vinca alkaloids (vincristine, vinblastine), cisplatin, paclitaxel (Taxol), docetaxel (Taxotere), vinorelbine (Navelbine), and bortezomib (Velcade). Neuropathic pain is often resistant to treatment and may require using multimodal therapy that includes combinations of various analgesic agents, as described.

2. **D.** Osseous lesions are not seen on plain radiographs until at least 50% decalcification has occurred. Thus, a bone scan (isotope scanning, scintigraphy) is preferred for evaluating potential bone metastases. However, with primary bone tumors, thyroid cancer, and multiple myeloma, plain films are considered to be more sensitive.

3. **C.** ECOG scores:
   0: Fully active, able to carry out all pre-disease performance without restriction.
   1: Restricted in physically strenuous activity but ambulatory and able to carry out light or sedentary work (e.g., light housework, office work).
   2: Ambulatory and capable of all self-care, but unable to work; up and about more than 50% of waking hours.
   3: Capable of only limited self-care, confined to bed or chair more than 50% of waking hours.
   4: Completely disabled, cannot carry on any self-care, totally confined to bed or chair.
   5: Dead

4. **B.** The cost of intrathecal therapy is initially high because of equipment costs, whereas the cost of implementing long-term epidural therapy is initially low. Studies evaluating the costs of these therapies identified a "break-even" point around 3 months of therapy.

5. **C.** In general, patients with a survival expectancy of longer than 3 months will be candidates for intrathecal

therapy with a permanent intraspinal catheter and an implanted pump.

6. **A.** Bone tumor infiltration or bone metastasis is cited as the most common cause of cancer pain and is most often seen with stage IV carcinoma of the prostate, breast, thyroid, lung, or kidney. Pain is often described as constant, dull, achy or deep, and intense with movement or weight bearing. Around 25% of patients with bone metastases experience pain.

7. **A.** The study by Klazen et al. reported significant pain control at 1 week and 1 month, but *not* at 3, 6, and 12 months. (Klazen C, Lohle P, de Vries J, et al. Vertebroplasty versus conservative treatment in acute osteoporotic vertebral compression fractures (Vertos II): an open-label randomized trial. *Lancet.* 2010;376(9746):1085-1092.)

8. **D.** Painful polyneuropathy occurs most commonly with vincristine (motor and sensory involvement), vinblastine, paclitaxel, docetaxel, platinum derivative (predominantly sensory involvement), vinorelbine, and bortezomib.

9. **A.** Involvement of organic structures by tumor accounts for approximately 65% of cancer-related pain. Therapy, including chemotherapy, radiotherapy, and surgery, can account for approximately 25% of cancer-related pain. The other approximately 10% of "cancer pain" is typically caused by common chronic pain syndromes (back pain and headaches), sometimes exacerbated by the ongoing growth or treatment of cancer.

10. **D.** Brachial plexopathy is most often caused by upper lobe lung cancer (Pancoast syndrome, or superior sulcus syndrome), breast cancer, or lymphoma, with the lower cord of the plexus (C8–T1) most frequently affected. Brachial plexopathies may respond better to pharmacologic therapy, whereas lumbosacral plexopathies may require earlier intervention with intrathecal therapy.

24 Neuropathic Pain Syndromes

QUESTIONS

1. Which of the following statements is **FALSE** regarding neuropathic pain?
   A. Neuropathic pain is defined as pain arising as a direct consequence of a lesion or disease affecting the somatosensory system.
   B. Neuropathic pain conditions include complex regional pain syndrome (CRPS), postherpetic neuralgia (PHN), and human immunodeficiency virus (HIV) sensory neuropathy.
   C. Opioid therapy is considered first-line in the treatment of neuropathic pain.
   D. The diagnosis of a neuropathic pain condition can be further confirmed using various diagnostic studies including MRI, CT, nerve biopsy, nerve conduction studies, and laboratory studies.
   E. All of the above are false.

2. Which of the following statements is **FALSE** regarding CRPS?
   A. CRPS type 2 is differentiated from type 1 by the presence of pain following a nerve injury.
   B. Fractures have been reported as the most common initiating injury for CRPS.
   C. To meet the Budapest criteria for CRPS, the patient must have a symptom in three of the four categories (sensory, vasomotor, sudomotor/edema, motor/trophic) and a sign in two of the four categories (sensory, vasomotor, sudomotor/edema, motor/trophic).
   D. CRPS has a higher incidence in younger individuals.
   E. All of the above are false.

3. Which patient with CRPS is most likely to have the worst outcome?
   A. Patient who had a fracture leading to CRPS
   B. Patient who had a nerve injury in the lower extremity with "warm" CRPS
   C. Patient who had a nerve injury in the upper extremity with "cold" CRPS
   D. Patient who had a nerve injury in the upper extremity with "warm" CRPS
   E. Patient who has depression and CRPS

4. Which of the following psychological factors have a positive correlation with CRPS?
   A. Depression
   B. Anxiety
   C. Personality disorder
   D. Schizophrenia
   E. None of the above

5. The major receptor type that is involved in central sensitization in the pathophysiology of CRPS is:
   A. μ-1
   B. GABA (γ-aminobutyric acid)
   C. NMDA (N-methyl-D-aspartate)
   D. Ca^{2+}
   E. Calcitonin gene-related peptide (CGRP)

6. Which of the following is most consistent with sympathetic nervous system dysfunction in complex regional pain syndrome?
   A. Allodynia
   B. Skin color changes
   C. Weakness
   D. Hyperalgesia
   E. Dystrophy

7. Which of the following therapies have been recommended for the treatment of CRPS?
   A. Bisphosphonates
   B. Membrane stabilizers (gabapentin, pregabalin)
   C. Physical therapy
   D. Spinal cord stimulator therapy
   E. All of the above

8. Which of the following is the most common location for postherpetic neuralgia?
   A. Facial
   B. Thoracic
   C. Ophthalmic
   D. Lumbar
   E. Cervical

9. Postherpetic neuralgia is the result of infection by which virus?
   A. Herpes simplex virus-1 (HSV-1)
   B. Herpes simplex virus-2 (HSV-2)
   C. Cytomegalovirus (CMV)
   D. Varicella zoster virus (VZV)
   E. None of the above

10. A 70-year-old female comes to your clinic complaining of right thoracic pain that travels along the fourth rib. Her pain was preceded by prodromal symptoms of fever and malaise followed by a maculopapular vesicular rash. Which of the following is most likely true about this patient?
    A. Her condition is a result of a decrease in her humoral immunity.
    B. She had less risk of developing postherpetic neuralgia compared with a 35-year-old male.
    C. Use of corticosteroids to treat her rash would have prevented her from developing chronic pain.
    D. She most likely did not receive the zoster vaccine.
    E. None of the above

11. Which of the following regarding diabetic neuropathy is true?
    A. Oxycodone is not effective in its treatment.
    B. Diabetic neuropathy can affect cranial nerves.
    C. The use of antioxidants has not been shown to be beneficial in the treatment of diabetic neuropathy.
    D. Diabetic neuropathy is more common with type 1 diabetics rather than type 2 diabetics.
    E. All of the above

12. Which of the following is **FALSE** regarding HIV-related sensory neuropathy?
    A. The two most common forms are distal sensory polyneuropathy and antiretroviral toxic neuropathy.
    B. HIV causes sensory neuropathy by infecting axons and Schwann cells.
    C. HIV neuropathy shows an axonal, length-dependent, sensory polyneuropathy on nerve conduction studies.
    D. The first step in treating HIV-related sensory neuropathy is removing or reducing the dose of antiretroviral medications when possible.
    E. All of the above are false.

13. Which of the following medications are **NOT** effective in the treatment of HIV-related sensory neuropathy?
    A. Lamotrigine
    B. Gabapentin
    C. Capsaicin
    D. Amitriptyline
    E. All are effective treatments.

ANSWERS

1. **C.** Opioid therapy is not considered first-line treatment for neuropathic pain conditions. Although some opioids may decrease pain scores in various neuropathic pain conditions, membrane stabilizers (gabapentin, pregabalin) are typically used as first-line treatments. Because of multiple side effects (constipation, drowsiness, respiratory depression) and risk of addiction, opioids are considered a last resort in the therapy for neuropathic pain.

2. **D.** The incidence of CRPS is higher in the older population. The average age is between 16 and 79 years (median, 41.6). Females also appear to be at higher risk of developing CRPS.

3. **C.** Outcomes of CRPS tend to be worse in patients with upper extremity injuries (rather than lower extremity injuries), injuries outside of fractures, and "cold" (commonly chronic) CRPS rather than "warm" (acute) CRPS.

4. **E.** Psychological factors have not been shown to correlate with CRPS, suggesting that there is no specific type of CRPS personality. However, the incidence of job-related injuries leading to CRPS tends to be high, which may indicate a psychosocial or secondary gain component.

5. **C.** The NMDA receptor is a major receptor involved in central sensitization. Its activation can lead to hyperalgesia and allodynia seen in CRPS. With CRPS, there are abnormalities in the somatosensory, sensory (central and peripheral sensitization), and sympathetic nervous systems.

6. **B.** In CRPS, there can be dysfunction within the sympathetic nervous system leading to excessive sympathetic outflow. This can result in vasoconstriction, which is thought to cause the cooler temperature, discoloration (blue), and pain in the affected limb.

7. **E.** There are a host of therapies that are recommended for CRPS. Physical therapy is one of the mainstays of therapy, which can help prevent the atrophy associated with disuse of the painful, affected limb. Although there are limited studies, membrane stabilizers and antidepressants are recommended for CRPS treatment. Bisphosphonates can be used to treat the bone resorption that can sometimes occur with CRPS. Sympathetic nerve blocks (stellate ganglion block for upper extremity and lumbar sympathetic block for lower extremity) can provide a significant reduction in pain with CRPS; however, the pain relief is typically short lived. Spinal cord stimulator therapy has also shown promise with CRPS, providing significant pain improvement for the first 2 years of therapy. Intravenous ketamine infusion has also been investigated for CRPS and has been shown to decrease levels of pain; however, patients can relapse with their pain reverting back to their baseline level.

8. **C.** The most common sites for postherpetic neuralgia (PHN) are ophthalmic (32%), thoracic (16.5%), and facial (16%) distributions.

9. **D.** Postherpetic neuralgia can occur in 10%–20% of people infected with herpes zoster (or shingles). Herpes zoster (HZ) is the result of reactivation of the

varicella zoster virus, which lies dormant within one of the sensory nerve ganglia after the initial chickenpox infection.

10. **D.** This patient's symptoms are suggestive of postherpetic neuralgia. Receiving the zoster vaccine has been shown to decrease the incidence of both HZ and PHN. Herpes zoster is a result of the reactivation of the varicella zoster virus, which can occur from a decrease in cell-mediated immunity, not humoral immunity. Risk factors for PHN include increased age, female gender, and greater severity of rash or pain. Antivirals such as acyclovir, famciclovir, and valacyclovir initiated within the first 72 hours of HZ are effective in increasing healing and decreasing pain. Corticosteroids have also been shown to decrease the intensity of the HZ pain; however, neither of these therapies has been shown to prevent the development of PHN definitively.

11. **B.** There are two main categories of diabetic neuropathy: generalized neuropathies and focal/multifocal neuropathies. Generalized neuropathies include acute sensory neuropathy and chronic sensorimotor distal polyneuropathy. Focal/multifocal neuropathies include cranial, truncal, focal limb, proximal motor neuropathy (amyotrophy), and chronic inflammatory demyelinating polyneuropathy. Diabetic neuropathy is more common in type 2 diabetics. Oxycodone has been shown to decrease pain from diabetic peripheral neuropathy (DPN) but is not recommended because of its side effect profile. Tight glycemic control can delay the onset and progression of DPN. Membrane stabilizers, antidepressants, capsaicin cream, and topical lidocaine are all effective in the treatment of DPN. The use of antioxidants (such as α-lipoic acid) may also have some beneficial effects with DPN.

12. **B.** HIV does not infect axons or Schwann cells. It is hypothesized that the axonal damage of HIV may be caused by cytokine-mediated effects, which leads to an inflammatory reaction in the nerve.

13. **D.** Gabapentin, capsaicin, and lamotrigine have been shown to be effective in the treatment of HIV-related sensory neuropathy, whereas amitriptyline, topical lidocaine, and pregabalin have failed to show any benefit over placebo.

Pain in Selected Neurologic Disorders

25

1. Regarding acute inflammatory demyelinating polyneuropathy (AIDP), which of the following statements is **FALSE?**
   A. Pain is more prominent in the later phases after destruction of small nerve fiber endings.
   B. It has an annual incidence of approximately 1.11 per 100,000 person-years, with a 20% increase every decade after the first decade of life.
   C. Paresthesias or dysesthesias proceed in an ascending pattern.
   D. Headaches and abdominal pain can be associated findings.
   E. Straight leg raise testing may be positive in the acute phase.

2. You are treating an HIV patient for peripheral neuropathy. The patient makes an urgent clinic visit for sudden, intense burning pain of the feet that started 2 weeks ago. Which of the following is the most appropriate course of action?
   A. Initiate morphine sulfate therapy.
   B. Discuss with the patient's infectious disease physician about possibly reducing or stopping the dose of a recently started antiretroviral drug.
   C. Admit the patient for concern for an opportunistic infection requiring IV antibiotics.
   D. Reassure the patient that their neuropathy will likely improve conservatively over the next 1–2 months.
   E. None of the above

3. Your patient with intense lightning pain of the lower extremities shows inflammatory infiltrates along the dorsal roots with degeneration of the posterior columns on spine MRI. Which condition is your patient most likely suffering from?
   A. Subacute sensory neuropathy
   B. Idiopathic sensory polyneuropathy
   C. Distal symmetrical polyneuropathy
   D. Tabes dorsalis
   E. Multiple sclerosis

4. Which of the following about spinal cord injury is true?
   A. Approximately 41% of patients will report pain 6 weeks after injury.
   B. The pain is usually less intense at the area of transition from complete sensory loss to normal sensation.

   C. Morphine and baclofen intrathecally offers superior pain relief in the majority of cases.
   D. The most dominant pain type following spinal cord injury is central neuropathic pain.
   E. Spinal cord injury always results in complete paralysis.

5. A 47-year-old patient presents to your clinic with complaints of left-sided facial pain of slow onset over the last few months. She reports being in a motor vehicle accident approximately 6 months ago, resulting in pain in the chest that progressed to the left arm, described as burning. X-ray examination of the chest and spine is negative. What is the most likely diagnosis?
   A. Prinzmetal angina
   B. Syringomyelia
   C. Multiple sclerosis
   D. Trigeminal neuralgia
   E. Intercostal neuralgia

6. Which of the following is a type of primary pain in multiple sclerosis (MS)?
   A. Chronic headaches
   B. Overuse syndrome
   C. Trigeminal neuralgia
   D. Myofascial pain
   E. All of the above

7. A 76-year-old male with a history of right-sided stroke 2 months earlier presents with right arm pain. He has preserved motor function but is avoiding use of the arm because of diffuse burning. He denies having spasticity. Which of the following would you advise?
   A. Obtain a surgical evaluation with an orthopedic surgeon
   B. Repeat the brain scan to look for a new stroke and evaluate for Wallenberg's syndrome
   C. Begin a regimen of regular exercises for the shoulder
   D. Try baclofen for pain control
   E. Attempt a spinal cord stimulator trial

8. Which of the following pharmacologic therapies would be **LEAST** appropriate in treating pain related to cervical dystonia?
   A. Gabapentin
   B. Botulinum toxin

C. Baclofen
D. Valium
E. Droperidol

9. In syringomyelia, dissociated sensory loss is described as:
   A. Loss of both dorsal column and spinothalamic function
   B. Loss of dorsal column function with intact spinothalamic tract function
   C. Partial dorsal column function loss
   D. Loss of spinothalamic function with intact dorsal column function
   E. None of the above

10. Which type of brainstem infarct may result in Wallenberg's syndrome and central neuropathic pain?
    A. Medial medullary infarct
    B. Lateral medullary infarct
    C. Pontine infarct
    D. Middle cerebral artery (MCA) infarct
    E. Anterior cerebral artery (ACA) infarct

11. Which of the following statements is **FALSE** regarding pain in Parkinson's disease?
    A. Pain often occurs in the "off periods" of rigidity, bradykinesia, and tremor.
    B. Pain is typically described as muscular tightness or cramping.
    C. Restless leg syndrome or peripheral dysesthesias are common sources of pain.

D. More than 50% of patients with Parkinson's disease have pain.
E. Dopaminergic agents are important for treating the sensory manifestations of pain.

12. All of the following can be used to treat dystonia **EXCEPT:**
    A. Benzodiazepines
    B. Muscle relaxants
    C. Dopaminergic agents
    D. Anticholinergic agents
    E. Anticonvulsants

13. Which of the following pain syndromes associated with HIV is commonly found in the intermediate stage of the disease?
    A. Acute inflammatory demyelinating polyneuropathy
    B. Autoimmune vasculitic mononeuropathy multiplex
    C. Cytomegalovirus polyneuropathy
    D. Neurosyphilis
    E. Cytomegalovirus mononeuropathy multiplex

14. Which of the following antibodies have been commonly associated with sensory neuropathy?
    A. Anti-Rho
    B. Anti-AB
    C. Anti-O
    D. Anti-Hu
    E. Anti-Duffy

ANSWERS

1. **A.** In AIPD, or Guillain-Barré syndrome, pain is more prominent in the early acute phases of the syndrome. Headaches and abdominal pain can result from autonomic dysfunction.

2. **B.** Sudden increase in neuropathic pain in an HIV patient likely results from antiretroviral medications. Reducing the dose or cessation will often improve the symptoms. This antiretroviral-induced polyneuropathy can be distinguished from HIV polyneuropathy in that it occurs more abruptly with more rapid progression and is often more painful. Antiretroviral polyneuropathy occurs in 26%–66% of patients.

3. **D.** Tabes dorsalis is a neurosyphilitic involvement of the dorsal root entry zone. It is characterized by "lightning" pain of the lower extremities but can also involve the trunk, thorax, and abdomen. Therapy involves standard antibiotic therapy to eradicate the Treponema pallidum organism.

4. **D.** The neuropathic pain in spinal cord injury emanates from the area of injury and extends variably into areas of sensory loss. It is the most dominant pain type and is considered a central neuropathic pain. Forty-one percent will report pain by 12 months. Addition of morphine to intrathecal baclofen has

shown variable results in controlling pain. The pain may be more intense at the transition zone known as "end-zone pain" or "transitional pain."

5. **B.** Syringomyelia can present after a trauma as a neuropathic pain. Extension of the syrinx into the upper cervical region may be associated with ipsilateral facial pain caused by involvement of the descending trigeminal tract and nucleus. Treatment may involve neurosurgical drainage. The condition is often refractory to medication therapy for pain.

6. **C.** The association of MS with trigeminal neuralgia is thought to be related to brainstem demyelination. Unlike idiopathic trigeminal neuralgia, MS-associated trigeminal neuralgia can be associated with a sensory loss. This pain is a type of primary pain. All other choices are secondary types of pain.

7. **C.** Central poststroke pain can be seen in 10% of patients after 1 year from a cerebrovascular accident. It is characterized as a neuropathic pain with concomitant sensory loss. Motor function can be spared or have a mild deficit. Attention should be paid to secondary disorders such as frozen shoulder and decubitus ulcers. A regimen of regular exercises for the shoulder can help avoid frozen shoulder. Antidepressants and antiepileptics can serve as

first-line analgesics for neuropathic pain. Centrally acting muscle relaxants have a role when there is muscular spasticity.

8. **A.** Dystonia is characterized by disordered control of muscle groups. Pain is a prominent feature, occurring as a result of sustained muscle contraction. Treatment includes dopaminergic agents, anticholinergic agents, muscle relaxants, and benzodiazepines. There is limited role for antiepileptic medications.

9. **D.** In syringomyelia, when there is loss of spinothalamic function but the dorsal column remains intact, this is known as dissociation of sensory function (loss of sensation of pain and temperature).

10. **B.** Infarcts involving the lateral medullary (Wallenberg's) areas of the brainstem may be associated with central neuropathic pain.

11. **E.** Dopaminergic agents are used for treatment of motor symptoms in Parkinson's. Anticonvulsants and tricyclic antidepressants are more appropriate to treat sensory manifestations of pain in Parkinson's.

12. **E.** Pain from dystonia is mediated by tissue acidosis, which occurs from sustained contraction of muscle. Regulation and relaxation of muscles is the pharmacologic target for therapy. Anticonvulsants are not typically used for the treatment of dystonia.

13. **B.** Acute inflammatory demyelinating polyneuropathy occurs in the early stages. Cytomegalovirus polyneuropathy, neurosyphilis, and cytomegalovirus mononeuropathy multiplex occur in the late stages. Autoimmune vasculitis mononeuropathy multiplex occurs in the intermediate stage of the disease.

14. **D.** Anti-Hu antibodies have been associated with sensory neuropathy. These antibodies attack cells of the dorsal root ganglia, resulting in ataxia, sensory loss, and painful dysesthesia, primarily of the lower extremities.

26 Phantom Limb Pain

1. Which of the following is true of phantom limb pain?
   A. It will not present after 1 year if no phantom pain is experienced in the first year.
   B. It is more frequent in the very young.
   C. Male gender and lower extremity amputation is associated with greater phantom pain.
   D. It typically presents in the first week after amputation.
   E. It is most common with congenital amputations.

2. All of the following are true regarding characteristics of phantom limb pain **EXCEPT:**
   A. Phantom pain is less frequent in very young children and congenital amputees.
   B. The appearance of phantom pain may be delayed for months or even years after amputation.
   C. The severity and intensity of phantom pain attacks generally increase with time.
   D. Phantom pain is usually intermittent and only a small subset of patients experience constant pain.
   E. Phantom pain is primarily localized to the distal parts of the missing limb.

3. Which of the following psychological factors is **LEAST** likely to impact phantom pain?
   A. Anger
   B. Depression
   C. Grief
   D. Catastrophizing
   E. Poor social support

4. A patient with recent leg amputation presents with pain at the site of the stump. Which of the following statements about stump pain is **FALSE?**
   A. The incidence of severe cases ranges from 5% to 10%.
   B. It is present in the majority of patients with phantom pain.
   C. It is present in the first week after amputation and always subsides with surgical healing.

   D. It can be associated with sensory abnormalities.
   E. Severe contractions of the stump can be observed.

5. Which of the following best describes the pathophysiologic mechanism involved in developing phantom limb pain?
   A. After injury, there is increased excitability of neurons where C fibers and A-delta afferents gain access to secondary pain-signaling neurons.
   B. Sensitization of ventral horn neurons is mediated by release of glutamate and neurokinins.
   C. Decreased persistent neuronal discharges with prolonged pain after stimulation (wind-up phenomena) occurs.
   D. A and B
   E. All of the above

6. All of the following have been described as mechanisms for phantom limb pain **EXCEPT:**
   A. Formation of neuromas leads to abnormal spontaneous and evoked activity after mechanical or chemical stimulation.
   B. After nerve injury, there is an increase in the general excitability of spinal cord neurons.
   C. With the loss of afferent input, sympathetic neurons begin to fire spontaneously, leading to hypersensitivity and pain.
   D. Loss of sensory input leads to substantial reorganization of the somatosensory cortex.
   E. Increased activation of the NMDA receptor system.

7. Which of the following has been best demonstrated to reduce development of chronic phantom pain most significantly?
   A. Preoperative epidural infusion
   B. Preoperative gabapentin
   C. Intravenous ketamine
   D. Aggressive perioperative pain control
   E. Postoperative epidural infusion

ANSWERS

1. **D.** Phantom pain has a wide variability in incidence and affects a range of ages. It typically presents in the first week after amputation but can be delayed up to several years. A recent study has shown a greater incidence in female gender and amputation involving the upper extremity. It is less frequent in the very young and with congenital amputations.

2. **C.** The severity and intensity of phantom pain subsides over time, with an average pain score of 22/100 on VAS at 6 months.

3. **A.** Psychological factors shown to influence phantom pain include depression, anxiety, grief, self-pity, catastrophizing, and poor social support.

4. **C.** Stump pain is typically present in the first week after amputation but can persist beyond the surgical stages of healing.

5. **A.** Sensitization at the spinal level occurs at dorsal, not ventral, horn neurons. Wind-up is characterized by increased persistent neuronal discharge after stimulation. There is increased excitability of secondary pain neurons mediated by C and A-delta afferent fibers.

6. **C.** The sympathetic system has not been shown to be involved in phantom pain. Neuroma formation, general excitability of spinal cord neurons, receptor activation of NMDA, and reorganization of the somatosensory cortex have been described as mechanisms.

7. **D.** The studies looking at various preventive interventions are controversial, and larger, well-designed studies are needed to better understand preventive therapies for phantom pain. A large study by Karanikolas et al. showed that aggressive perioperative pain control, whether with IV PCA or epidural infusion, was associated with lower incidence of phantom limb pain at 6 months. Memantine treatments also showed reduced phantom limb pain at 6 months, but these findings were not sustained at 12 months. (Karanikolas M, Aretha D, Tsolakis I, et al. Optimized perioperative analgesia reduces chronic phantom limb pain intensity, prevalence, and frequency: a prospective, randomized, clinical trial. *Anesthesiology* 2011;114:1144–1154.)

27 Central Poststroke Pain Syndrome

QUESTIONS

1. Injury to which major pathway is a key component to the pathophysiology of central poststroke pain (CPSP) syndrome?
   A. Corticobulbar pathway
   B. Dorsal column pathway
   C. Corticospinal pathway
   D. Spinothalamocortical pathway
   E. Spinocerebellar pathway

2. A 62-year-old female patient in a nursing home with a past medical history of diabetes and stroke presents to your clinic with a 2-day history of left leg and foot pain described as aching, deep, and squeezing. According to records, she had a right-sided thalamic stroke 1 month ago, resulting in numbness and sensory loss on her left side. What is the most appropriate next step in the management of this patient?
   A. No further tests are needed. Prescribe amitriptyline for treatment of CPSP.
   B. Order lower extremity ultrasound
   C. Order lumbar MRI
   D. Order a hemoglobin A1C and prescribe gabapentin for diabetic peripheral neuropathy
   E. Order an X-ray examination of her left leg

3. You diagnose a 50-year-old male patient with CPSP syndrome. He has a history of diabetes, hypercholesterolemia, and stroke. The patient is allergic to doxepin. In regard to pharmacologic management, what is the best initial choice?
   A. Amitriptyline
   B. Baclofen
   C. Mexiletine
   D. Duloxetine
   E. Pregabalin

4. Stimulation of which area of the brain by either epidural or noninvasive approach has been shown to provide the best pain reduction in CPSP syndrome?
   A. Motor cortex
   B. Sensory cortex
   C. Periventricular gray
   D. Ventroposterolateral thalamus
   E. Cerebellum

5. In patients with a history of stroke, what percentage develops CPSP syndrome?
   A. 1%
   B. 3%
   C. 8%
   D. 16%
   E. 24%

ANSWERS

1. **D.** For a diagnosis of CPSP, a lesion in the spinothalamocortical pathway is necessary and can develop after cortical, subcortical, thalamic, and lateral brainstem strokes. Both stimuli external and internal to the body and nociceptive and non-nociceptive stimuli are transmitted through this tract. There are multiple theories as to the pathophysiology of CPSP, but they all depend on this concept.

2. **B.** The diagnosis of CPSP syndrome is one of *exclusion*. There are many painful conditions that are common in the acute and subacute stages after a stroke, including gout, deep vein thrombosis (DVT), and musculoskeletal pain. The patient in the example has risk factors for DVT (recent stroke, nursing home patient) and, given the acute onset of her pain, a lower extremity ultrasound is warranted. Other diagnostic criteria include pain with a distinct neuroanatomically plausible distribution, a history suggestive of stroke, indication of a distinct neuroanatomic distribution by clinical examination, and indication of a relevant vascular lesion by imaging.

3. **E.** The five main classes of medications useful in treating CPSP are (preferred agent in bold) membrane stabilizers (**carbamazepine,** lidocaine, mexiletine), aminergic agents (**amitriptyline,** duloxetine), glutamate antagonists (ketamine, **lamotrigine**), GABA agonists (thiopental, propofol, **baclofen**), and N-type calcium channel blockers (**gabapentin, pregabalin**). Current recommendations for first-line treatment include amitriptyline, lamotrigine, and pregabalin,

or gabapentin. Baclofen and duloxetine and SSRIs may have a potential secondary role. Mexiletine was shown to improve pain but was poorly tolerated because of side effects. In this patient, amitriptyline is not the best choice, given her allergy to doxepin. Therefore, pregabalin is the best option.

4. **A.** Although it is not entirely clear why, stimulation of the motor cortex has been shown to reduce pain in patients with CPSP syndrome. The stimulating electrode can be implanted epidurally, or stimulation can be performed noninvasively. Studies have shown better pain relief compared with stimulation of the sensory cortex. Patients should be carefully selected. Both the periventricular gray and ventroposterolateral thalamus are targets for deep brain stimulation (DBS), but not for epidural or noninvasive stimulation. Studies have shown that stimulation of the motor cortex is more effective than DBS. The cerebellum is not in the pathway associated with CPSP.

5. **C.** CPSP occurs in about 8% of patients after stroke. Although it is uncommon, it is a major cause of central neuropathic pain, given the common occurrence of stroke.

28 Spinal Cord Injury Pain

QUESTIONS

1. A 26-year-old male quadriplegic suffered a spinal cord injury (SCI) at the level of T5 and now complains of excruciating pain at the level of his lower abdomen, hips, and lower extremities. Which of the following is true?
   A. This localization of pain is considered "central" and is typically the most difficult to treat.
   B. This type of injury puts him at risk of suffering from cerebral hemorrhage and seizures.
   C. His pain is most likely myofascial in nature.
   D. His injury most likely occurred in the last 4–6 months.
   E. His pain should resolve over the course of 3–6 months without treatment.

2. After SCI, pain above the level of the lesion is most likely caused by:
   A. Psychogenic pathology
   B. Musculoskeletal pathology
   C. Neuropathic pathology
   D. "True central pain"
   E. Visceral pain

3. Which of the following pharmacologic treatments are considered first-line therapy for neuropathic SCI-related pain?
   A. Methadone
   B. Gabapentin
   C. Duloxetine
   D. Memantine
   E. Baclofen

4. A 26-year-old male quadriplegic suffered an SCI at the level of T5 and now complains of pain in his lower extremities. On examination, the patient has developed allodynia. The patient and his family are excited about these symptoms since he could not feel or move his legs previously and they see the onset of pain as a sign of partial recovery of sensation in his legs. The following is true about this type of pain/injury:
   A. This type of pain has no association with stress or emotions.
   B. Changes in CNS are dynamic after SCI and progress rostrally only from the core of the lesion.
   C. This type of sensitization is thought to contribute to acute, but not chronic and persistent pain.
   D. This type of pain can be explained by a phenomenon called synaptic plasticity (rewiring).
   E. None of the above

5. Which of the following factors has been demonstrated to have an association with increased pain?
   A. Lack of acceptance of injury
   B. Completeness of injury
   C. Level of injury
   D. Level of family support
   E. All of the above

6. All of the following findings on neurometabolic imaging are consistent with central pain **EXCEPT:**
   A. PET scan showing an overall decrease in thalamic activity ipsilateral to the side of pain.
   B. SPECT study showing an increase in activity in the thalamus contralateral to the pain.
   C. SPECT study showing an overall increase in activity in the parietal cortex.
   D. Proton magnetic spectroscopy study showing abnormal concentrations of N-acetyl inositol and myoinositol.
   E. Cortical reorganization seen in the prefrontal and anterior cingulate cortex.

7. Which of the following is correct regarding shortest onset duration time of pain from SCI?
   A. At level pain 4.2 years; above level pain 1.3 years; below level pain 1.8 years; visceral pain 6 months
   B. At level pain 1.2 years; above level pain 1.8 years; below level pain 1.3 years; visceral pain 4.2 years
   C. At level pain 1.8 years; above level pain 4.2 years; below level pain 1.3 years; visceral pain 1.2 years
   D. At level pain 1.2 years; above level pain 1.3 years; below level pain 1.8 years; visceral pain 4.2 years
   E. None of the above

8. A patient has a T3 spinal cord injury that required spinal fusion at the time of injury. The spinal cord was found to be completely transected at the time of the operation. The patient is wheelchair bound and has been experiencing increased frustration and anger. After 2 years, the patient begins to experience intermittent burning pain in the abdomen and legs. Which of the following is most closely related to severity of pain?
   A. High thoracic SCI (as opposed to low thoracic or lumbar SCI)
   B. Spinal fusion around the injury site
   C. Experiencing anger
   D. Complete (as opposed to incomplete) transection of the spinal cord
   E. Being wheelchair bound

ANSWERS

1. **A.** Central pain occurs below the level of injury and is the most difficult to treat. It can range from 23% to 52% and is described as the most "severe or excruciating." Onset time for central pain is approximately 1.8 years.

2. **B.** Pain above the level of lesion is most likely related to musculoskeletal pathology. Above level pain often responds to appropriate treatment, once recognized. Examples include joint and muscle overuse, mechanical compression such as in use of crutches, and secondary changes resulting from fractures and fixation.

3. **B.** Opioids can have a role in treating SCI but should not be considered first-line therapy. There are several high quality studies showing the benefit of gabapentin, Lyrica, and tricyclic antidepressants (TCAs). These drugs should be considered first-line treatments. Mixed serotonin-norepinephrine reuptake inhibitors can also be quite effective in therapy when the gabapentinoids and TCAs are not effective or have intolerable side effects. NMDA receptor antagonists theoretically can provide analgesia, but data for this are lacking. Baclofen can be useful in treating associated spasticity symptoms, but benefit for neuropathic pain is questionable.

4. **D.** Below level pain is thought to be a result of a dynamic cascade of molecular, biochemical, anatomic ("plasticity"), and cellular responses. These events in turn produce physiologic changes at both the spinal and supraspinal level that contribute to the onset of dysesthetic sensations, prominently pain. It can be associated with stress and negative emotions. Changes of the CNS progress rostrally and caudally from the lesion. Central pain, when it occurs, is typically chronic and persistent.

5. **A.** In a study of 42 patients, anger, lack of acceptance of injury, and negative cognitions were associated with greater SCI pain.

6. **C.** SPECT studies show an overall hypoactivity of the parietal cortex in central pain. There is evidence showing an overall decrease in thalamic neuronal activity between bursts, but there seems to be a hyperactivity in the thalamus contralateral to the pain. Overall, changes seem to be occurring in the thalamus, anterior cingulate cortex, and the prefrontal cortex.

7. **D.** The shortest onset duration time of pain from SCI at level pain occurs at 1.2 years, above level pain at 1.3 years, below level pain at 1.8 years, and visceral pain at 4.2 years. The mean onset time for any type of SCI pain is 1.6 years.

8. **C.** Psychological factors, not physiologic factors, are more closely related to pain severity.

29 Chronic Widespread Pain

QUESTIONS

1. Which of the following physical examination findings was associated with the strongest validity for documenting myofascial pain syndrome?
   A. Eliciting local tenderness
   B. Palpating a taut band
   C. Documenting the local twitch response
   D. Reproduction and referral of pain to a zone of reference
   E. Erythema

2. When comparing trigger points of myofascial pain syndrome and tender points of fibromyalgia, all of the following are true **EXCEPT**:
   A. Tender points are symmetrically distributed throughout the body, whereas trigger points have a more random distribution.
   B. Tender points and trigger points are both associated with referred and radiating pain.
   C. Tender points are not limited to muscular locations but also include other soft tissue structures.
   D. Myofascial pain syndrome has been associated with the muscles of mastication, while fibromyalgia has not.
   E. All of the above are true.

3. To diagnose fibromyalgia using the 1990 American College of Rheumatology (ACR) Criteria for Research Classification, _____ out of _____ anatomically tender points should be identified.
   A. 11, 20
   B. 13, 18
   C. 10, 20
   D. 11, 18
   E. 13, 20

4. Which of the following meets the clinical diagnostic criteria for fibromyalgia based on the American College of Rheumatology?
   A. Widespread pain index (WPI) score of 3 and symptom severity (SS) score of 7
   B. WPI score of 3 and SS score of 8
   C. WPI score of 10 and SS score of 4
   D. WPI score of 10 and SS score of 5
   E. WPI score of 4 and SS score of 10

5. Which of the following clinical features is most common with fibromyalgia?
   A. Depression
   B. Fatigue
   C. Irritable bowel syndrome
   D. Urinary urgency
   E. Eczema

6. All of the following are associated with fibromyalgia **EXCEPT**:
   A. Sjögren's syndrome
   B. Tuberculosis
   C. Lyme disease
   D. Hepatitis C
   E. All of the above are associated with fibromyalgia.

7. Which region of the brain most consistently exhibits increased activity in fibromyalgia?
   A. Amygdala
   B. Thalamus
   C. Somatosensory cortex
   D. Hypothalamus
   E. Insula

8. Fibromyalgia patients have been found to have higher levels of which of the following?
   A. Glutamate
   B. Substance P
   C. 5-hydroxytryptamine (5-HT)
   D. Dopamine
   E. Both A and B

9. Which of the following is the **LEAST** effective as a monotherapy for fibromyalgia?
   A. Aerobic exercise
   B. Cognitive behavioral therapy
   C. NSAIDs
   D. Gabapentin
   E. All are effective.

10. All of the following medications are FDA-approved for the treatment of fibromyalgia **EXCEPT**:
    A. Pregabalin
    B. Gabapentin
    C. Milnacipran
    D. Duloxetine
    E. All are FDA approved for fibromyalgia treatment.

ANSWERS

1. **D.** For documenting myofascial pain syndrome, stronger reliability was associated with a tender spot (trigger point) in an affected muscle, referral of pain to a zone of reference, and reproducibility of the patient's usual pain.

2. **B.** Tender points of fibromyalgia do not refer or radiate to other locations; trigger points resulting from myofascial pain can radiate to another zone.

3. **D.** Eleven of 18 anatomically tender points should be identified for a diagnosis of fibromyalgia, according to the ACR criteria (1990). The ACR research criteria has a sensitivity and specificity of >80% for the diagnosis of fibromyalgia. Note that new ACR criteria were developed in 2010 by Wolfe et al. and later modified in 2011 and 2016 with the addition of the fibromyalgia symptom scale, which increased specificity and sensitivity to >85% each. New revisions have been made as of 2016. (Wolfe F, Clauw DJ, Fitzcharles MA, et al. 2016 revisions to the 2010/2011 fibromyalgia diagnostic criteria. *Semin Arthritis Rheum.* 2016;46(3):319-29.)

4. **E.** ACR clinical diagnostic criteria for fibromyalgia includes either a WPI score >7 and SS score >5 or WPI score of 4–6 with a SS score >9 based on the most recent (2016) revisions to the 2010/2011 criteria.

5. **B.** About 80% of patients with fibromyalgia complain of fatigue. Sixty percent of fibromyalgia patients experience urinary urgency and nocturia. Roughly 30%–50% of fibromyalgia patients suffer from irritable bowel syndrome and benign dyspepsia. Depression and anxiety are also seen in about 40% of fibromyalgia patients.

6. **E.** Secondary fibromyalgia can be seen in patients with rheumatoid arthritis, systemic lupus erythematosus, and Sjögren's syndrome. Infectious and inflammatory conditions associated with fibromyalgia include hepatitis C, tuberculosis, syphilis, and Lyme disease.

7. **E.** The insula has been shown consistently to exhibit increased activity in fibromyalgia and most other chronic pain states.

8. **E.** Both glutamate and substance P have been found to be elevated in patients with fibromyalgia. Dopamine and 5-HT levels appear to be lower in fibromyalgia patients.

9. **C.** NSAIDs have not been shown to be effective as monotherapy for fibromyalgia. Aerobic exercise, cognitive behavioral therapy, and gabapentin have been shown to be effective in the treatment of fibromyalgia.

10. **B.** Gabapentin has not been FDA approved for the treatment of fibromyalgia, but it has been shown to be effective. Pregabalin, duloxetine, and milnacipran have all been FDA approved for the treatment of fibromyalgia.

30 Headache Management

QUESTIONS

1. Which of the following about the epidemiology of migraine headaches is **FALSE**?
   A. It is more prevalent after puberty.
   B. It is more prevalent in females than males after puberty.
   C. Prevalence starts to decline after 40 years of age.
   D. The prevalence is lowest in Asians and highest in Caucasians.
   E. The incidence is directly proportional to household income.

2. A 22-year-old female college student with gradual onset of unilateral headaches presents to your clinic. She has associated nausea, vomiting, blurry vision, anxiety, and difficulty with concentrating on her schoolwork. Headaches can last several days at a time. She is worried she will not be able to graduate because of failing grades. Which of the following are consistent with migraine headaches?
   A. Unilateral headaches
   B. Nausea and vomiting
   C. Difficulty with concentration
   D. Anxiety
   E. All of the above

3. Which of the following is a migraine variant?
   A. Trigeminal migraine
   B. Basilar-type migraine
   C. Occipital migraine
   D. Vestibulocochlear migraine
   E. All of the above

4. Your patient is being evaluated for diagnosis and treatment of migraines. History is positive for coronary artery disease, diabetes, and asthma. Which of the following medications should be avoided in this patient?
   A. Acetaminophen
   B. Propranolol
   C. Valproic acid
   D. Topiramate
   E. Butterbur

5. You are evaluating a patient who has experienced migraine headaches on a regular basis for the last 2 years. The patient was initially using hydrocodone, ibuprofen, and acetaminophen sparingly, but progressively needed them daily. Which of the following interventions is most appropriate?
   A. Switch to a different class of opioid because of tolerance
   B. Abruptly discontinue all current medications and start indomethacin
   C. Wean the current regimen, give a medication holiday, and then initiate a prophylactic medication
   D. Send the patient to detoxification for opioid addiction
   E. Refer the patient for a psychiatric evaluation

6. A patient presents with mild bilateral temporal headaches that have been occurring for years. The headaches have a tightening quality not associated with any activity and occur 2–3 times per week, lasting approximately 12 hours each. Which of the following are characteristic of this type of headache?
   A. Nausea and vomiting
   B. Pulsating quality behind the eye unilaterally
   C. Flashing lights with the onset of headaches
   D. Excessive lacrimation
   E. None of the above

7. You evaluate a patient who describes an intense headache with multiple episodes of short but severe unilateral, orbital, supraorbital, or temporal pain. The headache is usually associated with nasal congestion, rhinorrhea, and facial sweating. Which of the following should be considered one of the first-line treatments to help treat an acute attack for this patient?
   A. Corticosteroids
   B. Calcium channel blockers
   C. Topical local anesthetics
   D. Inhaled oxygen 7–10 L/min for 10 minutes
   E. None of the above

8. Which of the following has been proposed as a mechanism for cluster headaches?
   A. Hypoactivation of the autonomic system at the level of the brainstem
   B. Dysfunction of the hypothalamus
   C. Dysfunction of the limbic system and connections with the trigeminal autonomic tract
   D. Dysfunction of the ocular neural pathways
   E. Cortical spreading

9. Which of the following is a diagnostic criterion of paroxysmal hemicrania?
   A. Attack prevented by indomethacin
   B. Ipsilateral nasal congestion and/or rhinorrhea
   C. Pressing or tightening quality
   D. Nausea or vomiting
   E. All of the above

ANSWERS

1. **E.** The incidence of migraines is inversely proportional to household income. The prevalence before puberty is 4% and increases to 17.6% in women and 6% in men after puberty. Migraines begin to decline after age 40 years. Asians have the lowest incidence, Caucasians have the highest incidence, and African Americans have intermediate incidence.

2. **E.** Migraines are typically unilateral but can progress to bilateral, generalized headaches. They have a gradual onset and a throbbing characteristic. Movement exacerbates the headaches. Nausea is almost always associated (90%), but vomiting is seen only one-third of the time. Other associated symptoms include sensory hypersensitivity, nasal stuffiness, anorexia, blurry vision, diarrhea, abdominal cramps, polyuria, facial pallor, and sweating. Psychological and mood changes such as anxiety, depression, irritability, nervousness, fatigue, and difficulty with concentration can also be seen.

3. **B.** Basilar-type migraines are characterized by brainstem-type symptoms such as vertigo, ataxia, nausea, tinnitus, nystagmus, dysarthria, paresthesia, and change in level of consciousness and cognition. Other variants include ophthalmoplegic and hemiplegic migraines.

4. **B.** Comorbidities should be reviewed carefully before initiating any therapy for migraines. Beta blockers should be used with caution in a patient with cardiac disease and asthma. Butterbur is a nutraceutical with evidence to support use for migraine prophylaxis. It can be associated with hepatotoxicity, specifically formulations with pyrrolizidine alkaloids.

5. **C.** Preventive/prophylactic medications are underutilized for migraine headache treatment. First-line medications include: divalproex, topiramate, beta blockers, and antidepressants. Evidence for calcium channel blockers is weak.

6. **E.** Tension-type headaches are the most common type of headaches. They are characterized by a nonpulsatile tension located bilaterally, which can be frontal, temporal, parietal, or occipital. There are typically no associated GI symptoms or auras. Migraine headaches can also be nonpulsatile and bilateral but are typically more severe.

7. **D.** Cluster headaches are characterized by multiple transient intense episodes of pain that are severe and unilateral, and often occur in the orbital, supraorbital, or temporal region. Inhaled oxygen at 7–10 L/min for 10 minutes is the first-line therapy and is 70% effective.

8. **B.** The mechanism behind cluster headaches is thought to be related to dysfunction of the hypothalamus causing alteration in the circadian rhythm. The trigeminovascular system and activation of the parasympathetic system are also thought to be mechanisms involved.

9. **A.** Paroxysmal hemicrania is similar to cluster headache and arguably in the same spectrum. What differentiates it most distinctly from cluster headache is response to indomethacin which can aid in diagnosis. Aspirin may also offer some relief, but this is typically not as robust as response to indomethacin.

31 Dental and Facial Pain

QUESTIONS

1. All of the following are true of burning mouth/tongue disorder (BMD) **EXCEPT:**
   A. Typically affects middle-aged and older men
   B. Can be associated with diabetes
   C. Can be associated with immune connective tissue disorders
   D. It is a neuropathic condition of a central origin.
   E. Can be associated with Sjögren's syndrome

2. A patient with chronic headaches, neck and shoulder pain, and bilateral jaw pain presents to your clinic. He is in a high-stress job and finds himself clenching his jaw throughout the day, which seems to exacerbate his pain. Which of the following would be the **LEAST** appropriate therapy for this patient's condition?
   A. Physical therapy for the neck and shoulder
   B. Placement of peripheral nerve stimulator
   C. Relaxation therapy
   D. A mouth guard
   E. Trigger point injection

3. If a patient has signs suggestive of trigeminal neuralgia, which diagnostic test should be performed?
   A. Complete blood count
   B. Cervical spine X-ray examination
   C. Computed tomography of the head
   D. Electrolyte panel
   E. Magnetic resonance imaging of the brain

4. A 29-year-old female presents with symptoms of right-sided selective V2-affected trigeminal neuralgia. You examined her for the first time 4 weeks ago and recommended gabapentin. She is currently on 600 mg orally three times a day and experiencing minimal benefit. The most appropriate next step is:
   A. Initiate oxcarbazepine along with gabapentin
   B. Add a low-dose NSAID to her regimen
   C. Offer a microvascular decompression
   D. Obtain a CT of her head
   E. Initiate opioid therapy

5. Which of the following is true of classic trigeminal neuralgia?
   A. It is associated with masseter muscle weakness.
   B. It is characterized by episodic bursts of bilateral severe, lancinating pain lasting 30–60 minutes.
   C. There is an absence of sensory deficits.
   D. Tricyclic antidepressants are considered first-line therapy.
   E. It is associated with visual changes.

6. An 83-year-old female presents with an 11-month history of intense, sharp pain over the left eye. You note healed vesicles over the left frontal area. Which of the following most accurately describes this patient's prognosis?
   A. Her pain will completely resolve with time.
   B. Her pain will transform to a dull sensation as nerve endings degenerate.
   C. Her condition will respond to high-dose antiviral medications.
   D. Her condition will respond poorly to antiepileptic drugs (AEDs) and surgical therapies.
   E. Her condition will eventually lead to paralysis in the distribution of the affected nerve root.

ANSWERS

1. **A.** BMD typically affects middle-aged and older women, not men. It can be associated with oral disorders such as Sjögren's disease, oral fungal infections, and systemic disorders such as diabetes mellitus, connective tissue disorders, vasculitides, and vitamin deficiencies. It is thought to be a neuropathic condition of central or peripheral etiology.

2. **B.** Treatment of temporomandibular disorders (TMDs) is multidisciplinary and is targeted to the mechanism of pain. With a myofascial component, muscle relaxants and trigger point injections with local anesthetic can be used. Other pharmacologic treatments include NSAIDs, antidepressants, and over-the-counter analgesics. In cases of psychological factors, biofeedback and relaxation techniques can be used. When there is a biomechanical disorder causing strain on adjacent structures, physical therapy and home therapy can be effective. Neck pathology can result in altered head position and myofascial pain that presents as facial pain, which can coexist with TMDs and should be treated appropriately.

3. **E.** Brain MRI and brain MR angiography can help differentiate "classic TN" from "symptomatic TN" and thus distinguish whether further surgical management is indicated.

4. **A.** Single AEDs can provide substantial relief from facial pain. The AED should be titrated to therapeutic effect. A second AED can be introduced if a single AED is not effective and may increase the chance for a therapeutic response. Baclofen has also been shown to be an effective treatment in addition to other AEDs such as carbamazepine, oxcarbamazepine, and lamotrigine.

5. **C.** Classic TN is typically associated with a normal sensory examination. Many patients have a small sensory trigger zone (< 10 mm) that can trigger the pain and is pathognomonic of TN. Pain is usually unilateral and momentary and patients are typically pain free between attacks. AEDs are usually considered first-line therapy.

6. **D.** Painful, posttraumatic trigeminal neuropathies such as postherpetic neuralgia have a poor response rate to AEDs and surgical therapies. The general approach is treatment with various neuropathic medications and analgesics, but this can be challenging. The inciting event is damage to a craniocervical nerve and ensuing pain that is continuous or recurrent. Other conditions in this group include inferior alveolar neuralgia (after mandibular third molar extraction) and infraorbital neuralgia (after maxillary trauma).

32 Visceral Pain

QUESTIONS

1. An 82-year-old male with pancreatic cancer presents with diffuse abdominal pain, anorexia, and nausea. Which of the following is true regarding visceral afferent pathways?
   A. Most abdominal visceral organs receive dual innervation.
   B. The spinothalamic tract relays information rostrally.
   C. Most visceral sensory neurons are polymodal.
   D. All of the above
   E. None of the above

2. Which of the following can produce acute visceral pain?
   A. Ischemia
   B. Burning
   C. Distension of hollow organs
   D. Chemical irritants
   E. A, C, and D

3. A 21-year-old female who was recently diagnosed with metastatic pancreatic cancer is admitted with uncontrolled abdominal pain. She has intense fear and anxiety associated with her pain and her diagnosis. Which of the following is true regarding the central processing of visceral sensation and pain?
   A. Vagal inputs are more closely linked to the emotional and autonomic responses triggered by pain.
   B. Spinal afferents project via the ventromedial thalamus to cortical areas and primarily serve discriminative functions.
   C. Visceral pain preferentially activates the perigenual portions of the anterior cingulate cortex, which potentially explains the stronger emotional response associated with painful visceral stimuli.
   D. Both A and C
   E. All of the above

4. Where is 95% of the body's serotonin located?
   A. Vesical epithelial cells
   B. The chemoreceptor trigger zone cells in the hypothalamus
   C. Enterochromaffin cells of the gut
   D. Epithelial cells in the airways
   E. Spinal cord (gray/white matter)

5. The transient receptor potential vanilloid-1 (TRPV1) is activated by:
   A. Acid
   B. Temperature
   C. Capsaicin
   D. Endogenous lipid mediators
   E. All of the above

6. Regarding neural ablation of the celiac plexus in upper abdominal visceral malignancies, which of the following is correct?
   A. Surgical neurolysis is superior.
   B. Unilateral chemical neurolysis of the splanchnic nerves has similar efficacy compared with bilateral neurolysis.
   C. It improves the quality of life.
   D. It decreases opioid requirements.
   E. All of the above

7. A 28-year-old female with widespread visceral and osseous metastases from breast cancer presents with neoplasm-related pain. She failed oral therapy and has an intrathecal drug delivery system with morphine. However, she continues to have intractable pain. A midline myelotomy is being considered. Which of the following is true regarding myelotomy?
   A. It should be considered as a last resort for visceral pain.
   B. Even though it offers complete and permanent relief, it should only be considered in patients with intractable pain with a terminal disease.
   C. It targets central sensitization, but relief is transient.
   D. It alters emotional responses to pain.
   E. It should be considered for pain secondary to osseous metastasis.

8. Visceral pain is often associated with abnormalities in organ function, such as constipation, nausea, cardiac failure, or dysuria. Serotonin antagonists can frequently be used to help with gastrointestinal pain management. Which of the following is correct?
   A. The ligand-gated 5-HT3 receptor has been found on vagal and spinal afferents and is involved in visceral sensation, including the perception of nausea.
   B. Ondansetron can be used to help treat nausea, vomiting, and visceral pain.
   C. Both the 5-HT3 antagonist alosetron and 5-HT4 antagonist tegaserod are available in the United States to treat visceral pain.
   D. A and B
   E. A and C

9. κ-Opioid receptors (KOR) are expressed in peripheral visceral afferents; thus, κ-agonists were developed. What is the reason for their limited utility?
   A. These medications will increase the likelihood of opioid addiction.
   B. These medications will increase the likelihood of nausea, vomiting, and constipation.
   C. These medications are incredibly costly.
   D. These medications cause significant dysphoria.
   E. All of the above

10. Most visceral sensory neurons respond to multiple stimuli such as endogenous and exogenous chemicals contained in the luminal contents, temperature, and stretch as a result of:
    A. Low and high threshold fibers (mechanosensitive spinal afferents)
    B. Their relation with the spinothalamic tract pathway
    C. Vagal afferents projected to the nucleus of the solitary tract
    D. The polymodal property of visceral sensory neurons
    E. All of the above

ANSWERS

1. **D.** Organs in the chest cavity and most viscera within the abdomen receive dual afferent innervation; vagal and spinal nerves convey sensory input to the central nervous system. The spinothalamic tract relays noxious stimuli rostrally. Most visceral sensory neurons are polymodal; they respond to multiple stimulus modalities, such as chemicals, temperature, and stretch sensations.

2. **E.** Traction on the mesentery, distention of hollow organs, strong contractions of muscle layers surrounding such hollow organs, ischemia, and chemical irritants can lead to visceral pain. However, cutting or burning (as in endoscopic procedures) are not felt when applied to viscera.

3. **D.** Visceral pain activates the perigenual portion of the anterior cingulate cortex (ACC) and nonvisceral pain, the midcingulate cortex. The structural closeness in areas that process visceral pain and emotion in the ACC may explain the increased emotional response to painful visceral relative to nonvisceral stimuli.

4. **C.** Serotonin is released from enteroendocrine (enterochromaffin) cells in the gastrointestinal tract (95% of the body's serotonin) when chemical or mechanical stimuli activate intrinsic and extrinsic neurons.

5. **E.** The capsaicin receptor/TRPV1 is an ion channel activated by capsaicin, temperature, acid, and endogenous lipid mediators. Hence, the hot, burning feeling upon application of capsaicin.

6. **D.** Splanchnic neurolysis decreases opioid requirements compared with pharmacotherapy, but not when compared with celiac plexus neurolysis. There are data to support a transient decrease in opioid requirements for these procedures targeted at the sympathetic axis, but not the superiority of one ablative approach over another.

7. **A.** Midline myelotomy is used to treat patients with refractory pain from visceral malignancies. The technique appears to provide only partial and transient pain relief and, without conclusive evidence, recommendations are that it be reserved for only patients with intractable pain resulting from terminal disease (thus answer choice B is partially true).

8. **A.** The ligand-gated 5-HT3 receptor exists on vagal and spinal afferents and is involved in both visceral sensations as well as the perception of nausea. Alosetron has been linked to ischemic colitis and it is therefore no longer readily available. Tegaserod has been associated with ischemic events and has also been removed from the market. Ondansetron, a 5-HT3 receptor antagonist, is used to treat severe nausea and vomiting but does not target visceral pain.

9. **D.** κ-agonists were developed to take advantage of κ-receptors (a subtype of the opioid receptor) in peripheral visceral afferents to increase analgesia while lowering the likelihood of adverse effects related to μ-opioid agonists. In studies of experimentally induced acute pain, administration of κ-agonists seem to raise the visceral pain threshold, but central effects with dysphoria limit their use.

10. **D.** Most visceral sensory neurons are polymodal and therefore respond to multiple stimulus modalities, including temperature, stretch, and chemicals.

33 Pediatric Chronic Pain Management

QUESTIONS

1. What is the most common cause of chest wall pain in children?
   A. Tietze's syndrome
   B. Slipping rib cage syndrome
   C. Costochondritis
   D. Myofascial chest wall pain
   E. None of the above

2. Which of the following is the most effective treatment for functional abdominal pain?
   A. Serial nerve blocks
   B. Amitriptyline
   C. Cognitive-behavioral therapy
   D. A and B
   E. None of the above

3. What is most common comorbid symptom that occurs with headaches in children?
   A. Sleep deprivation
   B. Dizziness
   C. Tachycardia
   D. Orthostatic hypotension
   E. Nausea

4. Which of the following children is most likely to develop complex regional pain syndrome (CRPS) Type 1?
   A. 2.5-year-old girl
   B. 5-year-old boy
   C. 7-year-old girl
   D. 11-year-old boy
   E. 13-year-old girl

5. Which of the following statements concerning headaches in children is true?
   A. An ultrasound-guided approach to the occipital nerve allows easier access to the C2 nerve root, providing a more robust blockade than an occipital nerve block.
   B. Delayed sleep causing sleep deprivation is a frequent cause, but not the most frequent cause, of headaches seen in children.
   C. A headache accompanied by nausea or vomiting is a common pattern seen in children and should not lead to overreaction in parents.
   D. Cranial circumference measurement can be misleading in children and is rarely used in the workup of headaches.
   E. None of the above

6. When treating an 8-year-old child for chronic chest pain, initial treatment will be most likely targeted to:
   A. Cardiac pathology
   B. Chest wall pathology
   C. Pulmonary pathology
   D. Gastrointestinal pathology
   E. Psychogenic causes

7. Which of the following has been shown to be an effective delivery medium of psychological treatment in children with chronic pain?
   A. Television-based
   B. Parent-directed
   C. Internet-based
   D. Biofeedback
   E. Hypnosis

8. What does quantitative sensory testing accomplish?
   A. Defines thresholds for allodynia
   B. Provides a comparison to standard abnormal values
   C. Useful for diagnosing factitious disorder
   D. Determines if there has been an axonal or demyelinating nerve injury
   E. Measures extent of neurodegeneration in CRPS

9. Which of the following is a useful assessment of chronic pain in children who have difficulty with self-report measures?
   A. Children's Comprehensive Pain Questionnaire (CCPQ)
   B. Varni/Thompson Pediatric Pain Questionnaire (VTPPQ)
   C. West Haven-Yale Multidimensional Pain Inventory (WHYMPI)
   D. Pain Catastrophizing Scale for Children (PSC-C)
   E. Pain behavior observation method

10. Which of the following therapies has been utilized in the management of pediatric CRPS?
    A. Intravenous regional anesthesia with guanethidine, bretylium, lidocaine, and ketorolac
    B. Continuous epidural analgesia
    C. Sympathetic chain blocks
    D. Sciatic nerve catheters
    E. All of the above

11. Eutectic mixture of local anesthetics (EMLA) cream has been used as an effective adjunct in children undergoing cancer-related treatment. What are the two local anesthetics in EMLA cream?
    A. Lidocaine and bupivacaine
    B. Ropivacaine and lidocaine
    C. Lidocaine and prilocaine
    D. Bupivacaine and prilocaine
    E. None of the above

12. Which of the following is cited as an advantage of epidural clonidine?
    A. Increased hemodynamic stability
    B. Improved circulation in cerebral, coronary, and visceral vasculature
    C. More cost effective than narcotic analgesics
    D. Can be administered without periodic monitoring
    E. Delayed respiratory depression

13. Your pediatric patient is in the preoperative holding area with multiple patches of EMLA on his arms to help decrease pain associated with intravenous access placement. The nurses also put some on his back in anticipation of the procedure. He has been feeling strange and his parents think he appears restless and agitated. His SpO_2 is noted to be 85%. What is the most likely explanation?
    A. Lidocaine toxicity
    B. Prilocaine-induced conformational change of hemoglobin
    C. The patient has a respiratory infection.
    D. The patient is anxious and needs to relax.
    E. Allergic contact dermatitis

14. Which of the following is a common cause of pediatric back pain?
    A. Spondylolysis
    B. Disk herniation
    C. Tumors of the spinal cord
    D. Sickle cell disease
    E. All of the above

15. Which of the following side effects of intrathecal opioids is dose dependent?
    A. Nausea
    B. Vomiting
    C. Pruritus
    D. Urinary retention
    E. Respiratory depression

ANSWERS

1. **C.** Chest wall pain is the most common cause of chest pain in children (greater than pulmonary, cardiac, abdominal, and psychogenic causes). Of the types of chest wall pain listed, costochondritis is the most common.

2. **C.** Functional abdominal pain (FAP) is abdominal pain with no identifiable organic cause and may have an affective component. Treatments with proven efficacy are cognitive-behavioral therapy with family-centered therapy. Amitriptyline has been used to treat FAP, although a randomized prospective trial showed no difference between amitriptyline and control. Serial nerve blocks are beneficial in neuropathic pain, but not for FAP.

3. **A.** Sleep deprivation is the most common comorbidity associated with headaches in children. Dizziness, tachycardia, and hypotension are also seen. New-onset headaches that awaken children from sleep or headaches with associated nausea/vomiting may necessitate a more in-depth neurologic assessment.

4. **E.** Although CRPS Type 1 has been reported in younger children, it is generally seen in those older than 9 years and more frequently in girls 11–13 years old. Prognosis of CRPS in children is more favorable than in adults and can resolve over time.

5. **A.** Trigeminal nerve blocks can be used for frontal headaches and occipital nerve blocks for occipital headaches in children. An ultrasound-guided approach to the occipital nerve allows access to the C2 nerve root, and injection of local anesthetic and a steroid at this location can provide a more robust blockade than peripheral subcutaneous injection.

6. **B.** Chest wall pain is the most common cause of chest pain in children.

7. **C.** Intensive inpatient/outpatient treatment, self-administered, school-based, home-based, internet-based, and CD ROM-based delivery of psychological interventions for recurrent or chronic pain in children has been shown to be effective. Although parental involvement is important, increased parental attention can exacerbate pain symptoms. Methods such as biofeedback and hypnosis can be safely used and are becoming more available to children; these aim to alter the sensory aspects of chronic pain and may be effective, but there is still limited evidence available.

8. **A.** Quantitative sensory testing (QST) compares pain detection thresholds for thermal and vibration sensations in patients with the same thresholds in healthy children. This allows measurement of dynamic allodynia and mechanical static allodynia and can aid in the diagnosis of CRPS in children.

9. **E.** Multiple assessment tools are available to assess pain, anxiety, stress, disability, quality of life, family functioning, and coping in children aged 4 years and older. The pain behavior observation method is a 10-minute observational pain behavior tool for children who have self-reporting difficulty because of age or cognition. The CCPQ and VTPPQ are standardized

interviews for school-age children and adolescents and their parents. Potential limitations include cultural or cognitive differences among children. The PSC-C assesses pain-specific coping strategies. The WHYMPI identifies clinical subgroups of adult chronic pain patients based on their ability to cope.

10. **E.** All of the therapies listed are regional anesthetic approaches for managing CRPS Type 1. Less invasive therapies also include psychological interventions, physical therapy, and pharmacologic therapy with: NSAIDs, tricyclic antidepressants, anticonvulsants, SNRIs, systemic vasodilators, and opioids. Neuromodulation and complementary therapies have also been used.

11. **C.** A eutectic mixture of lidocaine 2.5% and prilocaine 2.5% (EMLA) cream or patch can relieve pain in children undergoing cancer-related procedures. It should not be used in premature infants. Four percent tetracaine gel can also be useful for this purpose.

12. **B.** Clonidine is an alpha-2 agonist and can be used in the treatment of pain and for hypertension. Clonidine as an adjuvant in neuraxial preparations can reduce opioid requirements and opioid-related side effects, increase sedation and anxiolysis without increasing respiratory depression, and vasodilate the cerebral, coronary, and visceral vascular beds to improve circulation in these areas. Intravenous and topical routes can also play a role in pain management.

13. **B.** Plasma lidocaine levels of 4.5–7.5 µg/mL can cause restlessness, dizziness, blurred vision, or tremors, and at levels of > 7.5 µg/mL, it can produce generalized tonic-clonic seizures. However, this would not explain the patient's SpO$_2$ level, which is consistent with methemoglobinemia. With application of EMLA onto newly regenerated postburn or abraded skin, methemoglobinemia from prilocaine has been reported. Levels above 3% are associated with agitation.

14. **E.** Back pain is becoming more prevalent in children, especially with involvement in high-impact sports. All answer choices are common back problems in children. Alternative medicine is used extensively for management of pain in this population and is especially effective when there is a myofascial component.

15. **E.** Respiratory depression occurs with neuraxial opioid administration in a dose-dependent manner. Other opioid-related side effects such as nausea, vomiting, urinary retention, and pruritus are not dose dependent but are increased with intrathecal administration relative to epidural administration.

Management of Pain in Older Adults

QUESTIONS

1. Which of the following is true regarding physiologic changes in the geriatric population?
   A. Arterial hepatic blood flow increases.
   B. There is an increase in GABA synthesis in the lateral thalamus.
   C. Speed of processing nociceptive stimuli decreases.
   D. Total body fat decreases.
   E. Total body water increases.

2. All of the following are barriers to the assessment of pain in older adults **EXCEPT:**
   A. Presence of patient cognitive deficits
   B. Presence of patient sensory deficits, such as decreased hearing
   C. Provider belief that pain is an expected part of the aging process
   D. Multisystem complexity, leaving providers little time for pain evaluation
   E. Geriatric patients' readiness to admit to experiencing "pain"

3. All of the following are unidimensional pain scales **EXCEPT:**
   A. FACES pain scale
   B. Pain thermometer
   C. Verbal pain descriptor (none, mild, moderate, severe)
   D. Numerical rating scale
   E. McGill Pain Questionnaire (MPQ)

4. Which of the following pain assessment tools is intended for geriatric patients with cognitive impairment?
   A. DOLOPLUS
   B. PACSLAC (Pain Assessment Checklist for Seniors with Limited Ability to Communicate)
   C. Brief Pain Inventory
   D. A and B
   E. A, B, and C

5. Which of the following is true about nonopioid analgesics?
   A. Acetaminophen toxicity is the leading cause of acute liver failure in the United States.
   B. Acetaminophen is generally shown to be a more effective analgesic than ibuprofen.
   C. When compared with younger patients, geriatric patients are at lower risk of experiencing gastrointestinal complications such as peptic ulcer disease when using NSAIDs.
   D. COX-2 inhibitors are more efficacious for analgesia than nonselective NSAIDs.
   E. Preliminary evidence suggests that topical NSAIDs have the same toxicity profile as oral nonselective NSAIDs.

6. Tricyclic antidepressants (TCAs) are associated with which of the following problematic side effects in older patients?
   A. Bradycardia
   B. Increased urination
   C. Diarrhea
   D. Increased risk for falls
   E. Salivation

7. All of the following are nonpharmacologic pain management modalities useful in the management of chronic pain in geriatric patients **EXCEPT:**
   A. Cognitive behavioral therapy (CBT)
   B. Exercise program
   C. Nutritional supplements
   D. Patient education
   E. Limitation of physical movement

8. Which of the following is true regarding opioid use in the geriatric population for chronic non cancer pain?
   A. The geriatric age group is associated with a significant reduction in the risk of opioid misuse or abuse.
   B. Opioids have shown no efficacy for neuropathic pain conditions.
   C. Opioids are associated with a decreased risk of fractures.
   D. Opioids are associated with a decreased risk for all-cause mortality.
   E. No pain reduction with opioids has been shown in the setting of osteoarthritis.

9. Sensory impairments are commonplace in the geriatric population with approximately 30% experiencing visual impairments and 40% of patients above 75 years old experiencing hearing impairments. All of the following provider strategies can decrease the negative impact of these limitations **EXCEPT:**
   A. Use of good lighting in patient examination rooms
   B. Asking patients to wear eyeglasses and hearing aids to appointments
   C. Focusing on the computer screen while typing during the patient encounter
   D. Speaking slowly
   E. Speaking with a loud voice or using a handheld amplifier

10. Which of the following is true regarding pain management in cognitively impaired geriatric patients?
    A. Cognitively impaired geriatric patients generally receive significantly more pain medications than cognitively intact individuals.
    B. Cognitively impaired patients generally overreport their pain.
    C. Manifestations of pain in cognitively impaired geriatric patients vary from lethargy and physical aggression to grimacing and groaning.
    D. Providers are typically vigilant for pain in this challenging population.
    E. Limiting the administration of pain medication is encouraged in this patient population because of their inability to ascertain pain levels.

11. When providing pain care to a patient of an ethnic minority, all of the following should be kept in mind **EXCEPT:**
    A. Some ethnic minorities are less inclined to seek help for their pain.
    B. All cultures generally express pain in the same way.
    C. Varying attitudes exist to pain medication.
    D. Explanatory models for pain etiology are varying.
    E. Gender and time since migration are important factors in pain presentation.

12. A 90-year-old female with a history of severe constipation and peripheral edema presents with complaint of pain secondary to diabetic neuropathy. Your first-line treatment should be:
    A. Gabapentin
    B. Pregabalin
    C. Nortriptyline
    D. Duloxetine
    E. Fluoxetine

13. All of the following are risk factors for developing chronic pain in nursing home patients **EXCEPT:**
    A. Obesity
    B. Male gender
    C. Low income
    D. Depression
    E. Anxiety

14. A 78-year-old female with unstable angina, chronic renal insufficiency, and peptic ulcer disease presents with pain in her right knee secondary to osteoarthritis (OA). What is a reasonable first-line analgesic?
    A. Ibuprofen
    B. Diclofenac gel
    C. Acetaminophen
    D. Oxycodone
    E. Duloxetine

15. A patient arrives at your pain clinic with severe dementia and cognitive decline. Which of the following is the most useful pain assessment tool in this scenario?
    A. MPQ
    B. FACES pain scale
    C. DOLOPLUS-2
    D. Brief Pain Inventory
    E. Numerical rating scale

ANSWERS

1. **C.** Both hepatic and renal function often decline with age. There is a reduction in β-endorphin content and GABA synthesis in the lateral thalamus; speed of processing nociceptive stimuli and both C- and A-delta-fiber function decrease with age.

2. **E.** All of the choices are readily accepted barriers to geriatric pain assessment except answer choice E; geriatric patients are often averse to using the term "pain" and frequently choose to describe pain as an "ache" or "discomfort" instead.

3. **E.** Unidimensional pain scales assess pain intensity only. All of the choices belong to this category except the MPQ, which utilizes 78 descriptors to describe the pain experience more accurately.

4. **D.** The PACSLAC and DOLOPLUS are both intended for pain evaluation of geriatric patients with cognitive impairment.

5. **A.** Acetaminophen toxicity via unintentional overdose is the leading cause of acute liver failure in the United States. All of the other choices are false.

6. **D.** TCAs are often associated with anticholinergic side effects including dry mouth, urinary retention, and constipation; also problematic is an increased risk of falls.

7. **E.** Kinesiophobia (fear of movement secondary to worsening pain) often results in movement avoidance and reduced physical function, which tends to worsen pain in the long run. All of the other listed nonpharmacologic strategies are helpful for analgesia.

8. **A.** Opioid use in the geriatric population is associated with lower risk of misuse and abuse. Some comparative studies show an increased risk of fractures and all-cause mortality in opioid patients. Opioids have shown efficacy in the treatment of both osteoarthritis and neuropathic pain conditions.

9. **C.** Facing older patients directly during the visit to allow lip reading can be very helpful for those patients with hearing difficulty. Focusing on a computer screen limits this vital face-to-face interaction.

10. **C.** Round-the-clock analgesic administration is often encouraged in the cognitively impaired patient population; these patients express their pain in a broad array of symptomatology, including lethargy, anger, grimacing, and groaning.

11. **B.** There is considerable variation in how various cultures understand, manifest, and treat pain.

12. **D.** History of peripheral edema necessitates caution with both gabapentin and pregabalin. Constipation necessitates caution with TCA nortriptyline. Fluoxetine has no intrinsic analgesic qualities. Duloxetine is a reasonable first option in this patient.

13. **B.** Women suffer persistent pain more than men.

14. **C.** NSAIDs are contraindicated in this patient secondary to angina, renal insufficiency, and peptic ulcers. Oxycodone is not a first-line analgesic for OA. Acetaminophen is the most common first-line analgesic for OA in geriatric patients.

15. **C.** The DOLOPLUS and DOLOPLUS-2 are useful in patients with significant cognitive decline. Patient self-assessment may include simple scales such as the FACES pain scale, but not all patients with severe cognitive decline will be able to utilize this tool.

35 Managing Pain During Pregnancy and Lactation

QUESTIONS

1. What is the most critical period for minimizing maternal drug exposure?
   A. Conception to 10 weeks
   B. 10 weeks to 20 weeks
   C. 20 weeks to 30 weeks
   D. 30 weeks to 36 weeks
   E. Greater than 36 weeks

2. Which of the following medications has demonstrated improved birth weight and gestational age when given to an opioid-abusing parturient?
   A. Tylenol
   B. Methadone
   C. Gabapentin
   D. Buprenorphine
   E. Morphine

3. Which of the following antiepileptics, when given during the first trimester, is associated with neural tube defects, facial clefts, and possibly hypospadias?
   A. Gabapentin
   B. Lamotrigine
   C. Phenytoin
   D. Valproic acid
   E. Topiramate

4. Which of the following presentations is suggestive of round ligament hematoma?
   A. Pain in hypogastrium radiating to the pubic tubercle
   B. Severe localized pain often following a bout of sneezing
   C. Pain with raising the patient's head while in the supine position
   D. Pain worsened with Valsalva
   E. All of the above

5. A mother is receiving an epidural for labor. The anesthesiologist places 25 μg of fentanyl in the epidural and then tests the epidural with 3 mL lidocaine 1.5% and epinephrine 5 μg/mL. There is a positive test dose. Quickly after that, the patient's nurse notices that the fetal heart rate has lost its normal variability. Which of the following is the most likely explanation for the loss of fetal heart rate variability?
   A. Fetal hypoxemia
   B. Fentanyl administration
   C. Lidocaine administration
   D. Epinephrine administration
   E. Both A and B

6. Which of the following medications should be avoided in patients who prefer to breastfeed their infants?
   A. Methadone
   B. Ibuprofen
   C. Phenytoin
   D. Amitriptyline
   E. All of the above

7. Which of the following is true regarding migraine headaches during pregnancy?
   A. Migraine headaches typically improve during pregnancy.
   B. Migraine headaches typically worsen during pregnancy.
   C. One-third of migraine headaches improve during pregnancy, one-third get worse, and one-third stay the same.
   D. Migraine headaches rarely begin during pregnancy, but if they do, they typically occur during the second trimester.
   E. Postpartum headaches are more common in mothers who breastfeed infants compared with mothers who bottle-feed infants.

8. The risk of fetal malformation occurs at what radiation dosage?
   A. 10–15 Gy
   B. 0.1–0.15 Gy
   C. 0.1–0.15 Rads
   D. 1–10 Gy
   E. 1–10 Rads

9. A 39-year-old female has been taking buprenorphine 8 mg SL daily for chronic low back pain. She had a cesarean section 2 hours ago under spinal anesthesia and is now in severe pain. She has already received 30 mg of ketorolac and 1000 mg of acetaminophen IV. Which of the following is the next best step?
   A. Rotate to methadone 5 mg three times a day and increase as withdrawal symptoms begin
   B. Increase the buprenorphine dose by 50%
   C. Add short-acting opioids as needed
   D. Change buprenorphine 8 mg SL daily dose to 2 mg SL q6 hours
   E. Both C and D

10. A 28-year-old pregnant female presents complaining of new-onset back pain and radicular symptoms. Which of the following is true regarding back pain in pregnancy?
    A. Back pain is commonly considered a normal part of pregnancy.
    B. Estrogen production may cause pain by allowing an exaggerated range of joint motion.
    C. Imaging should always be performed before the administration of epidural steroids.
    D. The peak intensity of back pain occurs in the second trimester.
    E. The prevalence of lumbar disk abnormalities is increased in pregnancy.

11. All of the following statements are true regarding NSAID use in pregnancy **EXCEPT:**
    A. Fetal exposure is associated with premature narrowing of the ductus arteriosus.
    B. NSAIDs can interfere with implantation and placental circulation.
    C. There is an increased risk of miscarriage if NSAIDs are used for more than one week around the time of conception.
    D. Ibuprofen has a category D classification.
    E. If NSAIDs are used, the duration should be short (48 hours).

12. Most infants who undergo narcotic withdrawal are symptomatic by _____ postpartum.
    A. 48 hours

B. 3 days
C. 5 days
D. 7 days
E. 14 days

13. SSRIs during pregnancy are in FDA risk category _____.
    A. A
    B. B
    C. C
    D. D
    E. B and C

14. All of the following medications are considered pregnancy category C, **EXCEPT:**
    A. Ibuprofen
    B. Aspirin
    C. Gabapentin
    D. Sumatriptan
    E. Amitriptyline

15. Which of the following medications should not be consumed during lactation because there is strong evidence that serious adverse effects on the infant are likely with maternal ingestion of these medications?
    A. Ergotamine
    B. Atenolol
    C. Metoprolol
    D. Imipramine
    E. Cymbalta

ANSWERS

1. **A.** The most critical period for minimizing maternal drug exposure is during early development, from conception through the 10th menstrual week of pregnancy (the 10th week following the start of the last menstrual cycle). Drug exposure before organogenesis (before the fourth menstrual week) usually causes an all-or-none effect; the embryo either does not survive or develops without abnormalities. Drug effects later in pregnancy typically lead to single- or multiple-organ involvement, developmental syndromes, or intrauterine growth retardation.

2. **A.** Chronic opioid use in pregnancy is associated with low birth weight and decreased head circumference, although the contribution of comorbid conditions, including polysubstance abuse and smoking, is not clear. Enrollment and compliance with methadone therapy for opioid dependence improve birth weight and prolong gestation, thus supporting the role of therapy during gestation.

3. **B.** Exposure to valproic acid, especially in the first trimester, contributes to neural tube defects, facial clefts, and possibly hypospadias.

4. **A.** The round ligaments stretch as the uterus rises in the abdomen. If the pull is too rapid, small hematomas may develop in the ligaments. This usually begins at

16–20 weeks' gestation, with pain and tenderness being localized over the round ligament and radiating to the pubic tubercle. Treatment is bed rest and local warmth, along with oral analgesics in more severe cases.

5. **E.** Maternal administration of fentanyl or other opioids may cause loss of normal variability in fetal heart rate. Loss of fetal heart rate variability can signal fetal hypoxemia and the administration of opioids during labor may therefore cloud the picture.

6. **D.** The American Academy of Pediatrics has categorized medications in relation to the safety of ingestion by breastfeeding mothers. Although many common pain medications are listed as category 3 (compatible with breastfeeding), psychotropic medications such as amitriptyline, which are used frequently for the treatment of chronic pain, are category 2 (effects are unknown, and caution is urged).

7. **A.** Migraine headaches typically improve in the first trimester of pregnancy, related to a sudden and sustained increase in estradiol. 50%–80% of patients who suffer from migraines experience a significant reduction in frequency or total cessation of migraine attacks during pregnancy. Migraine headaches rarely begin during pregnancy, but if they do, they typically occur during the first trimester. Postpartum headaches

are frequent and can occur in 30%–40% of all women. Most take place in the first week after birth and about 50% of those who experience relief of their migraine during pregnancy have a recurrence a short time after delivery. In mothers of bottle-fed infants, the hormonal cycle is restored rapidly, which may contribute to the postnatal recurrence of migraine headaches.

8. **B.** Any increased risk of malformations is considered to be negligible unless radiation doses exceed 0.1–0.15 Gy (10–15 Rads), which is typically less than the amount of exposure that an embryo or fetus would probably receive from diagnostic procedures.

9. **E.** As a combined opioid agonist–antagonist, continued administration of buprenorphine can block the μ-mediated analgesic effect of additional short-acting opioids. Pain control options, in addition to nonopioid analgesics, include the following: (1) adding short-acting opioids with the realization that larger doses may be needed; (2) dividing the daily dose of buprenorphine into 6-hour intervals, which can take advantage of the short-term analgesic effect of buprenorphine; and (3) discontinuing buprenorphine and initiating methadone at 30 mg/day, with increasing titration in 5- to 10-mg intervals daily to alleviate withdrawal symptoms. In this way, short-acting opioids can be used for pain and methadone can be used to prevent withdrawal, with less direct antagonism at the μ-opioid receptor.

10. **A.** Fifty percent of women will experience low back pain during their pregnancy and it is commonly considered a normal part of pregnancy. In a third of pregnant women, back pain is a severe problem that compromises everyday activity. Relaxin, a polypeptide secreted by the corpus luteum, softens the ligaments around the pelvic joints and cervix to allow accommodation of the developing fetus and facilitate vaginal delivery; this laxity may cause pain by allowing an exaggerated range of motion. The onset of low back pain is usually around the 18th week of pregnancy, with peak intensity occurring between the 24th and 36th weeks. Pregnant women do not have an increased prevalence of lumbar disk abnormalities. The direct pressure of the fetus on the lumbosacral nerves or lumbar plexus has been postulated as the cause of radicular symptoms. In patients with a new onset of signs (e.g., unilateral loss of deep tendon reflex, sensorimotor change in a dermatomal distribution) and symptoms consistent with lumbar nerve root compression, it is reasonable to proceed with epidural steroid treatment before obtaining imaging studies.

11. **D.** NSAIDs are categorized within FDA risk category C until 30 weeks' gestation and category D after 30 weeks' gestation.

12. **A.** Most infants who undergo narcotic withdrawal are symptomatic by 48 hours postpartum, but there are reports of withdrawal symptoms beginning 7–14 days postpartum. Neonates with prenatal exposure to opiates for extended periods may require prolonged weaning (as slow as a 10% reduction every third day) to prevent withdrawal symptoms. The American Academy of Pediatrics considers methadone compatible with breastfeeding.

13. **E.** The SSRIs are category B or C and can be used with caution but should primarily be continued if comorbid depression is present. TCAs are typically in FDA category D.

14. **E.** Amitriptyline is rated risk category D by the FDA.

15. **A.** The American Academy of Pediatrics Committee on Drugs rates ergotamine as a category 1 medication, which should not be consumed during lactation. Category 2 medications have unknown effects on human infants. Category 3 medications are compatible with breastfeeding.

PART 5

PHARMACOLOGIC, PSYCHOLOGICAL, AND PHYSICAL MEDICINE TREATMENTS

Major Opioids and Chronic Opioid Therapy

36

QUESTIONS

1. A patient is taking high-dose Avinza for his chronic pain and Percocet for breakthrough pain. He is administered a random urine drug test. The patient reports the last dose for both was about 4 hours earlier. Which of the following is least likely to be detected in his urine?
   A. Morphine
   B. Hydrocodone
   C. Hydromorphone
   D. Oxycodone
   E. Oxymorphone

2. You decide to initiate opioid therapy in a patient who is also taking fluoxetine and tramadol. Which of the following is the best choice?
   A. Oxycodone
   B. Methadone
   C. Morphine
   D. Meperidine
   E. Fentanyl

3. You are seeing a patient in the hospital who has been on OxyContin 30 mg/day. The patient is starting to report decreased efficacy and continues to have issues with constipation. You decide to rotate him to a different opioid. Which of the following is the most appropriate equianalgesic dosage?
   A. Oxymorphone 60 mg/day
   B. Morphine 20 mg/day
   C. Morphine 60 mg/day
   D. Hydromorphone 30 mg/day
   E. Hydromorphone 10 mg/day

4. All of the following are true regarding methadone **EXCEPT:**
   A. Receptor activity includes μ- and δ- opioid agonism, NMDA antagonism, and serotonin reuptake blockade.
   B. Its long-acting property is based on compounding technology.
   C. It is a reasonable option in patients with renal failure.
   D. A potentially deadly complication is torsades de pointes arrhythmia.
   E. There is increased gastric absorption of methadone in patients taking proton pump inhibitors.

5. Patients typically develop a tolerance to all of the following opioid side effects **EXCEPT:**
   A. Pruritus
   B. Sedation
   C. Constipation
   D. Analgesia
   E. Nausea

6. A patient wants to discontinue use of a long-acting opioid that he has been taking for over a year. Which of the following interventions is **LEAST** likely to help manage withdrawal symptoms?
   A. Prescribe clonidine
   B. Prescribe naloxone
   C. Titrate down slowly by roughly 10%–20% every few days
   D. Prescribe propranolol
   E. Prescribe methadone

7. You are consulted on a patient who has been treated with MS Contin (sustained-release morphine) for chronic pain. She is now an inpatient after trauma and is

status post bowel resection. She has 150 cm remaining of the small intestine. The primary team has restarted her the long-acting opioid, but the patient is complaining of poor pain control. She has not been able to tolerate transdermal fentanyl because of skin irritation. Which of the following is the best option for continued long-acting opioid treatment of her chronic pain?

A. OxyContin (long-acting oxycodone)
B. Methadone
C. Transbuccal fentanyl
D. Exalgo (long-acting hydromorphone)
E. Opana ER (long-acting oxymorphone)

8. Which of the following is an appropriate treatment for the most common side effect of opioids?

A. Nalbuphine
B. Promethazine
C. Naloxone
D. Diphenhydramine
E. Methylnaltrexone

9. Which opioid is most likely to be considered safe in renal failure?

A. Morphine
B. Hydromorphone
C. Fentanyl
D. Methadone
E. Both C and D

10. Which of the following is a behavior more indicative of addiction?

A. Attempting to get prescriptions from more than one physician at a time
B. Taking someone else's pain medication
C. Requesting a specific opioid
D. Self-escalation of opioid dose
E. Drinking alcohol to relieve pain

11. What does the Federation of State Medical Boards note as a critical aspect of effective and safe opioid management?

A. Noting current functional status on initial evaluation and changes in function at each subsequent visit

B. Documenting visual analog scale (VAS) at each visit
C. Monitoring random urine drug screens at least every 3 months
D. Checking prescription drug databases for aberrant behavior at each visit
E. Pill counts at each visit

12. Which of the following statements about opioids is **FALSE?**

A. Some opioids have been shown to disrupt REM sleep.
B. Hormonal disruptions by opioids include testosterone, estrogen, and cortisol abnormalities.
C. They may cause immunosuppression.
D. Thirty percent of White individuals lack the 3A4 isoform of the CYP-450 system, making them "poor metabolizers" of oxycodone, hydrocodone, and codeine.
E. Tolerance to pruritus develops fairly quickly.

13. Which class of medications inhibits and induces the clearance of methadone and fentanyl respectively via the 3A4 isoform of the CYP-450 system?

A. Ketoconazole and protease inhibitors
B. Phenytoin and macrolides
C. Macrolides and phenytoin
D. Protease inhibitors and ketoconazole
E. Phenytoin and verapamil

14. All of the following opioids undergo metabolism by the CYP2D6 isoenzyme **EXCEPT:**

A. Hydrocodone
B. Codeine
C. Oxycodone
D. Fentanyl
E. Methadone

15. Which of the following does not have either an active or neurotoxic metabolite?

A. Morphine
B. Meperidine
C. Methadone
D. Hydromorphone
E. Oxycodone

ANSWERS

1. **B.** Avinza is a long-acting formulation of morphine, and Percocet is oxycodone with acetaminophen. Because the patient is actively taking his medications, both morphine and oxycodone should be present in the urine drug screen. Because oxycodone is metabolized into oxymorphone, this will likely be present. Hydromorphone is a minor metabolite of morphine, but can be seen in urine drug tests for patients receiving chronically high morphine doses. Hydrocodone is not a metabolite of morphine or oxycodone and therefore should not be present. The caveat to this is that there are reports of codeine contamination in the manufacturing of morphine, which metabolizes to hydrocodone and may lead to a positive hydrocodone result.

2. **C.** All of the choices have been shown to have serotonergic effects except morphine. Methadone, meperidine, and fentanyl exert their effects by inhibiting serotonin reuptake. Oxycodone interacts with other serotonergic medications (neuroleptics, tricyclic antidepressants, and SSRIs) through the CYP2D6 isoenzyme. Because the patient is already on an SSRI and tramadol, an opioid without serotonergic effects or interactions would be the best choice to minimize the risk of developing serotonin syndrome.

3. **E.** Equianalgesic dosages between opioids is an important concept when prescribing opioid medications. Poor understanding has led to medical

errors including overdoses and inadequate pain management. Equianalgesic dosages of opioids are based on morphine and relative potency. There is variability depending on the source, but 30 mg of oxycodone would be approximately 45 mg of oral morphine. Oxymorphone is more potent than its parent compound oxycodone; therefore, a higher dose of oxymorphone would not be appropriate (oxymorphone dose is about half of the oxycodone dose). The dose of hydromorphone is about one-fifth of morphine, which would be roughly 10 mg. In addition, the question asked for the most appropriate equianalgesic dosage; however, when performing an opioid rotation, especially on an opioid-tolerant patient, the patient may only need about half of the equianalgesic dose.

4. **B.** Methadone has many unique properties including receptor activity of μ- and δ-opioid agonism, NMDA antagonism, and serotonin reuptake blockade. It is also mainly eliminated in feces, which makes it a viable option for patients with renal failure. Unfortunately, methadone is associated with QT prolongation. Studies have shown that the magnitude may not be much different than that caused by other medications such as tricyclic antidepressants. Methadone absorption increases with decreased gastric pH, which can result from proton pump inhibitors. As for its long duration of effect, this is an intrinsic property from its slow elimination half-life rather than from a compounding technology.

5. **C.** Tolerance does not generally develop to constipation but develops fairly quickly to pruritus, sedation, and nausea. When opioid tolerance is discussed, it is referring to decreased analgesia at a fixed opioid dose or tolerance to the analgesic effect. The mechanisms of this are not completely understood, but the N-methyl-D-aspartate (NMDA) receptor is involved.

6. **B.** Patients on long-term opioid therapy will usually develop physical dependence, which can lead to a withdrawal syndrome if the opioid is abruptly stopped. This is not to be confused with addiction. Rather than abruptly discontinuing opioids, it is recommended to taper the dose gradually to prevent withdrawal symptoms. If withdrawal symptoms still develop, medications including alpha-2 agonists such as clonidine and beta-antagonists such as propranolol can attenuate many of the withdrawal symptoms. Methadone can prevent withdrawal symptoms given its long elimination half-life, specifically the beta elimination phase, which is the basis for using methadone for heroin detoxification. Naloxone is an opioid receptor antagonist and can precipitate withdrawal if given to patients taking opioids.

7. **B.** OxyContin, Exalgo, and Opana ER are all long-acting opioids that utilize a sustained-release matrix technology and are compounded using a short-acting opioid (oxycodone, hydromorphone, and oxymorphone respectively). The short-acting opioid is released slowly throughout the drug's passage through the gastrointestinal tract. In a patient with short gut syndrome, the medication will not remain in the gastrointestinal tract for a sufficient length of time to be completely absorbed. Transbuccal fentanyl has a very rapid onset and is used for acute breakthrough pain, mainly in cancer pain. Methadone is unique in that it has a long elimination half-life, making its long-acting property intrinsic to the medication. It does not rely on prolonged release of the medication in the GI tract.

8. **E.** Constipation is the most common side effect of opioids, thought to be caused by decreased gastric motility. There are highly concentrated opioid receptors in the antrum of the stomach and the proximal small bowel. Treatment includes an active laxative because stool softeners or bulking agents may be ineffective. Methylnaltrexone is a derivative of naltrexone but cannot cross the blood–brain barrier; therefore, it blocks the peripheral effects but spares the central analgesic effects. Nalbuphine is a μ-opioid antagonist and κ-opioid agonist that is used to treat pruritus. Promethazine is used to treat nausea caused by opioids, especially if the nausea is worse with ambulation. Naloxone is an opioid antagonist. Diphenhydramine is an antihistamine, which may be helpful for pruritus.

9. **E.** Fentanyl is metabolized in the liver to inactive metabolites; therefore, it can be used in patients with renal failure. Methadone is mostly eliminated in feces and therefore renal failure does not alter its excretion. Morphine and hydromorphone undergo hepatic metabolism via uridine diphosphate glucuronosyltransferase (UGT) enzymes into morphine 6-glucuronide (M6G), morphine 3-glucuronide (M3G), and hydromorphone 3-glucuronide (H3G). These metabolites are renally excreted, and patients with renal impairment are prone to the effects of metabolite accumulation. M3G and H3G in particular lack analgesic effect but may cause allodynia, hyperalgesia, myoclonus, and seizures.

10. **A.** Opioid addiction involves continued opioid use despite physical, psychological, and/or social dysfunction. It involves continued use of an opioid that is destructive to the patient's life. Tolerance and physical dependence are often confused with addiction. All of the options are behaviors of addiction; however, obtaining opioids from multiple providers without them knowing is more indicative of addiction. The other options are often seen in patients with undertreated pain, which should be distinguished from true addiction. The difference is that addiction behavior will continue despite receiving adequate analgesia.

11. **A.** The Federation of State Medical Boards indicates that documenting current functional status initially and throughout follow-up is a critical aspect of safe opioid management. Pain relief or scores as an end point are subjective and not a good marker for success or failure. Random drug screens, pill counts, and

querying prescription databases are useful in verifying compliance and checking for addiction behaviors, but they do not assess the success of treatment.

12. **D.** Up to 10% of White individuals lack the 2D6 isoform of the CYP-450 system, which is responsible for the biotransformation of codeine, oxycodone, and hydrocodone, thus making them "poor metabolizers." Opioids have been associated with immunosuppression, hormonal disturbances, and sleep disturbances.

13. **C.** Fentanyl and methadone are metabolized by the 3A4 isoform of the CYP-450 system. The metabolism can be induced or inhibited by other drugs/medications. Macrolide antibiotics inhibit the enzyme, which will increase levels of the parent compound. Anticonvulsants induce the enzyme, which will decrease levels of the parent compound by increasing clearance. Protease inhibitors, ketoconazole, and verapamil are all inhibitors of CYP3A4.

14. **D.** The 2D6 isoform of the CYP450 system is responsible for the metabolism of codeine, oxycodone, hydrocodone, and to a lesser extent, methadone. Fentanyl is metabolized by the 3A4 isoform.

15. **C.** Methadone does not have any known active or neurotoxic metabolites. Morphine metabolizes to morphine 3-glucuronide (M3G) and morphine 6-glucuronide (M6G). M3G is a μ- and δ-agonist, but M6G does not exhibit any analgesic effects. M6G may produce opposite effects such as allodynia and hyperalgesia as well as myoclonus and seizures. Meperidine metabolizes into normeperidine, which is neurotoxic, causing seizures. Hydromorphone 3-glucuronide is the metabolite of hydromorphone and is similar to M3G in that it does not have analgesic effects. It also may potentiate neurotoxic effects like M3G. Oxycodone metabolizes to oxymorphone, which is an active metabolite and 14 times more potent than oxycodone.

Minor and Short-Acting Analgesics, Including Opioid Combination Products

37

QUESTIONS

1. Which topical medication has a mechanism of action mediated by the activation of the TRPV1 receptor?
   A. Salicylates
   B. Capsaicin
   C. Camphor
   D. Both A and B
   E. Both B and C

2. Which of the following is not a sign or symptom of serotonin syndrome?
   A. Diaphoresis
   B. Tremor
   C. Elevated mood
   D. Decreased reflexes
   E. Diarrhea

3. How does menthol exert its analgesic effects?
   A. Metabolism of substance P
   B. Calcium channel blockade
   C. Weak mu receptor agonism
   D. COX-2 inhibition
   E. TRPV1 activation

4. According to the American College of Rheumatology, which of the following is the first-line therapy for mild osteoarthritis?
   A. NSAIDs
   B. Topical lidocaine
   C. Acetaminophen
   D. Tramadol
   E. Combination opioid analgesics (e.g., Codeine-APAP)

5. Topical capsaicin is limited in its efficacy because of:
   A. Poor absorption
   B. Patient adherence
   C. Rapid metabolism
   D. Expense
   E. None of the above

6. Oral steroids (glucocorticoids) are least likely to have a beneficial effect on pain for which of the following conditions?
   A. Rheumatoid arthritis
   B. Acute disk herniation with radicular complaints
   C. Complex regional pain syndrome
   D. Tumor-induced bone pain
   E. Polymyalgia rheumatica

7. What is the typical total systemic absorption from topical NSAID application compared with oral route?
   A. <1%
   B. 3%–6%
   C. 7%–10%
   D. 11%–15%
   E. >15%

8. Penetration of topical medications is primarily limited by which layer of the skin?
   A. Stratum granulosum
   B. Stratum basale
   C. Stratum spinosum
   D. Stratum corneum
   E. Dermis

9. Your chronic pain patient develops torsades de pointes. Which medication was she most likely taking?
   A. Propoxyphene
   B. Hydromorphone
   C. Oxycodone
   D. Tramadol
   E. Acetaminophen

10. Ten percent of acetaminophen undergoes _____, which is responsible for the formation of the potentially hepatotoxic and nephrotoxic metabolite _____. This metabolite is detoxified by conjugation with _____.
    A. Glucuronidation, glutathione, N-acetyl-p-benzoquinone imine (NAPQI)
    B. Glucuronidation, NAPQI, glutathione
    C. Oxidation, glutathione, NAPQI
    D. Oxidation, NAPQI, glutathione
    E. Sulfation, NAPQI, glutathione

11. All of the following are serotonergic drugs **EXCEPT:**
    A. Fentanyl
    B. Methadone
    C. Amphetamine
    D. Milnacipran
    E. Cyproheptadine

12. Which steroid has the largest glucocorticoid activity with the lowest mineralocorticoid activity?
    A. Cortisol
    B. Prednisone

C. Dexamethasone
D. Methylprednisolone
E. Triamcinolone

13. The mechanism of action of tramadol includes all of the following **EXCEPT:**
    A. COX-2 inhibition
    B. Increased norepinephrine levels
    C. Increased serotonin levels
    D. Mu opioid agonism
    E. Reduction of substance P

14. All of the following are side effects of long-term glucocorticoid therapy **EXCEPT:**
    A. Weight gain
    B. Bruising

C. Mood symptoms
D. Fatigue
E. Sleep disturbance

15. All of the following are differences between "topical" and "transdermal" agents **EXCEPT:**
    A. Both must traverse a major barrier of the skin to deliver treatment.
    B. Serum levels generally remain low with topical agents.
    C. Both should be applied to the area of pain.
    D. Transdermal agents have the goal of achieving similar therapeutic systemic levels, as do oral preparations.
    E. All are true.

ANSWERS

1. **E.** The vanilloid receptor (TRPV1) is a nonselective cation receptor in the transient receptor protein (TRP) channel family, which are thermosensation receptors. TRPV1 is activated by capsaicin, the pungent agent found in chili peppers. It is also activated by camphor, which comes from the wood of the camphor laurel tree. Salicylates have an unidentified mechanism of action and seem to be different from that of NSAIDs.

2. **D.** Serotonin syndrome or serotonin toxicity is a potentially life-threatening condition. It is a group of signs and symptoms that probably occur from overstimulation of $5-HT_{1A}$ and $5-HT_2$ receptors in the brain. Concomitant use of serotonergic medications such as tramadol, SSRIs, SNRIs, and MAOIs has been associated with this condition. The classic triad involves neuromuscular hyperactivity (tremor, myoclonus, hyperreflexia), autonomic hyperactivity (diaphoresis, fever, tachycardia), and altered mental status (agitation, excitement, confusion). Symptoms can also include diarrhea and elevated mood. As a side note, trazodone is primarily a $5-HT_{2A}$ antagonist and does not appear to exhibit serotonergic side effects or induce signs of serotonin toxicity.

3. **B.** Menthol is a topical cooling agent that comes from the Mentha species and gives the species the mint smell and flavor. Its analgesic effects are mediated through Ca^{2+} channel blockade via TRPM8. There may also be additional opioid analgesic effects via kappa opioid receptors. TRPV1 is a target for capsaicin and camphor.

4. **C.** The American College of Rheumatology and similar European professional colleges have recommended acetaminophen as first-line pharmacologic therapy for osteoarthritis.

5. **B.** The efficacy of capsaicin is limited most by patient adherence because of burning and pain on application. Although Qutenza, a high-concentration capsaicin (8%), may be costly, there are other lower-concentration formulations that are relatively inexpensive. The metabolism and absorption of capsaicin does not limit its efficacy.

6. **B.** Although common clinical practice, there is a scarcity of reports regarding the use of an oral steroid taper or burst for the treatment of acute disk herniation with radicular complaints. The studies that researched this did not show a significant reduction in pain compared with placebo. The other four conditions have all been shown to benefit from the use of corticosteroids.

7. **B.** In general, one benefit of topical medications is to administer medications to the target site without significant drug concentrations in the blood. Studies involving topical NSAIDs have shown peak plasma levels <10% (0.2%–8.0%) compared with oral dosing. Total systemic absorption was only 3%–6% of the oral route.

8. **D.** The layers comprising the epidermis include the stratum corneum, stratum lucidum (only in palms and soles), stratum granulosum, stratum spinosum, and stratum basale. The stratum corneum, which is a relatively dense layer of flattened dead cells or keratinocytes, is the major barrier to penetration of topical medications. The epidermis is avascular but contains cutaneous nociceptors (unmyelinated C fibers). The dermis is separate and deep to the epidermis. This layer also contains nociceptive fibers, fibroblasts, connective tissue, blood vessels, hair follicles, and glands. Features that make a topical agent effective in traversing the stratum corneum include a low molecular weight (<500 Da) and having a lipophilic component.

9. **A.** Torsades de pointes is a potentially fatal polymorphic ventricular tachycardia that can degenerate into ventricular fibrillation. It is associated with long QT syndrome, which can occur with propoxyphene. Its major metabolite is norpropoxyphene, which can accumulate in cardiac tissue. Local anesthetic effects in the heart can lead to prolonged action potentials and in some cases torsades de pointes. After a number of fatal overdoses and limited efficacy data, propoxyphene was removed from the United States market in 2011.

10. **D.** Acetaminophen is metabolized in the liver (up to 90%) by glucuronidation and sulfate conjugation to nontoxic metabolites. The remaining 10% undergoes **oxidative** metabolism by the CYP system to **N-acetyl-p-benzoquinone imine** (NAPQI), which is a potentially hepatotoxic and nephrotoxic metabolite. Increases in this minor pathway are caused by a number of factors including overdose (> 150 mg/kg), alcohol, isoniazid, and phenobarbital. NAPQI can be detoxified by conjugation with **glutathione**. Low glutathione levels, which can occur with chronic hepatitis C, malnourishment, human immunodeficiency virus infection, cirrhosis, and alcohol, may also lead to accumulation of NAPQI.

11. **E.** Cyproheptadine is an antiserotonergic medication that has been used to treat moderate to severe cases of serotonin syndrome. Fentanyl and methadone, along with tramadol and meperidine, are opioids that can inhibit serotonin reuptake. Milnacipran, venlafaxine, and duloxetine are all SNRIs that also inhibit serotonin reuptake. Amphetamine is classified as a serotonin releaser.

12. **C.** Corticosteroids can be divided into either glucocorticoids or mineralocorticoids. Glucocorticoids are anti-inflammatory and control carbohydrate, fat, and protein metabolism. Mineralocorticoids control electrolyte and water levels (sodium retention). Glucocorticoids act by inhibiting accumulation of inflammatory cells at sites of inflammation, macrophage phagocytosis, lysosomal enzyme relief and synthesis, and release of mediators of inflammation. Corticosteroids are often compared in terms of anti-inflammatory (or glucocorticoid) and mineralocorticoid activity relative to hydrocortisone, which has a relative potency of 1 for both glucocorticoid and mineralocorticoid activity. Of these choices, dexamethasone has the highest relative glucocorticoid activity (20–30) and the lowest relative mineralocorticoid activity (0). As a comparison, fludrocortisone, which is a mineralocorticoid, has a relative glucocorticoid activity of 15 and a relative mineralocorticoid activity of 150.

13. **A.** Tramadol is a unique analgesic with many mechanisms of action at central and peripheral sites. It has a weak affinity for the mu opioid receptor, which is about 10 times weaker than codeine. Tramadol also acts centrally by inhibiting serotonin and norepinephrine reuptake systems. It has also been noted to reduce substance P levels in human synovial fluid. Tramadol does not appear to have an effect on COX-2 inhibition.

14. **D.** There are minimal adverse effects with long-term physiologic glucocorticoid replacement and short-term supraphysiologic dosing; however, studies have found side effects associated with cumulative and average doses in a dose-dependent fashion. The most common side effects include weight gain (70%), skin bruising (53%), sleep disturbance (45%), mood symptoms (42%), cataracts (15%), acne (15%), and fractures (12%). Glucocorticoids often help relieve fatigue symptoms.

15. **C.** The delivery of medication to the skin can be differentiated by either "topical" or "transdermal." The goal of transdermal delivery is to achieve similar therapeutic systemic levels as active oral preparations but through percutaneous absorption. The target for topical delivery is the site of application, including the soft tissues and peripheral nerves underlying the site of application. They both must traverse the stratum corneum, which is a major barrier of skin delivery. Transdermal agents do not need to be applied to the area of pain or injury. In fact, transdermal agents are best placed in a flat, hairless area, free of any defects that may interfere with adherence.

38 Antidepressants as Analgesics

QUESTIONS

1. Which of the following is a common side effect of the tricyclic antidepressant (TCA) medications?
   A. Diarrhea
   B. Insomnia
   C. Pruritus
   D. Weight gain
   E. None of the above

2. Which of the following is an FDA-approved indication for venlafaxine?
   A. Diabetic peripheral neuropathy
   B. Postherpetic neuralgia
   C. Chronic musculoskeletal pain
   D. There are no pain-related indications.
   E. All of the above

3. Which of the following is a common side effect of the serotonin-norepinephrine reuptake inhibitor (SNRI) class of medications?
   A. Nausea
   B. Urinary retention
   C. Sedation
   D. Myalgias
   E. A and B

4. When compared with the antidepressant effects of TCAs, the analgesic effects:
   A. Manifest approximately 2 months after initiation of therapy
   B. Occur at higher serum levels
   C. Occur at lower doses
   D. Pose a greater risk of anticholinergic side effects
   E. None of the above

5. What is thought to be the primary mechanism of analgesia for TCAs?
   A. Serotonergic
   B. Noradrenergic
   C. Adenosine receptor effect
   D. Sodium channel blockade
   E. Anti-inflammatory effect

6. Which of the following SNRIs block serotonin (5-HT) and norepinephrine reuptake with almost equal efficacy?
   A. Duloxetine
   B. Venlafaxine
   C. Milnacipran
   D. Desvenlafaxine
   E. Fluoxetine

7. Which of the following antidepressants is associated with an increased risk of major fetal malformation?
   A. Fluoxetine
   B. Amitriptyline
   C. Citalopram
   D. Paroxetine
   E. None of the above

8. Which of the following drugs is most likely to cause driving impairment?
   A. Duloxetine
   B. Citalopram
   C. Nortriptyline
   D. Paroxetine
   E. None of the above

9. Sodium channel blockade may contribute to the analgesic efficacy of TCAs. Which TCA appears to be the most potent in its ability to block sodium channels?
   A. Desipramine
   B. Nortriptyline
   C. Amitriptyline
   D. Imipramine
   E. Cyclobenzaprine

10. Which of the following is a TCA that is most efficacious for postherpetic neuralgia and central poststroke pain?
    A. Nortriptyline
    B. Trimipramine
    C. Duloxetine
    D. Amitriptyline
    E. Gabapentin

11. A 54-year-old patient was recently started on fluoxetine but is also normally taking acetaminophen, oxycodone, tizanidine, and aspirin. Which of the following complications should you be most concerned about when initiating fluoxetine?
    A. Stroke
    B. Heart failure
    C. Peptic ulcer disease
    D. Delirium
    E. Sedation

12. A 65-year-old patient was recently started on venlafaxine for painful diabetic neuropathy. Which dose is most likely to alleviate the patient's pain?
    A. 25 mg/day
    B. 50 mg/day
    C. 75 mg/day
    D. 100 mg/day
    E. 150 mg/day

13. When prescribing an antidepressant, the potential for overdose and abuse should always be considered. Which of the following medication classes pose the lowest risk for suicide attempts by overdose?
    A. TCAs
    B. SSRIs
    C. SNRIs
    D. Opioids
    E. Antipsychotics

ANSWERS

1. **D.** Weight gain is a common side effect of antidepressants. When used for the management of depression, mood alteration may affect appetite. This is more prominent with TCAs compared with SSRIs (selective serotonin reuptake inhibitor) or SNRIs, and may affect compliance.

2. **D.** Venlafaxine is not currently approved by the FDA for any pain indication; however, it has been shown to be effective in the treatment of painful diabetic neuropathy (PDN) and other polyneuropathies, except for postherpetic neuralgia (PHN).

3. **A.** Nausea is one of the more common side effects of the SNRI class of medications. Lowering the dose can reduce this symptom. Also, nausea is self-limited in many patients and resolves within the first several weeks of use.

4. **C.** The analgesic effects of TCAs tend to occur more rapidly (within a week of initiating therapy), at lower serum levels, and at lower doses than required to exert their antidepressant effects. However, these effects vary for individual TCAs, accounting for the heterogeneity in their effectiveness.

5. **B.** TCAs have multiple mechanisms of analgesia, but noradrenergic effects appear to be the most prominent. Other mechanisms include serotonergic, opioidergic, adenosine receptor effect, sodium channel blockade, and even an anti-inflammatory effect.

6. **C.** Milnacipran blocks serotonin and norepinephrine reuptake with equal efficacy, whereas duloxetine has a 10-fold selectivity for serotonin and venlafaxine has a 30-fold selectivity for serotonin. Fluoxetine is an SSRI, not an SNRI.

7. **E.** Pharmacotherapy of any maternal drug during pregnancy warrants consideration of potential fetal consequences. Neither SSRIs nor TCAs appear to pose an increased risk for major fetal malformations, although poor neonatal adaptation has been reported.

8. **C.** TCAs have antihistaminic and anticholinergic effects that may initially cause acute somnolence or sedation, resulting in driving impairment. However, most individuals appear to adapt to this side effect within 1 week, with a return to normal driving performance. In addition, concomitant use of another sedative can significantly impair driving ability.

9. **C.** Amitriptyline appears to be the most potent TCA in its ability to block sodium channels, followed by doxepin and imipramine. Desipramine is less effective in this regard and nortriptyline is one of the least potent at sodium channel blockade. Cyclobenzaprine is a muscle relaxant that is structurally similar to TCAs.

10. **D.** Amitriptyline is widely considered the first-line agent for management of postherpetic neuralgia. Although amitriptyline has not been proven to be beneficial in pain associated with spinal cord injury, its utility has been demonstrated for central pain in poststroke patients.

11. **C.** Among the SSRIs, it appears that fluoxetine has the greatest propensity to cause gastrointestinal side effects including peptic ulcer disease. Patients taking an SSRI together with an NSAID, as in this case, can further increase this risk.

12. **E.** The analgesic effect of venlafaxine is seen at doses greater than or equal to 150 mg/day, which is the point that it starts behaving more like an SNRI. At lower doses, venlafaxine behaves like an SSRI.

13. **B.** The use of antidepressants can cause an increased risk of suicide in some patients. The number of deaths per million prescriptions of antidepressants is lowest for SSRIs.

39 Membrane Stabilizers for the Treatment of Pain

QUESTIONS

1. All of the following are true about neuropathic pain **EXCEPT:**
   A. Neural plasticity may result in peripheral nerve fibers communicating abnormal input to the central nervous system.
   B. Neural plasticity may result in enhanced pain signaling in the central nervous system communicating to the thalamus.
   C. Decreased pain inhibitory activity may result in enhanced pain processing.
   D. One specific mechanism underlies the hyperexcitability seen with neuropathic pain.
   E. Both sodium and calcium channels are thought to play a fundamental role in the propagation of neuronal hyperexcitability.

2. Which of the following is the correct pharmacodynamic action of both gabapentin and pregabalin?
   A. Sodium channel blockade
   B. Binding to the α2δ subunit of the L-type voltage-gated calcium channel
   C. Blockade of the P/Q-type calcium channel
   D. Agonism of the T-type calcium channel
   E. Antagonism the N-type calcium channel

3. All of the following are true of gabapentin **EXCEPT:**
   A. Gabapentin is generally administered in three divided daily doses gradually titrated up to 3600 mg/day.
   B. Gabapentin increases the reuptake of GABA intracellularly.
   C. The most common side effects are sedation and dizziness.
   D. Dose reduction is necessary in the setting of renal insufficiency.
   E. Slow titration is a drawback of the immediate-release formulation.

4. A patient with postherpetic neuralgia has had to titrate up nortriptyline to 50 mg orally each night to achieve analgesia. This dose, however, is associated with significant constipation. What is the most reasonable therapeutic option?
   A. Inform the patient that the constipation should be self-limited
   B. Recommend dose reduction of the nortriptyline to 25 mg nightly
   C. Recommend dose reduction of the nortriptyline to 25 mg nightly with addition of low dose gabapentin
   D. Discontinue nortriptyline and start gabapentin instead at low dose
   E. Increase the dose of nortriptyline and add a stool softener

5. All of the following are advantages of pregabalin over gabapentin **EXCEPT:**
   A. More rapid onset of analgesia
   B. More predictable, linear pharmacokinetics
   C. Fewer dose-related side effects allowing faster upward dose titration
   D. Lower cost
   E. Twice daily versus three times daily dose

6. A patient with chronic intractable pain is using ziconotide for analgesia. All of the following are true about ziconotide **EXCEPT:**
   A. Ziconotide is derived from the venom of a marine snail.
   B. Ziconotide enhances calcium influx into P-type calcium channels in the spinal cord dorsal horn, thereby flooding the dorsal horn with neural input until pain is reduced.
   C. Ziconotide is administered intrathecally via infusion.
   D. Ziconotide has no associated tolerance, dependence, or respiratory depression.
   E. Side effects are the main limiting factor of its usefulness for analgesia and include dizziness, ataxia, confusion, headache, and hallucinations.

7. All of the following therapeutic agents are sodium channel blockers **EXCEPT:**
   A. Phenytoin
   B. Carbamazepine
   C. Local anesthetics
   D. Levetiracetam
   E. Lamotrigine

8. You are treating a patient with refractory trigeminal neuralgia. You are considering initiating lamotrigine, given failure of oxcarbazepine, gabapentin, pregabalin, and nortriptyline. All of the following are true regarding lamotrigine **EXCEPT:**
   A. In addition to acting as a sodium channel blocker, the drug prevents release of glutamate, an excitatory transmitter involved in pain transmission.

B. Monitoring of laboratory values is not necessary.

C. The most concerning side effect is rash (including Stevens-Johnson syndrome), which occurs more often with rapid titration.

D. Lamotrigine upregulates P-450 liver enzymes.

E. Common side effects include dizziness, somnolence, and confusion.

9. All of the following are analgesic mechanisms of topiramate **EXCEPT:**
   A. Blockade of voltage-sensitive sodium channels
   B. Binding to GABA$_A$ receptors to enhance GABA activity
   C. Reduction of the activity of L-type calcium channels
   D. Blockade of AMPA-kainate glutamate receptors
   E. Partial agonism at the mu opioid receptor

10. Which of the following analgesics has the sometimes beneficial side effect of weight loss?
   A. Gabapentin
   B. Levetiracetam
   C. Topiramate
   D. Lamotrigine
   E. Lacosamide

ANSWERS

1. **D.** The development of neuropathic pain involves a complex array of mechanisms leading to hyperexcitability of the peripheral and central nervous system, resulting in enhanced pain signaling.

2. **B.** Both pregabalin and gabapentin bind to the α2δ subunit of the L-type voltage-gated calcium channel, resulting in decreased presynaptic release of glutamate, norepinephrine, and substance P.

3. **B.** Gabapentin has no effect on the GABA receptor or GABA reuptake.

4. **C.** Studies suggest either a synergistic or additive analgesic effect between gabapentin and TCA nortriptyline. Patients achieved greater pain relief with a combination of *low* dosages of both medications than with either medication given alone at high doses. The lower dosages resulted in fewer side effects from either medication.

5. **D.** Cost of pregabalin is higher than gabapentin. The other listed benefits of pregabalin over gabapentin are all correct.

6. **B.** Ziconotide blocks calcium influx into N-type calcium channels in the dorsal horn, thus preventing afferent conduction of pain signals and providing analgesia.

7. **D.** All of the listed medications are sodium channel blockers except levetiracetam, the analgesic mechanism of which has not been clearly established.

8. **D.** Importantly, lamotrigine has no effect on liver enzymes.

9. **E.** Topiramate is not known to possess any mu opioid receptor agonism.

10. **C.** Topiramate use is often associated with mild weight loss. This is a unique side effect amongst analgesics for neuropathic pain.

40

Nonsteroidal Antiinflammatory Drugs, Acetaminophen, and COX-2 Inhibitors

QUESTIONS

1. Which is the predominant eicosanoid released from the endothelial cells of small blood vessels and a key mediator of both peripheral and central pain sensitization?
   A. Thromboxanes
   B. Prostacyclin
   C. Prostaglandin E2 (PGE2)
   D. Prostaglandin E3 (PGE3)
   E. Leukotrienes

2. Which of the following medications is best avoided in a child with a viral illness?
   A. Acetaminophen
   B. Ibuprofen
   C. Aspirin
   D. Naproxen
   E. Ketorolac

3. All NSAIDs are likely to increase cardiovascular events in patients at risk. Which of the following is considered to pose the **LEAST** amount of cardiac risk at any dose?
   A. Diclofenac
   B. Meloxicam
   C. Ibuprofen
   D. Naproxen
   E. Celecoxib

4. What is the recommended maximum daily dosage for celecoxib?
   A. 200 mg
   B. 100 mg
   C. 400 mg
   D. 800 mg
   E. 250 mg

5. A 25-year-old male returns to clinic. He reports he failed ibuprofen but is willing to try another NSAID. Which of the following medications would be the best option to try next?
   A. Ketoprofen
   B. Naproxen
   C. Fenoprofen
   D. Flurbiprofen
   E. Diclofenac

6. Which of the following statements concerning COX-1 versus COX-2 is correct?
   A. COX-2 is constitutively expressed in tissues of the CNS and kidneys.
   B. COX-1 and COX-2 are structurally dissimilar.
   C. COX-2 is largely constitutively expressed.
   D. COX-1 is highly inducible.
   E. COX-2 is primarily involved in regulating physiologic processes.

7. Which of the following NSAIDs is capable of inhibiting anandamide hydrolase and NF-kB?
   A. Aspirin
   B. Naproxen
   C. Oxaprozin
   D. Meloxicam
   E. Meclofenamate

8. Which of the following NSAIDs is implicated in drug-induced aseptic meningitis?
   A. Ibuprofen
   B. Sulindac
   C. Tolmetin
   D. Naproxen
   E. All of the above

9. A patient with chronic low back pain is pregnant. Which of the following NSAIDs is best avoided to prevent neonatal jaundice?
   A. Aspirin
   B. Diclofenac
   C. Naproxen
   D. Meloxicam
   E. Ibuprofen

10. Celecoxib has been approved by the FDA for which of the following conditions?
    A. Osteoarthritis
    B. Rheumatoid arthritis
    C. Dysmenorrhea
    D. Familial adenomatous polyposis
    E. All of the above

11. A patient had a severe allergic reaction when taking glipizide for her diabetes. Which of the following NSAIDs is contraindicated in this patient?
    A. Celecoxib
    B. Timentin
    C. Ketorolac
    D. Oxaprozin
    E. Diclofenac

12. A patient took 325 mg of aspirin this morning prior to spinal fusion surgery and asks you what the effect will be on platelet function. You answer:
    A. It causes irreversible inhibition of platelet aggregation for the lifespan of the platelet, which is 7–10 days.
    B. It causes reversible inhibition of platelet aggregation for the lifespan of the platelet, which is 7–10 days.
    C. It causes irreversible inhibition of platelet aggregation for the lifespan of the platelet, which is 3–5 days.
    D. It causes reversible inhibition of platelet aggregation for the lifespan of the platelet, which is 3–5 days.
    E. None of the above

13. Which of the following medications inhibit prostaglandin synthesis in the central nervous system, but not in the peripheral tissue?
    A. Ibuprofen
    B. Acetaminophen
    C. Aspirin
    D. Indomethacin
    E. Celecoxib

14. What is true concerning the humoral induction of COX-2 by peripheral inflammation?
    A. Centrally acting COX-2 inhibitors are required.
    B. Topical NSAIDs are required to blunt this inflammatory pathway.
    C. It is the sole pathway in the induction of COX-2 centrally.
    D. Lipophilicity and ionization are minimal factors in the blockade of this process.
    E. It can be blocked by regional anesthesia.

15. You are seeing a 50-year-old male with a past medical history significant for a prior myocardial infarction and GERD. Which approach is recommended if NSAID therapy is required?
    A. Nonselective NSAID
    B. COX-2 inhibitor
    C. Nonselective NSAID with GI prophylaxis
    D. COX-2 inhibitor with GI prophylaxis
    E. None. All NSAIDs are absolutely contraindicated in the patient

ANSWERS

1. **C.** Eicosanoids include prostaglandins, thromboxanes, hydroxy acids, and leukotrienes, which are 20-carbon unsaturated fatty acids derived from arachidonic acid. The major eicosanoid released from endothelial cells of small blood vessels is PGE2. It is a key mediator in pain sensitization, both peripherally and centrally.

2. **C.** Reye's syndrome is a combination of seizures, coma, and sometimes death related to the use of aspirin in children during a viral illness. Of all the NSAIDs, Reye's syndrome has only been associated with aspirin.

3. **D.** The increased risk of cardiovascular events from taking NSAIDs is a major concern. All NSAIDs can lead to new onset or worsening hypertension. Many studies have shown a significant increase in risk for cardiovascular events associated with several NSAIDs. Naproxen, at any dose, had the least association with adverse cardiovascular events. This has been confirmed with multiple studies.

4. **C.** The maximum recommended dose of celecoxib for chronic pain is 400 mg/day. The recommended dose for acute pain is 400 mg, followed by 200 mg within the first 24 hours. As a side note, administration with aluminum- or magnesium-containing antacids can reduce plasma levels of celecoxib.

5. **E.** NSAIDs are compounds that are grouped together based on their antiinflammatory action. They are structurally diverse and have been broadly classified as salicylates, acetaminophen, acetic acid derivatives, propionic acid derivatives, and COX-2 inhibitors. Other groups include oxicam derivatives, pyrazolone derivatives, anthranilic acid derivatives,

and naphthylalkanones. The propionic acid derivatives include ibuprofen, naproxen, ketoprofen, fenoprofen, and flurbiprofen. Diclofenac is an acetic acid derivative. The knowledge of these subgroups is important because patients may respond differently depending on the class of NSAID.

6. **A.** Two main isoforms of cyclooxygenase, COX-1 and COX-2, while structurally similar, have significant differences that have led to the development of isoform-specific antagonists. COX-1 is constitutively expressed and helps regulate physiologic processes. COX-2 can be induced by neurotransmitters, growth factors, proinflammatory cytokines, and a number of other factors. While the constitutive versus inducible theory is generally true, there are some exceptions. For instance, COX-2 is constitutively expressed in central nervous system and kidney tissues.

7. **C.** Oxaprozin is a propionic acid derivative with strong analgesic properties and mechanisms of action unique to many NSAIDs. It inhibits both COX-1 and COX-2 isoenzymes, inhibits NF-κB activation in inflammatory cells, and modulates the endogenous cannabinoid system (inhibits anandamide hydrolase in neurons).

8. **E.** NSAIDs are the most frequently implicated class of drugs in hypersensitivity-induced aseptic meningitis. Specifically, ibuprofen, sulindac, tolmetin, and naproxen have been implicated. Symptoms usually begin within weeks of beginning therapy and include fever, headache, and stiff neck.

9. **C.** In general, NSAIDs are not recommended in the last trimester because of an increased risk of complications

in the newborn. Aspirin and indomethacin at term have been reported to cause serious pulmonary vascular disease in the newborn. Naproxen can cross the placenta in 20 minutes and cause neonatal jaundice. Some recommend not using NSAIDs in general when breastfeeding infants with jaundice.

10. **E.** Celecoxib, which was the first COX-2 inhibitor approved by the FDA, is approved for pain relief from osteoarthritis, rheumatoid arthritis, acute pain, dysmenorrhea, and familial adenomatous polyposis.

11. **A.** Celecoxib is contraindicated in patients with sulfonamide allergy or known hypersensitivity to aspirin or other NSAIDs. Many groups of medications have their basis in sulfonamides including antimicrobials, antidiabetic agents (sulfonylureas), diuretics, anticonvulsants, dermatologicals, antiretrovirals, and stimulants. Glipizide is a sulfonylurea used to treat diabetes.

12. **A.** PGG_2 and PGH_2 are converted to TXA2 in platelets by TXA2 synthase, but they are converted to PGI2 by PGI2 synthase in vascular endothelium. TXA2 is a platelet activator and vasoconstrictor, whereas PGI2 is a platelet inhibitor and vasodilator. The balance between TXA2 and PGI2 is important in platelet activity. Unlike most other cells, platelets cannot regenerate the COX enzyme, making them vulnerable to COX inhibition. Aspirin irreversibly acetylates the COX enzyme, which causes inhibition of platelet aggregation for 7–10 days, the lifespan of platelets. For other nonselective NSAIDs, the effect resolves after most of the drug is eliminated. As a side note, ibuprofen antagonizes the platelet inhibition induced by aspirin, and celecoxib does not interfere with platelet function.

13. **B.** Acetaminophen inhibits prostaglandin synthesis centrally but exhibits no significant peripheral prostaglandin synthase inhibition.

14. **A.** Both neural and humoral inputs from peripheral inflammation can induce COX-2 and prostaglandin E synthase in the central nervous system. While the neural input can be blocked by peripherally acting COX-2 inhibitors and neural blockade with local anesthetic, the humoral signal can be blocked only by centrally acting COX-2 inhibitors. In order for an NSAID or COX-2 inhibitor to be effective centrally, it must be able to traverse the blood–brain barrier through passive diffusion. Two factors that are critical determinants in this transfer are lipophilicity and ionization.

15. **C.** While the use of NSAIDs is associated with an increased risk of cardiovascular events and gastric enteropathy, there may be times when NSAID therapy is needed. For patients at risk for NSAID-induced GI complications, it has been recommended to prescribe a proton pump inhibitor for GI prophylaxis along with a traditional NSAID or COX-2 inhibitor. For patients with cardiovascular risk who require aspirin prophylaxis, COX-2 inhibitors should be avoided. Therefore, for patients with both cardiovascular and GI risk, a nonselective NSAID with GI prophylaxis should be used.

Skeletal Muscle Relaxants

41

QUESTIONS

1. A 43-year-old male presents after experiencing low back pain for 1 week. After evaluation, you decide to do a trial of NSAID and muscle relaxants for 1 week. Which of the following symptoms is of clinical importance to consider when treating with cyclobenzaprine?
   A. Dry mouth, urinary retention, constipation
   B. Sialorrhea, urinary incontinence, diarrhea
   C. Sedation, pruritus, priapism
   D. Muscle spasms, myoclonus, ototoxicity
   E. A and C

2. Research shows that there is little evidence to support the use of muscle relaxants in the management of pain associated with which of the following conditions?
   A. Multiple sclerosis
   B. Low back pain
   C. Rheumatoid arthritis
   D. Parkinson's disease
   E. Radicular leg pain

3. Which of the following agents are correctly matched to their proposed mechanism of action?
   A. Orphenadrine: CNS depressant
   B. Ativan: GABA agonist
   C. Tizanidine: central alpha-2 agonist
   D. Baclofen: GABA agonist
   E. All of the above

4. Which of the following is true regarding cyclobenzaprine?
   A. It is a GABA analog.
   B. The 5-mg dose is less effective than the 10-mg dose.

C. There is a potentially serious interaction with tramadol.
D. Time-limited diarrhea is common while titrating.
E. It acts directly on muscle tissue.

5. What needs to be routinely monitored when treating with metaxalone?
   A. Kidney function
   B. Heart function
   C. Liver function
   D. Immune function
   E. Intraocular pressure

6. The use of cyclobenzaprine is contraindicated in which of the following conditions?
   A. Acute/narrow-angle glaucoma
   B. Arrhythmia
   C. Immunosuppression
   D. Hypothyroidism
   E. Both A and B

7. A 53-year-old patient with multiple sclerosis presents with pain in bilateral lower extremities related to spasticity. Lioresal is being considered for treatment. All of the following are true of Lioresal **EXCEPT**:
   A. It produces its effects by inhibiting monosynaptic and polysynaptic transmission along the spinal cord.
   B. Diazepam has superior efficacy compared with Lioresal.
   C. It is a GABA-A agonist.
   D. The therapeutic range is 40–80 mg daily.
   E. If discontinued suddenly after long-term use, it can result in withdrawal seizures.

ANSWERS

1. **A.** Cyclobenzaprine is structurally related to TCAs; thus, clinicians must monitor for anticholinergic side effects (dry mouth, urinary retention, dizziness, hypotension, and constipation). Use of cyclobenzaprine is contraindicated in the setting of arrhythmias, congestive heart failure, hyperthyroidism, acute glaucoma, narrow-angle glaucoma, or acutely following myocardial infarction.

2. **C.** Two Cochrane reviews concluded that there is little evidence to support the use of muscle relaxants for the management of pain associated either with inflammatory arthritis or rheumatoid arthritis.

3. **E.** Classification of agents by proposed mechanism of action:
   - **CNS depressants**
     - Antihistamine: orphenadrine

- • Sedatives: carisoprodol, chlorzoxazone, metaxalone, methocarbamol
- • TCA-like: cyclobenzaprine
- • **Central alpha-2 agonists**
  - • Tizanidine
- • **GABA agonists**
  - • Baclofen, benzodiazepines (Ativan)

4. **C.** Cyclobenzaprine does not act directly on muscle tissue; animal data suggest that it acts primarily in the brainstem, resulting in decreased tonic somatic motor activity. Although no human evidence exists to support this mechanism, the newer 5-mg dose has yielded similar clinical efficacy with less sedation than the more sedating 10-mg dose. Cyclobenzaprine labeling suggests that concomitant use with tramadol may place patients at higher risk of developing seizures.

5. **C.** Though not common, hemolytic anemia, leukopenia, and impaired liver function have all been reported with the use of metaxalone. Metaxalone is contraindicated in patients who have severe renal or hepatic impairment.

6. **E.** Cyclobenzaprine is contraindicated in the setting of arrhythmias, congestive heart failure, hyperthyroidism, acute/narrow-angle glaucoma, or immediately after myocardial infarction.

7. **C.** Baclofen (Lioresal) is a GABA-B receptor agonist and produces its effects by inhibiting monosynaptic and polysynaptic transmission along the spinal cord. Studies have shown baclofen to have superior efficacy over diazepam. Baclofen has a therapeutic range of 40–80 mg daily. It should be tapered slowly after long-term use to avoid a withdrawal reaction, rebound phenomena, and potential withdrawal seizures that can occur with sudden cessation. It should be used with caution in older patients and patients with renal impairment.

Topical Analgesics | 42

1. Which of the following NSAIDs is FDA-approved for the topical treatment of acute pain from minor strains, sprains, and contusions?
   A. 1% diclofenac sodium gel (1% Voltaren gel)
   B. 1.3% diclofenac epolamine topical patch (Flector patch)
   C. 1.5% diclofenac topical solution (Pennsaid)
   D. Capsaicin 8% patch
   E. All of the above

2. All of the following are FDA-approved topical medications **EXCEPT**:
   A. Capsaicin
   B. Lidocaine patch
   C. Doxepin
   D. Lidocaine/chloroprocaine
   E. All are approved by the FDA

3. Topical capsaicin is hypothesized to reduce peripheral and central excitability because of the depletion of _____ in C fibers?
   A. Prostaglandins
   B. Thromboxanes
   C. Substance P
   D. Glutamate
   E. Bradykinins

4. Which topical agent has been shown in randomized, placebo-controlled studies to reduce pain in patients with chronic lateral epicondylitis or Achilles tendinopathy?
   A. Voltaren gel
   B. Lidocaine 5% ointment
   C. Capsaicin 8% topical (Qutenza)
   D. Topical glyceryl trinitrate
   E. EMLA cream

5. Which of the following is true of topical analgesics?
   A. Topical analgesics may have central nervous system effects.
   B. Topical analgesics have only limited clinical benefit in a small subset of chronic pain conditions.
   C. Topical analgesics are equivalent to transdermal analgesics.
   D. Use of a topical analgesic is likely to be associated with systemic side effects.
   E. Topical analgesics have been well studied in low back pain and are unequivocally beneficial for this condition.

6. A patient walks into the clinic with prior history of shingles and complains of a burning, sharp pain originating from her right lower back and wrapping around toward her belly button. She hates to take oral medications and asks you if there are any topical medications that are indicated for her symptoms. You prescribe:
   A. 5% lidocaine patches
   B. EMLA cream
   C. Capsaicin cream 0.1%
   D. Diclofenac cream
   E. Doxepin ointment

7. Which of the following is a tricyclic antidepressant topical agent currently FDA approved to treat pruritus associated with atopic dermatitis?
   A. Amitriptyline
   B. Nortriptyline
   C. Doxepin hydrochloride
   D. Imipramine
   E. Trimipramine

8. Capsaicin exerts its effects through the TRPV1 receptor on which fibers?
   A. A-beta fibers
   B. A-delta fibers
   C. A-gamma fibers
   D. C fibers
   E. A-delta and C fibers

9. Which of the following topical agents may provide sufficient analgesia and anesthesia for minor surgery?
   A. Lidocaine
   B. Lidocaine/prilocaine
   C. Diclofenac
   D. Doxepin
   E. Capsaicin

10. Which of the following requires systemic absorption for effectiveness?
    A. Lidocaine
    B. Fentanyl
    C. Diclofenac
    D. Doxepin
    E. Capsaicin

ANSWERS

1. **B.** Each of the topical treatments listed has different FDA-approved indications. The diclofenac epolamine topical patch is FDA-approved for the indications listed in the question: acute pain from minor strains, sprains, and contusions.

2. **D.** All the medications listed are FDA-approved topical medications except for the mixture of lidocaine and chloroprocaine. Lidocaine/*prilocaine* cream is FDA approved.

3. **C.** Capsaicin appears to be an agonist at the TRPV1 receptor on A-delta and C fibers. This results in release of substance P and CGRP. It is hypothesized that depletion of substance P in C fibers leads to reduced afferent input and decreased excitability and pain.

4. **D.** In a trial of 154 patients with lateral epicondylitis, topical glyceryl trinitrate (0.72 mg/day) provided statistically significant greater pain relief at 8 weeks compared with a placebo. In a separate trial of 52 patients with chronic Achilles tendinopathy, 3 years after treatment, those who received topical glyceryl trinitrate treatments for 6 months had less pain and improved function compared with a placebo.

5. **A.** Although topical analgesics are applied locally and have a peripheral mechanism of action, they may also create central nervous system effects. They have benefit for a wide range of pain conditions, though they have not been well studied in low back pain. They are often preferred because of their decreased systemic absorption and resultant better side effect profile relative to systemic analgesics.

6. **A.** Although there are limited studies regarding topical analgesics for low back pain, in one study of 120 patients, four 5% lidocaine patches applied to the most painful areas in the low back region provided at least a moderate degree of pain relief over 6 weeks for acute or chronic back pain.

7. **C.** Doxepin hydrochloride (Zonalon) is a topical antidepressant cream approved by the FDA for the short-term treatment of adults with pruritus from atopic dermatitis or lichen simplex chronicus. It has been used "off-label" as a topical analgesic.

8. **E.** Capsaicin appears to be an agonist at the vanilloid receptor (TRPV1) on A-delta and C fibers.

9. **B.** Controlled trials have shown that topical lidocaine/prilocaine (EMLA cream) can reduce pain associated with circumcision, venipuncture, and breast surgery.

10. **B.** Fentanyl is available in a *transdermal* preparation, which is distinctly different from *topical* preparations of analgesics. Transdermal preparations require systemic absorption through skin and systemic concentrations of the medication to be effective. Topical analgesics, in contrast, act locally and do not require systemic absorption to be effective.

Neuraxial Agents 43

QUESTIONS

1. All of the following neuropeptides are involved in pain transmission via A-delta and C fibers **EXCEPT:**
   A. Calcitonin gene-related peptide (CGRP)
   B. Substance P
   C. Vasoactive intestinal peptide (VIP)
   D. Beta natriuretic peptide (BNP)
   E. Somatostatin

2. All of the following mechanisms are involved in neuraxial binding of opioid receptors by its ligand **EXCEPT:**
   A. Inhibition of adenylate cyclase
   B. Activation of rectifying potassium channels
   C. Inhibition of rapid-acting sodium channels
   D. Inhibition of N- and L-type calcium channels
   E. All of the above are involved.

3. All of the following are risk factors for development of catheter tip granuloma for continuous intrathecal infusion of opioids **EXCEPT:**
   A. Drug lipophilicity
   B. Drug concentration
   C. Drug dose
   D. Duration of drug administered
   E. None of the above is a risk factor.

4. Which of the following opioid-related risk factors are increased with intrathecal administration compared to systemic administration?
   A. Pruritus
   B. Edema
   C. Constipation
   D. A and B
   E. B and C

5. Which of the following about intrathecal administration of ziconotide is true?
   A. It binds to L-Type calcium channel blockers.
   B. The incidence of side effects is reportedly >80%.
   C. The stability of the drug is enhanced when combined with other drugs such as opioids and baclofen.
   D. Tolerance can steadily build over time, requiring greater doses needed for analgesia.
   E. All of the above

6. Which of the following about GABA-B receptors is **FALSE?**

   A. Of all GABA receptors, GABA-B receptors are most involved in regulation of nociceptive transmission.
   B. Receptor antagonist binding to the GABA-B receptor blocks the release of glutamate, substance P, and CGRP from primary afferents and GABA from interneurons.
   C. GABA-B receptors are found in greatest abundance in the superficial dorsal horn of the spinal cord.
   D. GABA-B receptors are the sites of activity for baclofen, which then blocks peripheral C and A-delta nociceptive fibers.
   E. All of the above are true.

7. Which of the following has FDA approval for intrathecal administration?
   A. Midazolam
   B. Ziconotide
   C. Hydromorphone
   D. A and B
   E. B and C

8. Which of the following about intrathecal clonidine is true?
   A. Its antinociceptive properties exist through inhibition of excitatory neurotransmitters, substance P, and glutamate in the dorsal horn.
   B. It is FDA approved for intrathecal administration in chronic but not acute pain.
   C. It is not effective as a sole agent but can prolong and enhance intrathecal local anesthetics and prolong effects of intrathecal opioids.
   D. Doses of 300 µg administered epidurally are equal in terms of efficacy and side effect profile to 700-µg doses.
   E. None of the above

9. A woman with metastatic ovarian cancer refractory to many oral medications was given a single injection of intrathecal neostigmine. Which adverse side effect is she mostly likely to experience?
   A. Dry mouth
   B. Bradycardia
   C. Hypotension
   D. Pruritus
   E. Nausea

ANSWERS

1. **D.** The neuropeptides involved in pain transmission via A-delta and C fibers are substance P, CGRP, galanin, VIP, and somatostatin. BNP is not involved in pain transmission.

2. **C.** Opioid receptor activation by an agonist results in inhibition of cell excitability via inhibition of adenylate cyclase, activation of inward rectifying potassium channels, and inhibition of N- and L-type calcium channels. Inhibition of the sodium channels is not involved in opioid receptor activation.

3. **A.** Risk factors for catheter tip granuloma from continuous intrathecal opioid infusion include drug concentration, drug dose, and duration of intrathecal opioid therapy. The lipophilicity of the drug (lipophilic vs. hydrophilic) has not been identified as a risk factor.

4. **D.** Intrathecal opioid administration may increase pruritus, urinary retention, and edema. Constipation and sedation are typically decreased compared with systemic administration.

5. **B.** Ziconotide is a synthetic version of a peptide originally isolated from the marine cone snail, Conus magnus. It works by binding to N-type calcium channel blockers. The incidence of side effects is reported to be >80% and include abnormal gait, amblyopia, dizziness, nausea, nystagmus, pain, urinary retention, and vomiting. The stability of the drug deteriorates when combined with other drugs such as opioids and baclofen. Tolerance has not been observed to occur as evidenced by continued efficacy over time.

6. **B.** GABA-B receptors, of all GABA receptors, regulate nociceptive transmission to the greatest degree. Receptor *agonist* binding blocks the release of neurotransmitters in the pain signaling cascade. GABA-A and GABA-B receptors are found in greatest abundance in the superficial dorsal horn of the spinal cord. Baclofen, a central-acting muscle relaxer, binds to GABA-B receptors, blocking peripheral C and A-delta nociception.

7. **B.** Morphine, ziconotide, and baclofen are common medications with FDA approval for intrathecal administration. Hydromorphone is a common intrathecally administered opioid but is not FDA approved for such use. Midazolam does not have intrathecal FDA approval because there are safety concerns regarding neurotoxicity seen in animal models.

8. **C.** Clonidine is an effective analgesic medication when administered neuraxially in combination with either local anesthetics or opioids. Antinociceptive properties exist through activation of spinal cholinergic neurons. It does not have FDA approval for neuraxial administration but is still commonly used in this manner. Side effects are reduced when the dose is reduced to 300 µg versus 700 µg in the epidural space; this does not compromise efficacy.

9. **E.** Intrathecal neostigmine is associated with a high incidence of nausea. Interestingly, the same side effect profile is not seen when administered epidurally. Neostigmine does not have FDA approval for intrathecal administration.

Pharmacology for the Interventional Pain Physician

QUESTIONS

1. A referring provider asks you to use particulate steroids for an interlaminar lumbar epidural steroid injection. Which of the following steroids has the smallest particle size?
   A. Commercial methylprednisolone
   B. Betamethasone
   C. Triamcinolone
   D. Compounded methylprednisolone
   E. All are similar in size.

2. Which of the following steroids has the longest half-life?
   A. Methylprednisolone
   B. Triamcinolone
   C. Dexamethasone
   D. Prednisolone
   E. Prednisone

3. Which of the following steroids has the highest potency?
   A. Methylprednisolone
   B. Triamcinolone
   C. Betamethasone
   D. Dexamethasone
   E. They are all equipotent.

4. A patient treated with botulinum toxin is curious how the skeletal muscle will work after the toxin wears off. What do you tell them?
   A. The skeletal muscle remains paralyzed until new axons and synapses have formed.
   B. The skeletal muscle will return to normal function once the botulinum toxin is degraded by specific enzymes.
   C. The botulinum toxin has a high affinity for specific nerve endings. Once the toxin starts to compete with other antigens, it will eventually be overwhelmed and the skeletal muscle function will return to normal.
   D. Botulinum toxin is treated with a specific antidote to help muscle return to normal sooner if needed.
   E. None of the above

5. With regard to cortisol circadian pattern of secretion in humans, which of the following statements is true?
   A. Peak levels of ACTH and cortisol secretion occur between 4 a.m. and 8 a.m.
   B. Daily cortisol production (5–10 mg/day) is equivalent to 20–30 mg of hydrocortisone.

   C. Daily cortisol production (5–10 mg/day) is equivalent to 7 mg/day oral prednisone.
   D. All of the above
   E. None of the above

6. You are covering the acute pain service for the weekend and you are consulted on a patient who received high doses of prednisone for two weeks from an orthopedist to treat symptoms related to spinal stenosis. The patient has developed excruciating pain in their hip. A plain film of their right hip suggests avascular necrosis, but the diagnosis is not clear. A right hip MRI is pending. Which other pathology would be likely to coexist in this patient?
   A. Fatty liver degeneration
   B. Osteoarthritis of the hip
   C. Coarctation of the aorta
   D. Chronic obstructive pulmonary disease (COPD)
   E. None of the above

7. How does botulinum toxin exert its effect?
   A. Blocks presynaptic release of acetylcholine
   B. Fuses postsynaptic acetylcholine vesicles
   C. Irreversibly binds the light chain to SNAP-25
   D. Scavenges intrasynaptic calcium
   E. None of the above

8. Which of the following statements about corticosteroids is true?
   A. The longer the half-life, the higher the mineralocorticoid activity.
   B. Methylprednisolone has the highest anti-inflammatory activity of the corticosteroids.
   C. 0.75 mg of dexamethasone is equivalent to 5 mg of prednisone.
   D. Hydrocortisone is a long-acting steroid.
   E. None of the above

9. A 90-year-old woman presents with an L2 compression fracture secondary to osteoporosis. You are planning vertebroplasty at L2. Which of the following is correct with regard to kyphoplasty/vertebroplasty?
   A. Pain relief is expected to approach 50% in all cases.
   B. The risk of pulmonary cement embolization is less with vertebroplasty compared with kyphoplasty.
   C. The most severe reaction is anaphylaxis to the bone cement.

D. No more than two levels or 12 cc of polymethylmethacrylate (PMMA) should be injected at any one time to limit cardiotoxicity.
E. All of the above

10. A 69-year-old female presents with low back pain radiating to the posterior aspect of her right leg. Recent MRI shows L5–S1 right paracentral disk herniation contacting the descending S1 nerve root. You offer a transforaminal epidural steroid injection.

However, she is very anxious and afraid of getting a fungal infection from this procedure. Which of the following was associated with an outbreak of fungal infections from contaminated methylprednisolone in 2012?
A. Freshly compounded vials
B. Initial exposure
C. A small volume of injectate
D. Translaminar approach
E. None of the above

ANSWERS

1. **B.** Studies examining sizes of particles in steroid preparations have found that methylprednisolone has a significantly higher percentage of large particles, large enough to obstruct vessels and potentially lead to severe complications. One available formulation of betamethasone (Celestone Soluspan) was found to have the smallest particle size, with triamcinolone having the second smallest.

2. **C.** Dexamethasone is a long-acting steroid with a half-life of 36–54 hours, although it should be noted that half-life does not correlate with duration of action.

3. **C.** Betamethasone has a relative potency of 33 mg to hydrocortisone; dexamethasone is 27 mg.

4. **A.** Botulinum toxin leads to permanent chemical denervation; new nerve endings and synapses are required before recovery of skeletal muscle function.

5. **D.** Daily cortisol production (5–10 mg/day) is equivalent to 7 mg/day oral prednisone. Cortisol production varies throughout the day, with peak levels of adrenocorticotropic hormone (ACTH) and cortisol secretion occurring between the hours of 4 a.m. and 8 a.m. and trough levels between 8 p.m. and 12 a.m.

6. **A.** Aseptic necrosis can occur with glucocorticoid therapy; predisposing factors include alcoholism, systemic lupus erythematosus, fatty degeneration of the liver, altered lipid metabolism, and history of renal transplantation. Fat can deposit in terminal arterioles in bone, leading to necrosis.

7. **A.** Botulinum toxins block the presynaptic release of acetylcholine from cholinergic terminals of both motor and autonomic nerves. The commercially available form of botulinum toxin in the United States may also affect the central nervous system "neuroplasticity" and modulate pain transmission.

8. **C.** In terms of glucocorticoid dose equivalency, 0.75 mg of dexamethasone is equivalent to 5 mg of prednisone. Dexamethasone has the highest anti-inflammatory activity. Hydrocortisone's half-life is short relative to the others. Half-life duration is inversely related to mineralocorticoid activity.

9. **D.** Vertebroplasty and kyphoplasty are reportedly highly effective, with immediate and lasting relief observed in 80%–90% of cases. The most common injectable bone cement used in clinical practice is PMMA. This monomer is cardiotoxic and may lead to arrhythmias. Given these risks, 12 cc of PMMA total may be the upper recommended limit per surgical intervention. Leakage of cement to adjacent structures can result in nerve root impingement, cord compression, and pulmonary cement embolism resulting from liquid cement leaking into veins. The risk of embolism is lower with kyphoplasty than vertebroplasty.

10. **D.** *Exserohilum rostratum* fungal infections from epidural injections of contaminated methylprednisolone resulted from contaminated steroid out of the New England Compounding Company in Framingham, MA, USA. These resulted in a variety of neurological deficits ranging from local infection to meningitis, stroke, or cauda equina syndrome. Use of the translaminar approach, higher doses, older vials, and an increased number of procedures in the same individual increased risk of infection.

Psychological Interventions 45

QUESTIONS

1. Which of the following family stressors may develop with chronicity of pain?
   A. Family members suspect that patient complains of pain to receive attention.
   B. Family members suspect that patient is trying to avoid gainful employment.
   C. Family members suspect that patient is exaggerating pain symptoms to elicit sympathy.
   D. Family members suspect that patient is feigning pain to obtain mood-altering medications in an effort to escape daily challenges.
   E. All of the above

2. Which of the following is true about the psychogenic view of chronic pain?
   A. Many studies have confirmed the psychogenic view that chronic pain predominantly occurs in response to emotional distress.
   B. The psychogenic psychodynamic theory posits that patients with chronic pain possess compulsive and masochistic personalities and significant feelings of guilt.
   C. This theory holds that chronic pain patients have typically normal childhoods with minimal stress.
   D. The theory targets treatment toward pain itself rather than the underlying psychogenic mechanisms.
   E. Treatment is geared toward functional restoration.

3. Your 32-year-old male patient reports worsening back pain when he arrives home from work, although his strenuous job typically does not elicit pain itself. Upon arriving home, he is greeted by his solicitous spouse who offers him assistance to his favorite chair and encourages him to rest. This is an example of which behavioral model?
   A. Classical conditioning
   B. Operant conditioning
   C. Malingering
   D. Cognitive behavioral perspective
   E. Social learning model

4. Which of the following defines malingering by a patient?
   A. Subconsciously demonstrating pain behavior secondary to prior traumatic childhood experiences
   B. Consciously demonstrating pain behavior secondary to prior traumatic childhood experiences

C. Consciously and willfully feigning pain for some secondary gain
   D. Consciously speaking about pain in a spiteful, negative manner
   E. Subconsciously experiencing diffuse pain complaints secondary to anxiety

5. Your 31-year-old female patient with fibromyalgia grew up in a home where her mother also suffered with chronic pain but coped with it by maintaining an active lifestyle and positive attitude. Your patient adopts a similar attitude as part of her therapeutic approach. This situation is characteristic of which behavioral model?
   A. Operant conditioning model
   B. Classical conditioning model
   C. Social learning model
   D. Cognitive behavioral model
   E. Gate control model

6. A chronic pain patient complains to her psychologist that she feels powerless in the face of her pain. The psychologist, in turn, helps the patient shift her thinking from self-defeating to active coping thoughts and teaches her relaxation and distraction strategies. This is an example of:
   A. Social learning approaches
   B. Operant conditioning
   C. Cognitive behavioral therapy
   D. Biofeedback
   E. Meditation

7. Your patient originally injured his lower back while walking on a treadmill. Since that time, he has avoided the treadmill, fearing similar reinjury. The psychologist has recommended a graded, progressive exercise program on the treadmill. This is an example of which coping strategy?
   A. Classical or respondent conditioning
   B. Operant conditioning
   C. Cognitive behavioral therapy
   D. Biofeedback
   E. Social learning therapy

8. All of the following are assumptions of the cognitive behavioral perspective **EXCEPT:**
   A. People are actively rather than passively processing information.

B. Behavior is determined by both individual and environmental factors.

C. People can learn more adaptive ways of thinking, feeling, and behaving.

D. People should be actively involved in changing their negative thought patterns and behaviors.

E. Well-entrenched, negative, helpless thoughts should be extinguished through appropriate positive reinforcement.

9. In the motivational paradigm of behavior change, the stage in which chronic pain patients have *not* yet begun to consider a personal active role but rather wait for others to prescribe treatment is known as:

A. Precontemplation stage

B. Contemplation stage

C. Postcontemplation stage

D. Preparation stage

E. Action stage

10. All of the following are true about meditation **EXCEPT:**

A. Long-term meditation by Westerners has shown increased cortical thickness in brain areas involved in the integration of cognition and emotion.

B. Transcendental meditation focuses on one of the senses such as repeating a silent word or phrase with the goal of transcending ordinary experience.

C. Mindfulness meditation involves nonjudgmental observation of ordinary thoughts or sensations as they arise in the present moment.

D. Meditators have demonstrated EEG changes including higher alpha brain wave activity, which is thought to promote a general sense of well-being.

E. Mindfulness meditation has not been shown to increase healing speed but does decrease pain symptoms and improve mood.

ANSWERS

1. **E.** All of these thoughts and feelings may occur with chronicity of pain, creating significant family stressors for the chronic pain patient.

2. **B.** The psychogenic view argues that patients with chronic pain possess compulsive and masochistic personalities and significant feelings of guilt that promote development of and maintenance of chronic pain.

3. **B.** The operant conditioning model holds that pain behavior is often maintained because of reinforcing environmental factors, as in the case of an oversolicitous spouse.

4. **C.** Malingering involves the conscious, purposeful, and willful feigning of pain for a secondary gain.

5. **C.** The social learning model is demonstrated here, wherein patients acquire responses and strategies through the observation of others in similar situations.

6. **C.** Cognitive behavioral therapy builds on the premise that patients can gain control over their maladaptive thought processes to cope better with their pain.

7. **A.** The classic or respondent conditioning model involves repeated exposure to feared or avoided activities, resulting in less pain than the patient anticipated, to extinguish the prior associated link between the activity and pain.

8. **E.** Focusing on extinction of negative behavior or thoughts by withdrawal of attention or providing positive reinforcement is intrinsic to operant approaches to treatment.

9. **A.** The initial stage of behavior change in which patients assume a passive role is known as the *precontemplation* stage. Once patients assume responsibility for their pain and inactivity, they enter the *contemplation* stage. The *preparation* stage follows when they are ready to implement change, followed by the *action* stage when the patient engages in new positive behaviors.

10. **E.** Mindfulness meditation has interestingly been shown to increase healing speed as well as to have multiple analgesic benefits, including stress reduction and improved mood.

Physical Medicine Techniques in Pain Management

46

QUESTIONS

1. All of the following are contraindications to superficial therapeutic heat **EXCEPT:**
   A. Malignancy
   B. Ischemia
   C. Acute inflammation
   D. Demyelinating disease
   E. Metallic implants

2. All of the following are considered superficial heat modalities **EXCEPT:**
   A. Paraffin bath
   B. Fluidotherapy
   C. Whirlpool bath
   D. Ultrasound
   E. Hydrocollator packs

3. You suspect that your 20-year-old male patient has biceps tendonitis and wish to prescribe a physical treatment modality using heat. Which of these would be most appropriate for treatment of this patient's condition?
   A. Paraffin bath
   B. Hydrocollator pack
   C. Ultrasound
   D. Fluidotherapy
   E. None of the above

4. Which of the following is true?
   A. EMG is more sensitive than MRI in diagnosing radiculopathy.
   B. EMG is equally sensitive to MRI in diagnosing radiculopathy.
   C. EMG is less specific than MRI in diagnosing radiculopathy.
   D. EMG is more specific than MRI in diagnosing radiculopathy.
   E. None of the above

5. Common nerves that are studied for nerve conduction study (NCS) include all of the following **EXCEPT:**
   A. Tibial
   B. Sural
   C. Femoral
   D. Median
   E. Ulnar

6. All of the following are contraindications to therapeutic cold **EXCEPT:**
   A. Raynaud's phenomenon
   B. Peripheral vascular disease
   C. Cryoglobulinemia
   D. Malignancy
   E. Paroxysmal cold hemoglobinuria

7. The application of firm but gentle pressure in a rhythmic fashion while gently grasping the underlying tissues and lifting and squeezing them describes which type of massage?
   A. Stroking/effleurage
   B. Petrissage
   C. Friction massage
   D. Tapotement
   E. Thai massage

8. What is an example of an isometric exercise?
   A. Wall squat
   B. Dumbbell curl
   C. Box jump
   D. Bench press
   E. Pushup

9. Which of the following conditions may be worsened by lumbar traction?
   A. Disk protrusion
   B. Disk pressure
   C. Hemorrhoids
   D. Muscle spasms
   E. Nerve root pressure

10. Which of the following is a contraindication to cervical neck traction?
    A. Space-occupying lesion
    B. Localized infection
    C. Rheumatoid arthritis (RA)
    D. Pregnancy
    E. Muscle spasms

11. Which of the following disorders is associated with a normal NCS?
    A. Demyelinating polyneuropathy
    B. Plexopathy
    C. Radiculopathy
    D. Mononeuropathy multiplex
    E. None of the above

12. All of the following are evidence-based indications for the use of transcutaneous electrical nerve stimulation (TENS) **EXCEPT:**
    A. Post-tubal ligation pain
    B. Primary dysmenorrhea
    C. Post-thoracotomy pain
    D. Acute neck pain
    E. All of the above have indications and high-quality evidence for TENS therapy.

13. All of the following are contraindicated in TENS therapy **EXCEPT:**
    A. Pregnancy
    B. Demand-type cardiac pacing
    C. Placement across the chest
    D. Placement over the carotid sinus or eyes
    E. All of the above are contraindications.

14. The role of an occupational therapist includes:
    A. General aerobic conditioning
    B. Balance and coordination
    C. Strengthening of core and limb muscles
    D. Energy and conservation techniques and posture training
    E. Traction and spinal manipulation

15. Which modality is safe for use in pregnancy?
    A. Microwave diathermy
    B. Ultrasound
    C. TENS
    D. Fluidotherapy
    E. Electrical stimulation of acupuncture points

ANSWERS

1. **E.** Contraindications to therapeutic heat include insensate or atrophic skin, inability to communicate or respond to pain, acute inflammation, malignancy, ischemia, growth plates, peripheral vascular disease, and demyelinating disease. Shortwave diathermy is contraindicated in the setting of metallic implants because of the risk for excessive heating, but *superficial* therapeutic heat is not contraindicated in this setting.

2. **D.** Superficial therapeutic heat modalities include hot packs, heating pads, heat lamps, paraffin and whirlpool baths, and fluidotherapy. Deep heating agents include ultrasound, shortwave, and microwave diathermy.

3. **C.** Ultrasound treatment is considered a safe, noninvasive treatment for tendonitis. It uses high-frequency sound waves to deliver energy to the target tissue, which is absorbed more effectively at muscle–bone interfaces, resulting in higher tissue temperatures in these areas. Ultrasound is more effective in heating tendons and ligaments than muscle, which absorbs ultrasound relatively poorly.

4. **D.** The sensitivity of EMG in the diagnosis of radiculopathy is lower than that of MRI, but its specificity is significantly better. EMG helps identify both the nerve that is involved as well as the severity and chronicity of the lesion.

5. **C.** The median and ulnar nerves are often studied in the upper extremities. Common nerves studied using NCSs in the lower extremity include the sural, tibial, and deep peroneal nerves. NCS of the femoral nerve is difficult, especially in overweight patients, who are predisposed to the development of femoral neuropathy.

6. **D.** Contraindications to therapeutic cold include insensate skin, peripheral vascular disease, Raynaud's phenomenon, cold urticaria, cryoglobulinemia, and paroxysmal nocturnal hemoglobinuria. Malignancy is not a known contraindication.

7. **B.** Petrissage refers to massage movements with applied pressure, which are deep and compress the underlying muscles. Wringing, skin rolling, pick-up-and-squeeze are the petrissage movements. Kneading lifts, squeezes, and moves larger amounts of tissue than petrissage does.

8. **A.** Isometric exercises involve exertion of force against a fixed object or a muscle contraction that holds an object in one position and are best exemplified by wall squats.

9. **C.** Lumbar traction is contraindicated in the setting of hemorrhoids and intraabdominal conditions that may be affected by increased intraabdominal pressure.

10. **C.** Cervical traction should be avoided in patients with RA and significant vertebral or carotid artery disease. RA affecting the spine is associated with ligamentous instability, which might lead to dislocation of the cervical spine when traction forces are applied.

11. **C.** In patients with radiculopathy, nerve conduction studies are typically normal and the electrodiagnosis is established on needle EMG. The main reason to perform a nerve conduction study is to exclude other conditions that may mimic radiculopathy, especially entrapment neuropathy and plexopathy.

12. **D.** There is evidence that high-intensity TENS can reduce postoperative analgesic requirements after inguinal herniorrhaphy, laparoscopic tubal ligation, and thoracotomy, and it has been found to be of value in the treatment of primary dysmenorrhea. However, there is insufficient evidence to support the use of TENS for various musculoskeletal conditions, including acute shoulder pain, acute neck pain, and low back pain.

13. **E.** TENS involves the application of electrical stimulation across the skin to the peripheral nerves. Many acute and chronic pain syndromes have been treated with TENS because of its ease of use and relatively low side effects. Contraindications include all of the listed options.

14. **D.** For pain patients, occupational therapists are helpful in teaching conservation techniques. They can help patients function in their work by instructing them in ergonomics, work simplification, and energy conservation. Another important aspect that they address is proper posture, which can result in a significant reduction in pain if put into practice daily.

15. **D.** Among the listed options, fluidotherapy (as well as other superficial forms of heat therapy) is the only management that is safe during pregnancy.

47 Physical Rehabilitation for Patients With Chronic Pain

QUESTIONS

1. All of the following tests of daily activities are included in the Back Performance Scale **EXCEPT:**
   A. Fingertip-to-floor test
   B. Pick-up test
   C. Roll-up test
   D. Walking test
   E. Sock test

2. According to The Joint Commission, all of the following require documentation when assessing pain **EXCEPT:**
   A. Duration
   B. Intensity
   C. Location
   D. Plan
   E. Social history

3. Cognitive behavioral modification can be accomplished via all of the following ways **EXCEPT:**
   A. Discussing beliefs
   B. Participating in a "reward system"
   C. Listening to feedback from other patients on their behavior
   D. Avoiding activities that cause pain

   E. Increasing the number and duration of usual activities

4. The difference between a "third wave CBT (cognitive behavioral therapy) approach" that includes the "Acceptance Commitment Therapy" (ACT) and regular CBT is:
   A. ACT teaches people how to control their thoughts, feelings, and sensations better.
   B. ACT teaches people to "just notice," accept, and embrace life events.
   C. ACT teaches people to treat their painful conditions on their own.
   D. ACT and regular CBT are the same and only differ in treatment of acute versus chronic pain.
   E. There is no difference between the two.

5. What is the goal of ergonomics?
   A. To improve workplace efficiency
   B. To prevent work-induced injuries
   C. To treat workplace injuries
   D. To improve morale at the workplace
   E. To encourage exercise at the workplace

ANSWERS

1. **D.** The Back Performance Scale is a condition-specific performance measure of activity limitation for patients with back pain. Activities that require mobility of the trunk are often limited in patients with back problems. Therefore five tests (sock test, pick-up test, roll-up test, fingertip-to-floor test, and lift test), all requiring sagittal plane mobility, are performed, and the test scores are combined in this scale to obtain a performance measure of mobility-related activities.

2. **E.** The Joint Commission requires that all patients have the right to an adequate pain assessment, including documentation of pain location, intensity, quality, onset/duration/variations/rhythms, manner of expressing pain, pain relief, exacerbating factors, effects of pain, and a pain plan.

3. **D.** Rather than avoiding those activities that trigger pain, cognitive behavior modification is accomplished by gaining exposure to avoided activities. Pain-related

   fear is closely linked with chronic pain disability; behavioral methods such as graded activity and graded exposure treatment have been shown to be effective in reducing disability.

4. **B.** ACT differs from traditional CBT in that the objective is not elimination of difficult feelings; rather, it is to be present with what life brings us and to "move toward valued behavior." ACT has been described as acknowledgment of unpleasant feelings, then learning not to act upon them and not avoiding situations where they are invoked. Its therapeutic effect is meant to be a positive spiral where feeling better leads to a better understanding of the truth.

5. **B.** The goal of ergonomics is to ensure that the workplace is designed to prevent work-induced injuries. Several factors, including suboptimal postures and activities and manual handling and lifting, are all risk factors for work-related musculoskeletal disorders.

Acupuncture 48

QUESTIONS

1. Stimulation of the _____ acupuncture point is used to treat nausea and vomiting from surgery and/or chemotherapy.
   A. CV 17
   B. LR 13
   C. GB 34
   D. PC 6
   E. LI 4

2. Electroacupuncture at 100 Hz accelerates release of which of the following opioid peptides?
   A. Enkephalin
   B. Beta-endorphin
   C. Endomorphin
   D. Dynorphin
   E. None of the above

3. The unit of measurement used to determine the locations of acupuncture points on the body is called:
   A. Centimeter
   B. Foshan
   C. Tsun
   D. Zhang men
   E. Increments

4. Which of the following is the most serious reported complication of acupuncture?
   A. Bruising
   B. Hyperalgesia
   C. Pneumothorax
   D. Infection
   E. Headache

5. In blinded randomized controlled trials for acupuncture, what percentage of study subjects may respond positively to placebo?
   A. 20%
   B. 30%
   C. 40%
   D. 50%
   E. 60%

6. There are more than _____ identifiable acupuncture points in the human body. _____ connect these acupuncture points to each other. _____ is the functional, dynamic force that resides in living creatures.
   A. 10, Qi, Meridians
   B. 50, Tsun, Qi
   C. 100, De Qi, Qi
   D. 300, Meridians, Qi
   E. 500, Qi, Nei guan

7. Which of the following is the most commonly reported adverse event associated with acupuncture according to the World Health Organization?
   A. Needle pain
   B. Bruising
   C. Fainting
   D. Nausea, vomiting
   E. Allergic reaction

8. The locations of acupuncture points are strongly correlated to the locations of which of the following?
   A. Major nerve groups
   B. Lymph nodes
   C. Tendons
   D. Blood vessels
   E. Trigger points

9. Based on currently available evidence, acupuncture would be most effective for which of the following conditions?
   A. Temporomandibular joint dysfunction
   B. Headaches
   C. Neck pain
   D. Neuropathic pain
   E. Postoperative pain

10. The analgesic effects of acupuncture may be blocked by which of the following?
    A. Memantine
    B. Naloxone
    C. Flumazenil
    D. Oxytocin
    E. Aprepitant

ANSWERS

1. **D.** Acupoint stimulation at PC 6 (Nei guan "internal gate") at a deep depression between the tendons of the long palmar muscle and radial flexor muscle of the wrist has been shown to have beneficial results in 27 of 33 RCTs for treatment of nausea and vomiting.

2. **D.** Electrical stimulation at 100 Hz accelerates the release of dynorphin. Acupuncture stimulation at 2–4 Hz accelerates the release of the other endorphins and enkephalins listed. A combination of both electrical frequencies together can increase simultaneous release of all four opioid peptides, maximizing therapeutic effect.

3. **C.** The *tsun* (also sometimes spelled "cun") is the unit of measurement for acupuncture points related to the patient's own anatomy, rather than a standard metric system. The definition of a tsun is variable but is often thought of as the width of the patient's thumbnail or the distance between the distal interphalangeal joint and proximal interphalangeal joint on the middle finger. It is important to note that acupoints and their relative positions are related to the patient's own size and anatomical landmarks.

4. **C.** Major adverse reactions with acupuncture are rare when performed by a competent acupuncturist. Although needle pain, bruising, bleeding, and mild drowsiness can occur, the most common *serious* adverse event reported with acupuncture is pneumothorax. Use of sterile, disposable needles has significantly reduced the risk of infection.

5. **B.** Thirty percent may respond to placebo. Sham acupuncture, which involves needling the skin at non-acupuncture points, is often used as a placebo control, but needle insertion itself may have a physiologic effect that can lead to pain reduction. Thus, it is difficult (though not impossible) to find adequate placebo controls for acupuncture.

6. **D.** There are about 365 identifiable acupuncture points. These points are found along pathways called meridians. *Qi* is thought to be a type of energy flowing along these meridians. Disease processes are thought to manifest because of blockage of this energy flow, and needling of acupuncture points is used to restore its flow.

7. **C.** Syncope (fainting) can occur in approximately 60% of first-time acupuncture users. According to reviews that include studies performed in China, this is the most commonly reported adverse event. (Zhang J, Shang H, Gao X, Ernst E. Acupuncture-related adverse events: a systematic review of the Chinese literature. *Bull World Health Organ* 2010;88(12):915-921C).

8. **E.** In one randomized controlled study, a 71% correlation between trigger points and acupuncture points was noted. Acupuncture has been shown in several studies to be effective for the treatment of myofascial pain.

9. **B.** Cochrane Database Systematic Reviews have been performed regarding the use of acupuncture in several painful conditions. These have shown that acupuncture is at least as effective and potentially more effective than prophylactic pharmacologic treatments for migraines, with fewer side effects and at least a 50% reduction in headache frequency, pain intensity, and analgesic use. Acupuncture is thus a useful nonpharmacologic tool for migraine and tension headaches. Acupuncture may also be beneficial in the other conditions listed, but further studies are needed to determine whether the effects of acupuncture are greater than placebo in these conditions.

10. **B.** Many of acupuncture's analgesic effects are shown to occur through the endogenous opioid pathway. Naloxone can block these effects by acting as a competitive antagonist at the μ-opioid receptor.

Integrative Approaches to Pain Management

49

QUESTIONS

1. The _____ is a physical state or reaction that counteracts the physiologic and emotional responses to stress and is essentially the opposite of the fight-or-flight response.
   A. Meditation response
   B. Relaxation response
   C. Anxiolytic response
   D. Tai chi
   E. Qi gong

2. Extracts of *Boswellia serrata* plant have powerful anti-inflammatory activity through its inhibition of the _____ enzyme.
   A. 5-Lipoxygenase
   B. CYP250
   C. COX-2
   D. IL-6
   E. Thiamine synthase

3. Which of the following forms of yoga is usually practiced at temperatures between 95°F and 100°F?
   A. Bikram
   B. Iyengar
   C. Ashtanga
   D. Vinyasa
   E. Hatha

4. Osteopathic manipulation has been shown to be beneficial with all the following **EXCEPT:**
   A. Decreasing pain intensity of migraine headache
   B. Decreasing pain intensity of neck pain
   C. Decreasing length of disability from neck pain
   D. Decreasing low back pain symptoms for at least 3 months
   E. Decreasing pain intensity from pelvic floor pain

5. Which of the following is a contraindication to massage therapy?
   A. Thrombosis
   B. Active infection
   C. Metastatic lesion
   D. Bleeding disorder
   E. All of the above

6. Omega-3 fatty acids have been shown to reduce pain in which of the following conditions?
   A. Neck pain
   B. Dysmenorrhea
   C. Neuropathic pain
   D. Inflammatory bowel disease
   E. All of the above

7. A patient presents complaining of neck pain and headache. They report that they have been under a lot of stress at work recently. You provide a technique that encourages the generation of specific mental images to evoke a state of relaxation or physiologic change. Which form of mind–body medicine have you prescribed?
   A. Concentrative meditation
   B. Guided imagery
   C. Hypnosis
   D. Mindfulness meditation
   E. Tai chi

8. All of the following biologically based products have evidence for use in the treatment of pain **EXCEPT:**
   A. *Boswellia serrata*
   B. Glucosamine and chondroitin
   C. S-adenosylmethionine
   D. Omega-3 fatty acids
   E. St. John's wort

9. Which of the following mind–body techniques has been shown to prevent falls and improve bone density, cardiopulmonary fitness, balance, quality of life, and self-efficacy?
   A. Progressive muscle relaxation
   B. Yoga
   C. Tai chi and qi gong
   D. Meditation
   E. Hypnosis

10. Which of the following differentiates hypnosis from guided imagery?
    A. Hypnosis involves concentrating attention intensely on a specific image.
    B. Hypnosis involves blocking out distractions.
    C. Hypnosis involves offering a health-inducing suggestion.
    D. Hypnosis can be performed with a therapist or by the patient alone.
    E. Hypnosis has been shown to be beneficial in the perioperative period.

ANSWERS

1. **B.** The relaxation response essentially counteracts the fight-or-flight response to stress. Eliciting this response can lead to health-inducing physiologic effects; it is elicited by focusing the mind and learning to not respond to one's thoughts.

2. **A.** *B. serrata* has been an important treatment for pain used in Ayurvedic medicine over thousands of years. It has been shown to have anti-inflammatory activity via inhibition of the 5-LOX enzyme, and of five randomized controlled trials conducted on this plant, all showed significant analgesic effects.

3. **A.** Yoga is used to improve strength, flexibility, and relaxation through a combination of breathing, mindfulness, and physical movements. Each style of yoga has different intentions. Bikram is commonly practiced in a heated room.

4. **E.** Osteopathic manipulation is a type of manual therapy that intends to decrease pain and restore normal movement. There is evidence that it may be beneficial in all of the conditions listed, although it has not been well studied in pelvic floor pain.

5. **E.** Massage is typically safe in healthy individuals, but is contraindicated in certain conditions, including severe osteoporosis, metastatic lesions, active inflammatory conditions, thrombosis, bleeding disorders, infections, and wounds.

6. **E.** Omega-3 fatty acids (alpha-linolenic acid, eicosapentaenoic acid, docosahexaenoic acid) are thought to modulate autoimmune disorders and have been shown to reduce pain associated with inflammatory conditions (rheumatoid arthritis and inflammatory bowel disease), neck and back pain, neuropathic pain, and dysmenorrhea. There is a potential interaction with anticoagulant medications, but no significant toxicities have been associated with use of these supplements.

7. **B.** Guided imagery takes advantage of mind–body links and the imagination to induce physiologic changes such as relief of pain. It can be especially helpful in the perioperative period.

8. **E.** St. John's wort has been used in the treatment of depression. All of the other natural substances listed have been shown to produce pain-relieving effects in clinical trials.

9. **C.** All answer choices listed are mind–body therapies, but only tai chi/qi gong has been found to have all of the purported benefits listed. Tai chi and qi gong are used to improve balance, relieve stress, and reduce pain through combining breathing techniques with a series of physical movements and meditation. In a review of medical literature including more than 6000 patients undergoing this alternative exercise practice, the most compelling evidence was found for the health benefits listed in the question stem (cardiopulmonary, fall prevention, balance, bone density, etc.).

10. **C.** Although hypnosis and guided imagery are both mind–body therapies that can be practiced alone or with a therapist, the key difference is the introduction of a hypnotic suggestion with hypnosis. Both can be beneficial for anxiety and pain.

Pain and Addictive Disorders: Challenges and Opportunities

50

QUESTIONS

1. How do substances of abuse (such as heroin, cocaine, etc.) primarily cause pleasure on a neurobiological level?
   A. Decrease dopamine release in the ventral tegmental area
   B. Decrease serotonin reuptake
   C. Increase dopamine in midbrain
   D. Increase norepinephrine levels
   E. None of the above

2. How does addiction occur on a neurobiological level?
   A. Positive reinforcement is the major contributor associated with addiction (increased dopamine level from substance causing a pleasurable state).
   B. With addiction, there is a recruitment of antireward systems with consequent negative reinforcement that furthers continued addiction.
   C. Dysfunction of the medulla causes loss of impulse control.
   D. With addiction, there is an increase in reward systems, as there is more dopamine released with continued use.
   E. All of the above

3. Which of the following is true regarding urine drug testing?
   A. Tetrahydrocannabinol (THC) does not show up as positive simply from being in a room with significant marijuana smoke.
   B. Cocaine may show up as positive after eating poppy seeds.
   C. Testing only those patients who are suspected of using drugs will apprehend the majority of abusers.
   D. Hair sampling is very accurate and can even detect recent (<1 week) drug use.
   E. None of the above

4. When treating an opioid-addicted patient with acute pain:
   A. Buprenorphine should be started to mitigate addictive potential while controlling pain.
   B. There is a wider therapeutic window because these are opioid-tolerant patients.
   C. It is better to err on the side of inadequate analgesia than administer opioids in the setting of recovery from an elective procedure.

   D. Continuing the baseline maintenance medication while starting additional forms of analgesia as needed is a reasonable treatment strategy.
   E. All of the above

5. Identify the order in which tolerance develops to opioid effects (from earliest onset to latest):
   A. Constipation, pruritus, sedation
   B. Sedation, constipation, analgesia
   C. Nausea, analgesia, constipation
   D. Analgesia, pruritus, constipation
   E. Analgesia, constipation, nausea

6. Which of the following brain structures is believed to most contribute to the denial and lack of impulse control that underlie addiction?
   A. Nucleus accumbens
   B. Substantia nigra
   C. Ventral thalamic nuclei
   D. Prefrontal cortex
   E. Cerebellum

7. What is believed to be the purpose of establishing universal precautions in pain medicine?
   A. Screening for potential opioid misusers
   B. Mitigating risk to provider and patient
   C. Establishing cost controls to run a pain practice
   D. Ensuring that all patients have access to multiple modes of analgesia
   E. None of the above

8. Which of the following medications is thought to have the highest risk for addiction?
   A. Transdermal fentanyl
   B. Morphine extended release
   C. Oxycodone immediate release
   D. Hydrocodone
   E. Tramadol

9. Hair testing is able to detect substance use accurately in this timeframe:
   A. 1 day up to 2 months
   B. 3 days up to 3 months
   C. 1 week up to 3 months
   D. 3 days up to 2 months
   E. 1 hour up to 1 month

10. A long-standing patient comes to your clinic writhing in pain. They just recently injured themselves in a car accident and are begging you to increase oxycodone dose. The patient is typically very appropriate and you are alarmed by this aberrant behavior. What state is your patient most likely displaying?

A. Tolerance
B. Addiction
C. Pseudoaddiction
D. Withdrawal
E. None of the above

ANSWERS

1. **C.** Substances of abuse (such as heroin, cocaine, oxycodone) cause increases in midbrain dopamine. Important or pleasurable activities also naturally increase dopamine; consequently, the brain is hardwired to experience pleasure from these substances of abuse.

2. **B.** The brain reward system is implicated in both the positive reinforcement produced by exposure to drugs of abuse as well as negative reinforcement produced by drug dependence. Neuropharmacological studies in animal models of addiction have provided evidence for the recruitment of brain-stress systems (i.e., corticotropin [CRF], dynorphin, and norepinephrine) in the extended amygdala, which drives the negative motivational states associated with drug dependence. After the transition to addiction, negative reinforcement is the major driver—people use drugs not so much to feel good as to avoid feeling bad.

3. **A.** Second-hand exposure to cannabis smoke cannot be imputed in the setting of a positive toxicology screen for THC. A finding of THC is a reliable marker for use. On the other hand, spurious results can result from the consumption of legal substances, such as poppy seeds (which contain morphine) and some nasal inhalers (may contain l-methamphetamine). Hair testing is very accurate in detecting substances; however, it can miss recent use because it takes about 1 week for hair to grow to a length that can be collected.

4. **D.** A scheduled maintenance regimen of baseline opioids is recommended with supplemental multimodal analgesia, including short-acting opioids, local anesthetics, and adjuvant NSAIDs. A PCA is also effective in this setting. Undertreatment of acute pain is suboptimal medical treatment. Acute analgesia with opioids may be more hazardous in tolerant than in nontolerant patients. This is because tolerance develops differentially to the analgesic versus the sedating and respiratory depressant effects of the drug.

5. **C.** With chronic opioid use, most side effects subside because tolerance seems greater to side effects than to analgesic effects. Common side effects such as nausea usually subside during chronic treatment. Constipation is an exception and there appears to be no tolerance to opioids' bowel effects; constipation remains a high risk throughout opioid therapy and usually requires treatment.

6. **D.** Dysfunctional activity in the prefrontal cortex (PFC) is thought to impair impulse control. PFC dysfunction could also underlie patients' lack of awareness of their addiction despite overwhelming evidence. This decreased awareness, or "denial," is a hallmark of addiction and a significant barrier to treatment.

7. **B.** The term "universal precautions" originated from an infectious disease model that addressed an approach to patients when there was a deficiency of significant risk assessment information. Past behavior was not a reliable indicator of safe and reasonable approaches, especially with at-risk patients. In 2005, Gourlay et al. proposed the 10 steps of universal precautions in pain medicine. The rationale is that providing the same standard of care to all patients minimizes risk to both patient and provider. (Gourlay DL, Heit HA, Almahrezi A. Universal precautions in pain medicine: a rational approach to the treatment of chronic pain. *Pain Med.* 2005;6(2):107-112.)

8. **D.** In a study by Mironer et al., comparing the frequency of opioid prescriptions with the frequency of abuse, a relative risk of misuse was generated. Among the choices listed, hydrocodone was found to have the highest relative risk (RR = 1.61). (Mironer YE, Brown C, Satterthwaite J, et al. Relative misuse potential of different opioids: a large pain clinic experience. *Paper presented at a meeting of the American Pain Society*, Atlanta, GA; 2000.)

9. **C.** Hair testing is extremely accurate and virtually impossible to dispute but is susceptible to time variation depending on the growth rate of hair. Typically, drug use can be detected for up to 3 months or more. Recent use will be missed because it takes about 1 week for the hair to grow from the follicle to a length where it can be collected.

10. **C.** This patient's behavior is suggestive of pseudo-addiction. They sustained injuries in a recent car accident that has increased their pain. Their current analgesic dose is inadequate, leading to a behavior that mimics addictive behavior. With pseudoaddiction, drug-seeking behavior improves when the pain is controlled.

51

Issues Associated With Opioid Use

QUESTIONS

1. John is 26 years old and suffers from chronic lumbar back pain. During his last appointment, he was given a 30-day supply of opiate medication, but he returns to the clinic 15 days after his last appointment, claiming he had to take more medication than prescribed to control his pain. After the prescribed dose of opiate medication is increased, he is compliant with the medication as prescribed. His actions are characteristic of a patient with:
   A. Addiction
   B. Physical dependence
   C. Tolerance
   D. Pseudoaddiction
   E. Diversion

2. After initiating treatment with an opioid medication 8 months ago, a patient states that they have been arrested three times while attempting to obtain more pain medication off the streets. Additionally, they are in the process of divorce because the spouse does not understand that they need pain medications. They describe a persistent desire to quit using medication, but cannot stop. When they try to quit, they start feeling full-body malaise and pain. Under the *DSM-5*, the patient can be diagnosed with:
   A. Abuse
   B. Dependence
   C. Obsessive compulsive disorder
   D. A and B
   E. None of the above

3. What is the condition in which patient not genetically predisposed to abuse are prescribed opioids that lead to addiction?
   A. Tolerance
   B. Physical dependence
   C. Pseudoaddiction
   D. Aberrant behavior
   E. Iatrogenic addiction

4. Which of the following is an acceptable way to monitor for signs of problematic opiate use and aberrant behavior?
   A. Requiring police reports for stolen medications
   B. Using prescription drug monitoring programs
   C. Random pill counts
   D. Increasing the number of office visits
   E. All of the above

5. A patient with a 3-year history of pancreatic cancer status post resection and now with recurrence has been taking OxyContin 10 mg twice a day and oxycodone 5 mg q6h PRN for breakthrough pain over the last 12 months. The patient presents to the clinic weekly, complaining of inadequate pain control and requesting a higher dose of pain medicine. Over the last month, they have forged a prescription and used their sister's pain medications multiple times. You decide to increase the dosage and over the next 6 months, the patient follows all protocols required with no signs of opioid misuse. How would you best describe the aberrant behavior?
   A. Opioid tolerance
   B. Opioid addiction
   C. Pseudoaddiction
   D. Physical dependence
   E. Iatrogenic addiction

6. Which of the following risk factors is the most consistent predictor for opioid misuse or abuse in non–cancer-related pain?
   A. History of depression
   B. History of alcohol and heroin addiction
   C. Prior drug convictions
   D. History of bipolar mood disorder
   E. Citations for driving under the influence of alcohol

7. Which of the following is considered the cutoff for a high score on the Opioid Risk Tool (ORT), indicating increased risk for aberrant drug-related behavior?
   A. 6 or higher
   B. 7 or higher
   C. 8 or higher
   D. 9 or higher
   E. 10 or higher

8. All of the following are symptoms of abuse **EXCEPT:**
   A. Role impairment
   B. Hazardous use
   C. Legal problems
   D. Social problems
   E. Tolerance

9. Which of the following is the most validated screening tool for opioid misuse or abuse?
   A. CAGE questionnaire
   B. Screening Tool for Addiction Risk (STAR) questionnaire

C. Substance Use Questionnaire
D. Current Opioid Misuse Measure (COMM)
E. ORT

10. Which of the following is **NOT** one of the "four Cs"
that suggests addiction?

A. **C**oncurrent abuse of alcohol or illicit drugs
B. Adverse **c**onsequences as a result of use
C. Impaired **c**ontrol over use
D. **C**ompulsive use
E. Preoccupation with use because of **c**raving

ANSWERS

1. **D.** Pseudoaddiction results in patients seeking additional opioids as a result of inadequate dosing. These behaviors may appear to be addiction but resolve with an increased opioid dose once adequate analgesia is provided.

2. **D.** The patient has signs of abuse (social problems and legal problems), which is diagnosed when at least one of the abuse criteria is present. Dependence is diagnosed when at least three criteria for dependence occur within the same year. This patient has exhibited a persistent desire to quit, has spent excessive amounts of time using, and has shown signs of withdrawal. They arguably show other signs of dependence as well. Thus, they qualify for diagnoses of both opioid abuse and dependence.

3. **E.** In iatrogenic addiction, patients without a genetic predisposition for abuse become addicted because of physician prescribing patterns. These claims can place physicians at risk of medical malpractice.

4. **E.** Measures that can be taken by a prescribing physician to identify and modulate aberrant behavior include all methods listed as well as others (random urine drug screens and avoiding early prescriptions, or replacement of lost or stolen prescriptions).

5. **C.** Although the patient initially showed signs of abuse and addiction, the resolution of aberrant behaviors with an increase in opioid medication indicates pseudoaddiction. In this patient, the recurrence of cancer and likelihood of increasing cancer-related pain justifies an increase of the patient's opioid medication. However, physicians must be careful regarding the diagnosis of pseudoaddiction because they risk

supporting a patient's true addiction, leading to the risk of intentional or accidental overdose. Forging prescriptions and using another person's medication is extremely concerning. In this scenario, the prescribing physician would have been justified in refusing to prescribe further narcotics given the patient's inappropriate behavior, even though the patient has cancer-related pain.

6. **B.** The most consistent predictor of opioid abuse identified in multiple studies is a personal or family history of addiction, especially with multiple substances (as opposed to alcohol alone, which is suggested by answer choice E).

7. **C.** The ORT is a screening tool for opioid abuse or misuse and is based on a number of factors that include age, gender, history of childhood sexual abuse, psychiatric comorbidities, and personal or family history of drug or alcohol abuse. The ORT categorizes patients into low (≤ 3), moderate (4–7), or high (≥ 8) risk of opioid abuse or misuse.

8. **E.** Tolerance is a criterion for dependence, not abuse. The others are criteria for abuse.

9. **D.** The COMM is a well-validated tool for screening opioid misuse or abuse. The other tools listed are less validated but still may be useful in clinical practice.

10. **A.** The "four Cs" are a short list of patterns that may suggest addiction. These include (1) adverse **c**onsequences, (2) impaired **c**ontrol, (3) **c**ompulsive use, and (4) **c**raving.

PART 6

NERVE BLOCK TECHNIQUES

Nerve Blocks of the Head and Neck

52

QUESTIONS

1. A middle-aged woman presents complaining of chronic upper neck pain and headaches. You suspect cervicogenic headaches. Which of the following joints is the first joint where an intervertebral disk exists?
   A. C0-1
   B. C1-2
   C. C2-3
   D. C3-4
   E. C5-6

2. A 43-year-old female is diagnosed with cluster headaches and elects to undergo a sphenopalatine ganglion radiofrequency ablation after failing multiple medications. During the procedure, she becomes bradycardic. Which of the following is the most likely cause?
   A. Aschner–Dagnini reflex
   B. Bezold–Jarisch reflex
   C. Konen reflex
   D. Oculocardiac reflex
   E. Oculocephalic reflex

3. The sphenopalatine ganglion block is useful for the treatment of all of the following **EXCEPT:**
   A. Acute migraine headaches
   B. Acute cluster headaches
   C. Chronic cluster headaches
   D. Facial neuralgias
   E. Cervicogenic headaches

4. Which of the following is true regarding the location of the vertebral artery relative to the upper cervical joints?
   A. It is medial to the atlanto-occipital joint.
   B. It is lateral to the atlanto-axial joint.
   C. It is lateral to the atlanto-occipital joint.

D. It is medial to the atlanto-axial joint.
   E. A and B

5. The inferior alveolar nerve exits the mental foramen at the level of the _____ tooth.
   A. First incisor
   B. Third molar
   C. Second molar
   D. First molar
   E. Wisdom

6. What is the only factor predicting success of radiofrequency (RF) of the third occipital nerve (TON), measured by >50% pain reduction lasting at least 6 months?
   A. Facet joint pain
   B. Paraspinal tenderness
   C. Negative Spurling's test
   D. Pain with extension
   E. Pain with flexion

7. When performing pulsed RF of the sphenopalatine ganglion, correct placement of the tip of the RF needle adjacent to the sphenopalatine ganglion is confirmed most accurately when paresthesia is felt at which location?
   A. Root of the nose
   B. The second upper molar
   C. The anterior zygomatic arch
   D. The lateral zygomatic arch
   E. Down the jaw

8. The maxillary division of the trigeminal nerve exits at the _____.
   A. Foramen ovale
   B. Foramen rotundum

C. Foramen magnum
D. Sphenopalatine foramen
E. Mental foramen

9. Which nerve block may be helpful in treating a painful tumor in the posterior third of the tongue and pharynx?

A. Maxillary nerve block
B. Facial nerve block
C. Glossopharyngeal nerve block
D. Mandibular nerve block
E. Auriculotemporal nerve block

ANSWERS

1. **C.** The C2–3 joint is the first joint with an intervertebral disk and true joint capsule. The C1–2 (AA) joint lacks an intervertebral disk and posterior articulation and therefore is not a true zygapophyseal joint.

2. **C.** The Konen reflex is a bradycardic reflex that can occur with pulsed or conventional radiofrequency therapy of the sphenopalatine ganglion. The bradycardic response can be avoided by pretreatment with glycopyrrolate or atropine.

3. **E.** Sphenopalatine ganglion block has been used in the treatment of acute migraine headaches, acute and chronic cluster headaches, post-traumatic headaches, and facial neuralgia. It is not used for cervicogenic headaches.

4. **E.** The vertebral artery is medial to the atlanto-occipital joint and lateral to the atlanto-axial joint.

5. **C.** The inferior alveolar nerve is a distal branch of the mandibular nerve, originating from the trigeminal nerve. It exits from the mental foramen at the level of the second molar, where it can be blocked.

6. **B.** According to a 2007 study by Cohen, pain on palpation of the paraspinal muscles is the only factor predicting success of RFA of the TON. (Cohen SP, Bajwa ZH, Kraemer JJ, et al. Factors predicting success and failure for cervical facet radiofrequency denervation: a multi-center analysis. *Reg Anesth Pain Med.* 2007;32:495-503.)

7. **A.** The sphenopalatine ganglion is located just posterior to the middle turbinate. Conventional or pulsed RF is used for the treatment of various headaches and facial neuralgias. Correct needle placement adjacent to the nerve is verified by stimulation felt at the root of the nose.

8. **B.** The ophthalmic division of the trigeminal nerve exits at the superior orbital fissure. The maxillary division exits at the foramen rotundum. The mandibular division exits at the foramen ovale. The distal branch of the mandibular nerve, the inferior alveolar nerve, exits at the mental foramen.

9. **C.** The glossopharyngeal nerve provides sensory innervation to part of the tongue, mouth, and pharynx. It can be blocked to provide analgesia for glossopharyngeal neuralgia and tumors of the posterior third of the tongue and mucous membranes of the mouth and pharynx.

Upper Extremity Blocks 53

53

QUESTIONS

1. When compared with traditional opioid-based postoperative analgesia, single-injection regional anesthesia techniques have all of the following benefits **EXCEPT:**
   A. Superior analgesia
   B. Reduced opioid-related side effects
   C. Faster rehabilitation or return to work
   D. Improved patient satisfaction
   E. Reduced number of unplanned admissions

2. The infraclavicular approach blocks the brachial plexus at the level of:
   A. Roots
   B. Trunks
   C. Divisions
   D. Cords
   E. Branches

3. While performing brachial plexus block, using an infraclavicular approach, the posterior cord is stimulated. Which motor response is most likely observed?
   A. Wrist extension
   B. Shoulder abduction
   C. Forearm flexion
   D. Finger flexion
   E. Thumb opposition

4. Upper extremity block can be clinically assessed using the "four Ps" tool. The median nerve can be tested by asking the patient to:
   A. Extend the forearm against resistance
   B. Flex the forearm against resistance
   C. Pinch the palmar base of the index finger
   D. Pinch the palmar base of the little finger
   E. All of the above

5. When performing brachial plexus block, 0.5% bupivacaine is equipotent to:
   A. 0.75% ropivacaine
   B. 0.5% ropivacaine
   C. 0.25% ropivacaine
   D. 1% ropivacaine
   E. None of the above

6. Adding epinephrine to local anesthetic has the following advantages **EXCEPT:**
   A. The duration of block is prolonged.
   B. The onset of block is faster.

C. Systemic uptake of local anesthetic is decreased.
D. It is a marker for intravascular injection.
E. All of the above are advantages of adding epinephrine.

7. Which of the following statements about alkalinization of local anesthetics for brachial plexus blocks is true?
   A. Facilitates faster onset of the block
   B. Reduces block intensity
   C. Increases block duration
   D. Effects are similar to epidural alkalinization
   E. Leads to burning sensation

8. Interscalene block is most appropriate for surgery on:
   A. Elbow
   B. Shoulder
   C. Medial aspect of upper arm
   D. Forearm
   E. Hand

9. Axillary blocks are ideal for:
   A. Shoulder surgery
   B. Upper arm surgery
   C. Surgery on the humerus
   D. Forearm surgery
   E. Placing perineural catheters

10. All of the following are warning signs for serious nerve injury after upper extremity block **EXCEPT:**
    A. Paresthesia
    B. Complete absence of nerve function immediately after surgery
    C. Motor deficit
    D. Worsening symptoms over time
    E. Failure to show early signs of resolution

11. Local anesthetic systemic toxicity is relatively common with brachial plexus regional anesthesia because:
    A. There is a chance of unintentional injection into arteries that directly supply the brain.
    B. It is an extremely challenging procedure to perform.
    C. The brachial plexus is highly vascular.
    D. There is high chance of intrathecal injection.
    E. None of the above

12. After receiving an interscalene block, a patient develops bilateral upper and lower extremity block associated with hypotension, bradycardia, and apnea. What is the most likely complication that has occurred?
    A. Unintentional vascular injection
    B. Unintentional intrathecal injection
    C. Unintentional epidural injection
    D. Excess volume of local anesthesia
    E. Pneumothorax

13. A patient with chronic obstructive pulmonary disease is scheduled for elbow open reduction internal fixation. He is requesting regional anesthesia. Spirometry results show that he will be unable to withstand a 25% or greater reduction in pulmonary function. Which block should be avoided?
    A. Interscalene block
    B. Supraclavicular block
    C. Axillary block
    D. A and B
    E. All of the above

ANSWERS

1. **C.** When compared with traditional opioid-based postoperative analgesia for outpatient shoulder, arm, or hand surgery, single-injection regional anesthesia techniques provide superior analgesia, reduce opioid-related side effects, improve patient satisfaction, and reduce the number of unplanned admissions. Although these benefits are generally limited to the day of surgery, they nevertheless represent a valuable alternative to general anesthetic and postoperative opioid techniques. What remains unclear is whether these techniques substantially improve economic outcomes such as faster rehabilitation or return to work.

2. **D.** Brachial plexus approaches are directed toward its various anatomic divisions. For example, the interscalene approach is directed toward the level of the distal roots and proximal trunks, whereas the infraclavicular approach is directed toward the level of the cords.

3. **A.** Stimulation of the posterior cord during the infraclavicular approach causes wrist **extension** (the little finger moves posteriorly). As stimulation moves proximally along the brachial plexus, it yields muscle movements of a mixed nature. As an example of this concept, electrical stimulation of the superior trunk during the interscalene approach results in mixed muscle stimulation that produces shoulder elevation.

4. **C.** Asking the patient to pinch the palmar base of the index finger can test the median nerve.

5. **A.** Potency studies of long-acting local anesthetics applied to the brachial plexus suggest that 0.5% bupivacaine is equipotent to 0.75% ropivacaine. This equivalence is important because a tendency to use more ropivacaine to obtain the same effect as bupivacaine will probably negate the lower cardiotoxic properties of ropivacaine. When considering the total mass (dose) of a local anesthetic, decisions are best skewed toward using a lower volume, concentration, and dose.

6. **B.** Epinephrine, 2.5 μg/mL (1:400,000), prolongs the duration of local anesthetic blockade, acts as a marker of intravascular injection through its associated tachycardia, and decreases systemic uptake of local anesthetic. The ability of epinephrine to prolong a local anesthetic block is a consequence of reduced clearance from the injection site and is unlikely to involve a significant alpha-2 adrenergic agonist effect. The onset of block is not affected.

7. **B.** Alkalinization of intermediate-acting local anesthetics facilitates faster onset of the block **during** epidural anesthesia but does not have the same effect at the brachial plexus. Onset is not hastened by adding sodium bicarbonate to plain local anesthetic or to local anesthetic freshly mixed with epinephrine; animal models have shown that alkalinization of local anesthetic reduces block intensity and duration.

8. **B.** For an interscalene block, the brachial plexus is approached at the level of its distal roots or proximal trunks. The most consistent local anesthetic distribution resulting from this approach involves the shoulder and upper part of the arm. The inferior trunk (C8, T1) is unaffected by local anesthetic in approximately 50% of cases. Therefore an interscalene block is not recommended for surgeries involving the medial aspect of the upper part of the arm, the forearm, and the hand. Ultrasound-guided approaches are also likely to spare the lower trunk distribution, although some investigators describe targeting these nerves.

9. **D.** The axillary block anesthetizes the brachial plexus at the level of the four terminal nerves: the radial, ulnar, median, and musculocutaneous nerves. It is indicated for surgeries distal to and including the elbow. With the exception of very proximal approaches high in the axilla, the axillary block is not as ideally suited for continuous catheter techniques as are the infraclavicular approach and approaches above the clavicle.

10. **A.** Permanent nerve injury after an upper extremity block is extremely rare and probably occurs in less than 16 per 10,000 patients (95% confidence interval [CI]). Nerve dysfunction, particularly persistent paresthesia or numbness, is relatively common (up to 19%) immediately after surgery, but the vast majority of these symptoms resolve within 4 weeks. Warning signs that an injury may be particularly worrisome include complete absence of nerve

function immediately after surgery (indicative of nerve transection or ischemia), motor deficit, worsening symptoms over time, or failure to show early signs of resolution. Early neurologic consultation in these cases is recommended to rule out reversible causes, establish baseline function, and coordinate further diagnostic workup and rehabilitation.

11. **A.** Brachial plexus blocks have a relatively low risk of delayed local anesthetic systemic toxicity (LAST) when compared with epidural or intercostal blocks, but there are no reliable data to support the maximum recommended doses of local anesthetic in this block. The risk for seizure secondary to intravascular injection is five times higher with peripheral nerve blocks than with epidural blocks. This risk is particularly relevant to brachial plexus regional anesthesia because of the proximity of the vertebral, carotid, and subclavian (via retrograde flow) arteries to direct injection during placement of an interscalene or supraclavicular block.

12. **C.** One of the most serious complications of brachial plexus block is when local anesthetic is unintentionally placed near the neuraxis and causes epidural or spinal anesthesia during attempted interscalene anesthesia. The C6 foramen is only 23 mm from the skin in the average patient, therefore it is easy to conceive how excessively deep needle placement could result in this complication. Neuraxial injection of local anesthetic is manifested by the rapid (total spinal anesthesia) or delayed (massive epidural anesthesia) appearance of a bilateral upper and lower extremity block, which is often associated with hypotension, bradycardia, and apnea. This complication must be diagnosed and treated rapidly with airway control, volume expansion, and early provision of exogenous epinephrine to counteract blockade of the cardioaccelerator fibers and absent vascular tone.

13. **D.** Hemidiaphragmatic paresis (HDP) occurs in all patients who undergo an interscalene block via the traditional techniques, and about one in four of these patients will have a 25%–32% reduction in spirometric measures of pulmonary function. Ultrasound-guided interscalene blocks that use low volumes of local anesthetic (5–10 mL) result in a reduced incidence and severity of HDP, but the side effect still occurs unpredictably. The incidence of HDP is less (95% CI = 14%–86%) in patients undergoing a supraclavicular block. Although healthy volunteers experienced no diminution in pulmonary function during the supraclavicular approach, this may not hold true for patients with underlying pulmonary disease. A low-volume supraclavicular block performed under ultrasound guidance reduces the incidence of HDP to almost zero. Nevertheless, it is recommended that any patient unable to withstand a 25% or greater reduction in pulmonary function not be given an above-the-clavicle brachial plexus block, even when using ultrasound guidance.

54 Lower Extremity Nerve Blocks

QUESTIONS

1. All of the following are advantages of lower extremity blocks (LEBs) **EXCEPT:**
   A. LEBs may decrease the incidence of postoperative pain syndromes.
   B. LEBs are beneficial in patients with complex regional pain syndromes.
   C. LEBs do not usually require ultrasound use.
   D. LEBs are used for patients with peripheral vascular diseases.
   E. None of the above are advantages.

2. The femoral nerve is formed by:
   A. The anterior divisions of L2–4
   B. The posterior divisions of L2–4
   C. The anterior divisions of L3–5
   D. The posterior divisions of L3–5
   E. The anterior and posterior divisions of L3–5

3. Which nerve provides motor innervation to the adductor muscles?
   A. Lateral femoral cutaneous nerve
   B. Iliohypogastric nerve
   C. Femoral nerve
   D. Ilioinguinal nerve
   E. Obturator nerve

4. A lumbar plexus block (LPB) can provide anesthesia or analgesia to all **EXCEPT:**
   A. The anterolateral and medial aspects of the thigh
   B. The knee
   C. The medial portion of the leg below the knee
   D. The lateral portion of leg below the knee
   E. It provides analgesia to all of the above.

5. Patients with known coagulopathy receiving lumbar plexus block are at risk of:
   A. Psoas hematoma
   B. Subcapsular renal hematoma
   C. Retroperitoneal hematoma
   D. All of the above
   E. None of the above

6. Which of the following statements about the anatomy of the lateral femoral cutaneous nerve (LFCN) is correct?
   A. LFCN is 1–2 cm lateral and inferior to the anterior superior iliac spine (ASIS).
   B. LFCN lies beneath the fascia lata.
   C. LFCN is just medial to the sartorius muscle.
   D. LFCN lies beneath the fascia iliaca.
   E. LFCN lies lateral to the tensor fasciae latae muscle (TFLM).

7. The advantage of fascia iliaca block is that:
   A. It blocks both femoral nerve and LFCN.
   B. It blocks the femoral nerve, obturator nerve, and LFCN.
   C. It requires lower volume of local anesthesia.
   D. Both B and C
   E. All of the above

8. Which nerve provides sensation to the posterior aspect of the thigh?
   A. Popliteal nerve
   B. Sciatic nerve
   C. Posterior femoral cutaneous nerve
   D. Lateral femoral cutaneous nerve
   E. Obturator nerve

9. All of the following are clinical applications of sciatic nerve block **EXCEPT:**
   A. Foot and ankle surgery
   B. Surgery on medial leg
   C. Ischemia-induced pain in lower extremity
   D. Treatment of pressure ulcers
   E. Knee and hip flexor spasticity

10. What is the location of the sciatic nerve relative to the popliteal artery?
    A. The sciatic nerve is medial and deep to the artery.
    B. The sciatic nerve is lateral and superficial to the artery.
    C. The sciatic nerve is lateral and deep to the artery.
    D. The sciatic nerve is medial and superficial to the artery.
    E. None of the above

ANSWERS

1. **C.** LEBs may decrease the incidence of postoperative pain syndromes, including chronic postamputation phantom limb pain. In addition to surgical applications, LEBs have also been reported to be beneficial in patients with complex regional pain syndrome, chronic cancer pain, peripheral vascular diseases (ischemia, Raynaud's disease, peripheral embolism), intractable phantom limb pain, and spasticity. Several reports have suggested that ultrasound guidance results in more precise needle and catheter placement during LEBs than do blocks performed with nerve stimulator or landmark techniques.

2. **B.** The femoral nerve is formed by the posterior divisions of L2–4. The nerve descends from the plexus lateral to the psoas muscle. The femoral nerve innervates the rectus femoris, vastus medialis, vastus intermedius, and vastus lateralis muscles. It also provides cutaneous sensory innervation to much of the anterior and medial aspects of the thigh, as well as the medial part of the leg distal to the knee.

3. **E.** The lateral femoral cutaneous nerve is formed from the L2 and L3 nerve roots and, as its name indicates, is a cutaneous sensory nerve. It provides sensation to the lateral aspect of the thigh. The obturator nerve (L2–4) provides sensory innervation to a variable portion of the leg proximal to the knee, as well as motor innervation to the adductor muscles. The iliohypogastric and ilioinguinal nerves are primarily sensory nerves that arise from L1 and supply innervation to the skin of the suprapubic and inguinal regions. The genitofemoral nerve arises from the L1 and L2 roots and supplies motor innervation to the cremasteric muscle and additional sensory innervation to the inguinal area.

4. **D.** An LPB can provide anesthesia or analgesia to the anterolateral and medial aspects of the thigh, the knee, and the medial portion of the leg below the knee. Common indications include anesthesia and analgesia following total hip arthroplasty, total knee arthroplasty, and anterior cruciate ligament reconstruction, as well as for treatment of chronic hip pain. The sacral plexus supplies the lateral portion of leg below the knee.

5. **D.** Care should be taken to avoid major vascular structures and the lower pole of the **kidney** because cases of subcapsular renal hematoma have been reported. The reported cases of delayed retroperitoneal hematoma after LPB in the absence of anticoagulation underscore the need for caution in patients treated with anticoagulants. Although there are no clear guidelines on the safety of LPB in the presence of anticoagulation, it is prudent to consider alternative anesthetic plans for patients with known coagulopathy.

6. **D.** The LFCN is typically blocked 1–2 cm medial and inferior to the ASIS. At this location, the nerve lies beneath the fascia iliaca, just lateral to the sartorius muscle and medial to the TFLM.

7. **A.** A fascia iliaca block is an alternative approach to a femoral nerve block in which local anesthetic is injected underneath the fascia iliaca at a distance from the femoral nerve. Functionally, the technique is similar to a femoral block except that the large volume of local anesthetic used has a greater chance of also blocking the LFCN in addition to the femoral nerve.

8. **C.** Sensation to the posterior aspect of the thigh is provided by the posterior femoral cutaneous nerve, which also originates from the sacral plexus and follows a similar course as the sciatic nerve in the thigh, but is not formally part of the sciatic nerve. If blockade of the posterior femoral cutaneous nerve of the thigh is desired (such as for surgical anesthesia for above-knee amputation), a block of the sciatic nerve at the subgluteal level or above is indicated.

9. **B.** The primary indications for sciatic nerve blockade are for foot and ankle surgery. However, the other areas listed are also covered, except for the medial leg. The medial leg is supplied by the saphenous nerve, not the sciatic nerve. The saphenous nerve is a branch of the femoral nerve.

10. **B.** The sciatic nerve is lateral and superficial to the artery. A transducer should be placed at the level of the popliteal crease and the popliteal artery located at this level. The sciatic nerve can then be located as a hyperechoic round or oval structure lateral and superficial to the artery.

55 Truncal Blocks

QUESTIONS

1. Which of the following statements about paravertebral blocks is true?
   A. The block targets nerves at the level where the spinal nerves exit the intervertebral foramina.
   B. The block produces somatic but not sympathetic blockade.
   C. The block is limited to the level of injection.
   D. It is often associated with cardiovascular or respiratory effects.
   E. All of the above

2. What is the most likely complication when performing a large-volume single-injection thoracic paravertebral block?
   A. Nausea and vomiting
   B. Hypotension
   C. Epidural spread of the solution
   D. Pneumothorax
   E. Nerve injury

3. Which dermatomes should be blocked for most breast surgeries?
   A. T4–10
   B. T1–6
   C. T1–10
   D. T4–6
   E. T1–4

4. What is the needle target when performing an ultrasound-guided intercostal nerve block (ICB)?
   A. Visceral pleura
   B. Internal intercostal muscle
   C. Parietal pleura
   D. Ribs
   E. Transverse process

5. Transverse abdominal plane (TAP) block requires placement of local anesthetic between:
   A. Subcutaneous tissues and the external oblique muscle
   B. External oblique and internal oblique muscles
   C. Internal oblique and transverse abdominis muscles
   D. Transverse abdominis muscle and peritoneal cavity
   E. Anterior superior iliac spine and rectus abdominis

6. All of the following statements regarding blockade of the ilioinguinal (II) and iliohypogastric (IH) nerves are true **EXCEPT:**
   A. The classic approach has a high success rate.
   B. The IH nerve is close (<1 cm) to the II nerve.
   C. The needle is inserted between the obliquus internus abdominis and transversus abdominis muscles.
   D. The volume of the local anesthetic dose required is much smaller than those recommended with the "blind" technique.
   E. All of the above are true.

7. Which of the following statements regarding paravertebral blocks for thoracic surgery is true?
   A. Chronic pain after thoracotomy is significantly reduced when early and effective paravertebral block is provided.
   B. Continuous paravertebral analgesia is considered the "gold standard" for postoperative analgesia after thoracic surgery.
   C. Catheter insertion under direct visualization by the surgeon before wound closure has been shown to be more efficacious than when the catheter is inserted blindly by the anesthesiologist.
   D. Paravertebral block is associated with more risks than epidural analgesia.
   E. None of the above is true.

8. All of the following are complications of paravertebral blocks **EXCEPT:**
   A. Pneumothorax
   B. Hypotension
   C. Epidural hematoma
   D. Toxic seizures
   E. Horner's syndrome

9. The intercostal nerves are distributed to the following **EXCEPT:**
   A. Neck
   B. Thoracic pleura
   C. Abdominal peritoneum
   D. Upper limb
   E. Groin

10. Which nerve supplies the superomedial aspect of the thigh?
    A. Ilioinguinal nerve
    B. Iliohypogastric nerve
    C. Femoral nerve
    D. Obturator nerve
    E. Lateral femoral cutaneous nerve

ANSWERS

1. **A.** Paravertebral blockade consists of injecting local anesthetic close to the vertebra at the level where the spinal nerves exit the intervertebral foramina. This induces an ipsilateral somatic and sympathetic blockade that extends, most of the time, longitudinally above and below the injected vertebral level. It is indicated for acute as well as chronic unilateral pain. It is not associated with major cardiovascular or respiratory effects.

2. **C.** Some studies suggest that a single-injection technique is as effective as a multiple-injection one (average of five dermatomes blocked) as long as the total volume of 0.3 mL/kg is used. These results were confirmed in a thermographic study by Cheema and coworkers. However, it seems preferable to use a "multiple-injection" technique when an extensive spread of local anesthetic is required because of the risk for bilateral or epidural spread associated with a single large-volume injection. (Cheema SP, Ilsley D, Richardson J, Sabanathan S. A thermographic study of paravertebral analgesia. *Anaesthesia* 1995;50(2):118-121.)

3. **B.** At the thoracic level, breast surgery requires blockade of the T1–6 dermatomes, whereas thoracotomy requires lower dermatomal blockade (T4–10). At the lumbar level, an extensive block (T10–L2) is required.

4. **B.** With direct visualization of the ribs and pleura, ultrasound guidance allows the anesthesiologist to perform an ICB proximal to the scapula, where the intercostal nerve can be blocked before its division to ensure adequate anesthesia of the pleura. In addition, ultrasound guidance allows visualization of injection of the local anesthetic into the intercostal space, thereby enabling the provider to adjust the trajectory and depth of the needle to ensure an adequate spread of anesthetic and avoid pleural puncture. The needle target is the internal intercostal muscle.

5. **C.** Ultrasound allows direct visualization of the external oblique, internal oblique, and transverse abdominal muscles, thus allowing accurate placement of the local anesthetic solution within the relevant plane (i.e., between the internal oblique and transverse abdominis muscles).

6. **A.** The classic approach can have a failure rate as high as 20%–30%. The ultrasound examination allows the II nerve to be best visualized immediately medial to the anterior superior iliac spine. It is located at a mean distance of 6 mm from this bony landmark. The IH nerve is close (< 1 cm) to the II nerve and both nerves are located close to the peritoneum. With an out-of-plane approach, the needle is inserted between the obliquus internus abdominis and transversus abdominis muscles. The volume of local anesthetic

required to anesthetize both nerves is 0.075 mL/kg in children and 0.2 mL/kg in adults, doses much smaller than those recommended with the "blind" technique. The ultrasound-guided technique resulted in a 96% success rate and significantly reduced the risk for complications such as an intestinal puncture.

7. **A.** Although thoracic epidural analgesia is still considered the "gold standard" for postoperative analgesia after thoracic surgery, continuous paravertebral analgesia is as effective as epidural analgesia. Such efficacy occurs whether the catheter is inserted blindly by the anesthesiologist or under direct visualization by the surgeon before wound closure. Moreover, a paravertebral catheter avoids the potential risks observed with epidural analgesia, including epidural hematoma, infection, and spinal cord injury. Chronic pain after thoracotomy occurs in 20%–50% of patients. The occurrence of this syndrome is significantly reduced when early and adequate postoperative pain treatment (e.g., epidural analgesia, paravertebral block) is provided.

8. **C.** The incidence of complications after paravertebral blocks varies between 2% and 5%. The common complications are pneumothorax (0.5%–1.5%), hypotension, vascular puncture (6%), intrathecal spread (1%), toxic seizures, Horner's syndrome, and epidural spread. The incidence of hypotension requiring a low dose of vasopressors (e.g., ephedrine) is 4%. The hypotension may result from either sympathetic blockade (unilateral or bilateral) or a vasovagal event during the procedure. Horner's syndrome is caused by cephalad spread of the local anesthetic after a high thoracic paravertebral block. With regard to epidural spread, dye injection studies have shown the incidence of unilateral epidural spread to be up to 70% when using the blind approach. However, its clinical effects are negligible because of the small amount of local anesthetic injected.

9. **A.** The intercostal nerves are the anterior divisions of the thoracic spinal nerve from T1 to T11. They are distributed mainly to the thoracic pleura and abdominal peritoneum. The first two nerves supply fibers to the upper limb in addition to their thoracic branches; the next four are limited in their distribution to the parietal pleura of the thorax, and the lower five supply the parietal pleura of the thorax and abdomen. The 7th intercostal nerve terminates at the xiphoid process, the 10th intercostal nerve terminates at the umbilicus, and the 12th (subcostal) thoracic nerve is distributed to the abdominal wall and the groin.

10. **A.** The ilioinguinal nerve supplies the skin region of the superomedial aspect of the thigh, as well as the anterior region of the scrotum in males or the mons pubis and labia majora in females.

56 Peripheral and Visceral Sympathetic Blocks

QUESTIONS

1. Which of the following conditions is least likely to respond to a stellate ganglion block (SGB)?
   A. Sympathetically mediated pain
   B. Phantom pain
   C. Posttraumatic stress disorder
   D. Cervical radiculopathy
   E. Cardiac arrhythmias

2. All of the following are expected to occur with a successful SGB **EXCEPT:**
   A. Horner's syndrome (ptosis, miosis, anhidrosis)
   B. Increased skin temperature
   C. Metallic taste
   D. Increased skin blood flow
   E. Numbness

3. All of the following are true regarding the SGB **EXCEPT:**
   A. The stellate ganglion is situated at the lateral border of the longus colli muscle.
   B. Ultrasound is the preferred technique when performing a stellate ganglion block.
   C. An important landmark with SGB is Chassaignac's tubercle (anterior tubercle of the transverse process at the C6 level).
   D. Hematoma following an SGB is likely because of damage to the vertebral artery.
   E. All of the above are true.

4. All of the following are true in regard to a celiac plexus block **EXCEPT:**
   A. The celiac plexus is typically located at the T12–L1 level anterior to the aorta.
   B. The celiac plexus receives parasympathetic supply from the vagus nerve.
   C. The T10 preganglionic fiber constitutes the least splanchnic nerve.
   D. There is level I evidence for celiac plexus neurolysis for neoplasm-related pain of the abdomen.
   E. All of the above are true.

5. Which of the following organs will be least affected by the celiac plexus block?
   A. Kidney
   B. Adrenal gland
   C. Testes
   D. Descending colon
   E. Spleen

6. What is the most common adverse effect of a celiac plexus neurolysis?
   A. Orthostatic hypotension
   B. Postprocedural pain
   C. Diarrhea
   D. Bradycardia
   E. Pneumothorax

7. What is the recommended sympathetic block to treat the pain associated with endometriosis?
   A. Celiac plexus block
   B. Superior hypogastric plexus block
   C. Ganglion impar block
   D. Pudendal nerve block
   E. Stellate ganglion block

8. You are planning to perform a superior hypogastric plexus neurolysis for metastatic rectal cancer. What is your target level for the block?
   A. T12–L1
   B. Middle of L3
   C. Lower third of L5 to upper third of S1
   D. Sacrococcygeal joint
   E. None of the above

9. Where is the ganglion impar commonly found?
   A. Anterior to the sacrococcygeal junction or the lower coccygeal vertebral bodies
   B. Anterior to the aorta and crus of the diaphragm
   C. Anterior to the fifth lumbar vertebral body and first sacral vertebral body
   D. In the caudal epidural space
   E. None of the above

10. You are seeing a patient who is suffering from coccygodynia and has already failed conservative therapy. Which procedure is most likely to alleviate this patient's pain?
    A. Lumbar medial branch blocks
    B. Sacral lateral branch blocks
    C. Ganglion impar block
    D. Lumbar sympathetic block
    E. Transforaminal epidural steroid injection

ANSWERS

1. **D.** The SGB has been suggested to be effective in treating multiple conditions including sympathetically mediated pain, vascular insufficiency of the upper extremity, phantom pain, postherpetic neuralgia, cancer pain, cardiac arrhythmias, orofacial pain, vascular headache, cerebral vasospasm, hot facial flushes, and posttraumatic stress disorder. The pain of cervical radiculopathy is managed with cervical epidurals.

2. **C.** A patient who has undergone a successful SGB will typically have Horner's syndrome (ptosis, miosis, anhidrosis), increased skin temperature, and increased skin blood flow. At times, spillage of local anesthetic onto nerves and nerve roots in the area may lead to numbness in the distribution of those nerves as well. Patients should not sense a metallic taste because this could be an indication of intravascular injection and an early sign of local anesthetic systemic toxicity.

3. **D.** Hematoma following an SGB is likely because of damage to the inferior thyroid artery.

4. **C.** The T10 and T11 preganglionic fibers constitute the lesser splanchnic nerve, while T12 forms the least splanchnic nerve.

5. **D.** The celiac plexus block will affect the following visceral organs: diaphragm, liver, stomach, spleen, adrenal glands, kidneys, ovaries/testes, small intestine, and colon up to the splenic flexure. Pain at the descending colon is not affected by the celiac plexus block.

6. **B.** The most common adverse effect from a celiac plexus neurolysis is postprocedural pain (90% of patients). This pain usually subsides in 24–48 hours. Orthostatic hypotension and transient diarrhea occur in roughly 40% of patients. Administering intravenous fluid (about 500 mL) with the block can minimize the hypotension. Rare complications associated with the block include retroperitoneal hematoma, pneumothorax, renal and intestinal injury, and paraplegia.

7. **B.** The superior hypogastric plexus block can be effective in treating pain originating from the pelvic viscera secondary to endometriosis and cancers in this area; it has also been reported to provide relief with postprostatectomy penile pain, urethral pain, and post uterine artery embolization pain.

8. **C.** The superior hypogastric plexus block is usually located at the lower third of the fifth vertebral body and can extend caudally to the upper third of the first sacral body.

9. **A.** The ganglion impar is located at the anterior surface of the sacrococcygeal junction to the lower coccygeal vertebral bodies.

10. **C.** The ganglion impar block has been shown to alleviate pain from sympathetically mediated pain in the anus, distal rectum, urethra, and vagina; it can also be helpful with coccygodynia.

57 Intraarticular Analgesia

QUESTIONS

1. Use of steroids intra-articularly following arthroscopy can lead to a _____ incidence of postoperative infection.
   A. 0.25%
   B. 2%
   C. 5%
   D. 8%
   E. 20%

2. Hypotension can be a problem when greater than _____ of clonidine is administered intra-articularly.
   A. 5 µg
   B. 15 µg
   C. 50 µg
   D. 100 µg
   E. 150 µg

3. What is the most frequently seen side effect with intra-articular tramadol of > 100 mg?
   A. Nausea/vomiting
   B. Numbness/tingling
   C. Vision
   D. Seizures
   E. Diarrhea

4. Which of the following is a rare but serious complication of intra-articular injection of bupivacaine in higher concentrations?
   A. Chondrotoxicity
   B. Bleeding
   C. Seizures
   D. Nausea/vomiting
   E. Hypotension

5. Which of the following medications given intra-articularly has been shown through studies to be most efficacious for postoperative pain management as a single agent?
   A. Ketamine
   B. Ketorolac
   C. Morphine
   D. Bupivacaine
   E. Fentanyl

6. Which drug class when injected intra-articularly in combination with other medications may have a synergistic analgesic effect?
   A. Clonidine combined with local anesthetic
   B. Neostigmine combined with local anesthetic
   C. Ketamine combined with local anesthetic
   D. NSAID combined with local anesthetic
   E. All of the above

7. A patient undergoes a total knee arthroplasty and is complaining of pain with postoperative physical therapy. Which of the following types of pain is she experiencing?
   A. Hyperalgesia
   B. Sensitization
   C. Breakthrough pain
   D. Dynamic pain
   E. Static pain

8. The analgesic effect of adrenaline is exerted through which receptor?
   A. Alpha-1 receptors of the substantia gelatinosa
   B. Alpha-2 receptors of the substantia gelatinosa
   C. Beta-1 receptors of the substantia gelatinosa
   D. Beta-2 receptors of the substantia gelatinosa
   E. Dopaminergic receptors of the substantia gelatinosa

ANSWERS

1. **B.** Use of steroids intra-articularly following arthroscopy can lead to a 2% incidence of postoperative infection.

2. **E.** Hypotension can be a problem when 150 µg of clonidine is injected intra-articularly.

3. **A.** Nausea and vomiting was the most frequent side effect in a dose response study involving 20 mg versus 50 mg versus 100 mg of intra-articular tramadol.

4. **A.** Chondrotoxicity is a concern with intra-articular injection of bupivacaine in higher concentrations

and over longer periods based on histological studies. Systemic toxicity is usually not seen even with intra-articular injection of high dose concentration of bupivacaine as measured by plasma concentrations.

5. **B.** Several studies show that intra-articular NSAIDs are more effective in reducing postoperative pain than systemic NSAIDs, suggesting peripheral intra-articular receptor mediated pain relief. There is concern about poorer bone healing with intra-articular NSAIDs in animal models, but this has not been clearly shown in human studies.

6. **D.** The NSAIDs, when injected in combination with local anesthetic or with morphine or both, seem to have a greater effect than either drug as a sole agent. Overall, few studies compare combination medications injected intra-articularly.

7. **D.** Dynamic pain is pain on provocation. Examples include pain on coughing or pain on movement. Static pain is pain on rest that occurs even without provocation.

8. **B.** The analgesic effect of epinephrine (adrenaline) is thought to be exerted at the alpha-2 receptors of the substantia gelatinosa. A clear intra-articular mechanism of analgesia is not defined.

58 Chemical Neurolytic Blocks

QUESTIONS

1. Neurolytic therapy remains a therapy of last resort. However, for the appropriate patient, it can result in significant improvement in the quality of life and possibly improved function. All of the following are criteria for the use of neurolytic therapy **EXCEPT:**
   A. Pain is relieved by diagnostic blocks using local anesthetic.
   B. Pain is unremitting, diffuse, and not well localized.
   C. The patient is unable to function and perform their ADLs because of pain.
   D. The patient has failed all conservative medical management.
   E. No undesirable effects appear during the local anesthetic blockade.

2. Neurolytic agents available in the United States for common use include ethanol and phenol. Glycerol is a colorless, odorless, viscous, liquid, polyol compound. What type of neurolytic block is glycerol primarily used for?
   A. Gasserian ganglion
   B. Iliohypogastric
   C. Stellate ganglion
   D. Intercostal nerve
   E. Celiac plexus

3. A 31-year-old female with complex regional pain syndrome of the right upper extremity for 6 months presents to a pain clinic. She has failed conservative treatment with physical therapy and medications, including NSAIDs, gabapentin, nortriptyline, and lidocaine ointment. A decision is made to proceed with an SGB. The needle is inserted under ultrasound guidance at the C6 level, posterolateral to the prevertebral fascia on the surface of the longus colli muscle. The vertebral artery enters the vertebral foramen _____ to the anterior tubercle of C6 and _____ to the transverse process of C7.

A. Posterior, lateral
B. Posterior, anterior
C. Medial, inferior
D. Posterior, superior
E. Medial, anterior

4. When using ethanol as a neurolytic agent, which of the following medications may cause a disulfiram-like effect?
   A. Clindamycin
   B. Furosemide
   C. Hydrochlorothiazide
   D. Metronidazole
   E. Vancomycin

5. All of the following are characteristics of phenol as a neurolytic agent **EXCEPT:**
   A. Absorbs water with air exposure
   B. Hyperbaric relative to cerebrospinal fluid
   C. Painless, warm feeling upon injection
   D. Prepared at a concentration of 4%–8%
   E. Unstable at room temperature

6. A 54-year-old male presents with intractable pain of the left jaw secondary to oral cancer. A decision is made to proceed with the gasserian ganglion block and possible neurolysis. The needle is inserted approximately 2.5 cm lateral to the side of the mouth and advanced, perpendicular to the middle of the eye, in a cephalad direction toward the auditory meatus. When contact is made with the base of the skull, the needle is withdrawn and "walked" posteriorly toward the foramen ovale. Which of the following would be expected when performing a gasserian ganglion block/neurolysis?
   A. Free flow of cerebrospinal fluid
   B. Hemorrhage in the temporal fossa
   C. Permanent lateral rectus palsy
   D. Spinal anesthesia
   E. Subscleral hematoma of the eye

ANSWERS

1. **B.** Neurolysis can be considered in patients with severe visceral or well-localized somatic pain when less invasive techniques have failed. Before neurolysis, there should be pain relief with a diagnostic local anesthetic blockade and no undesirable effects following the block.

2. **A.** Glycerol causes myelin disintegration and axonolysis in both myelinated and unmyelinated fibers; it is now primarily restricted to neurolysis of the gasserian ganglion.

3. **B.** The vertebral artery passes over the stellate ganglion and enters the vertebral foramen posterior to the anterior tubercle of C6. The bony foramen is often absent at C7, and the vertebral artery often courses unprotected anterior to the C7 transverse process.

4. **D.** There have been case reports of a disulfiram-like effect and acetaldehyde syndrome when ethanol/alcohol was used as a neurolytic agent for celiac plexus in a patient taking moxalactam (a beta-lactam antibiotic that inhibits aldehyde dehydrogenase) and in a patient taking 1-hexyl carbamoyl-5-fluorouracil (an anticancer drug). Symptoms include flushing, hypotension, tachycardia, and diaphoresis. Medications that may cause disulfiram-like effects include chloramphenicol, beta-lactams, metronidazole, tolbutamide, chlorpropamide, and disulfiram; caution should be taken when neurolysis with alcohol is planned on patients taking these medications.

5. **A.** Phenol is poorly soluble in water and, at room temperature, forms only a 6.7% aqueous solution. It has a shelf life of approximately one year if refrigerated and shielded from light exposure. When exposed to room air, it oxidizes and turns a reddish color. Concentrations of 4%–10% are typically used for neurolysis. It is frequently prepared with contrast and sterile water, sterile saline, or glycerin. When phenol is prepared in glycerin, it has a specific gravity of 1.25, making it hyperbaric and limiting its spread. Unlike alcohol, phenol injection has an initial local anesthetic effect.

6. **A.** The gasserian ganglion bathes in CSF, and a free flow of CSF is usually noted when performing a gasserian ganglion block. Possible complications include spinal anesthesia, hematoma of the face and subscleral hematoma of the eye, hemorrhage in the temporal fossa, problems with mastication, diplopia, and strabismus caused by oculomotor palsy, and lateral rectus palsy from blockade of the abducens nerve.

59 Neurolysis of the Sympathetic Axis for Cancer Pain Management

QUESTIONS

1. A 69-year-old male with locally advanced anorectal mucosal melanoma, now status post neoadjuvant chemotherapy and sphincter-preserving (limited) surgery, presents with worsening anal pain described as aching, deep, sharp, and constant. The pain is aggravated with sitting and alleviated by lying on one side. The patient is unable to drive from pain and sedation due to pain medication. His pain is 9/10 on a numerical pain rating scale and improves to 5/10 with opioids. He has tried gabapentin, tramadol, NSAIDs, and extended-release morphine in the past without adequate relief. The pain is deemed most likely to be visceral from the remaining disease burden. A ganglion impar block is considered. The ganglion impar receives visceral afferents innervating all of the following structures **EXCEPT:**
   A. Anus
   B. Rectum
   C. Distal urethra
   D. Distal third of the vagina
   E. Testicles

2. A celiac plexus neurolysis is performed for a 54-year-old female with pancreatic cancer who presented with upper abdominal pain. Her past medical history is significant for hypothyroidism and anxiety. She reports that she is completely pain-free in the recovery room and is discharged home. Three days later, she calls the clinic with the complaint that when she tried to get out of the bed, she felt extremely dizzy and fell. Luckily, she was able to grab on to the furniture and did not hit her head, and feels OK now sitting in a recliner. Orthostatic hypotension can occur up to how many days following a celiac plexus block?
   A. 2 days
   B. 4 days
   C. 5 days
   D. 7 days
   E. 10 days

3. In addition to pharmacologic therapy, neurolytic blocks of the sympathetic axis are also effective in controlling visceral cancer pain. They should be considered as important adjuncts to pharmacologic therapy for the relief of severe visceral pain. What is the average duration of pain control with a neurolytic block?
   A. 12 months
   B. 8 months
   C. 6 months
   D. 2 months
   E. 1 months

4. Mrs. Jones is a 55-year-old female with metastatic pancreatic cancer. She has just received a celiac plexus block for abdominal pain related to her tumors. In the PACU, she complains of back pain and is noted to be hypotensive. What is the next best step in her medical management?
   A. Provide IV fluids and discharge her home
   B. Check a hematocrit in the patient and, if within normal limits, discharge home
   C. Reassure the patient that pain is likely due to needle insertion and hypotension is due to sympathectomy
   D. Admit the patient to the hospital for serial hematocrit monitoring
   E. Check two hematocrits 1 hour apart; if stable, discharge the patient home

5. A genitourinary oncologist asks you if there is any procedure you can offer his 58-year-old male patient with bladder cancer and multiple pelvic metastases who has intractable hypogastric pain. You explain that pelvic pain associated with cancer and chronic nonmalignant conditions may be alleviated by blocking the superior hypogastric plexus. Analgesia of the organs in the pelvis is possible because the afferent fibers innervating these structures travel in the sympathetic nerves, trunks, ganglia, and rami. What is the incidence of neurologic complications reported with superior hypogastric neurolysis?
   A. 1 in 100
   B. 1 in 1000
   C. 1 in 5000
   D. 1 in 10,000
   E. None of the above

ANSWERS

1. **E.** The ganglion impar contains visceral afferent fibers from the perineum, distal part of the rectum, anus, distal end of the urethra, vulva, and distal third of the vagina.

2. **C.** Orthostatic hypotension may occur up to 5 days after the celiac plexus block. It disappears after compensatory vascular reflexes are fully activated. Treatment is conservative and includes bed rest, avoidance of sudden changes in position, and replacement of fluids.

3. **D.** Neurolytic blocks of the sympathetic axis can be used for control of chronic upper abdominal pain or pelvic pain in patients with cancer. Research shows that even in the best-case scenario, the duration of full pain control is two months.

4. **D.** A patient who develops backache and orthostatic hypotension after a celiac plexus block might have a retroperitoneal hemorrhage, which is a rare complication of the block. These patients should be admitted to the hospital for serial hematocrit monitoring to rule out hemorrhage.

5. **E.** In a multicenter study done by Plancarte et al. of over 200 patients who received hypogastric plexus block, there were no neurologic complications noted. (Plancarte R, de Leon-Casasola OA, El-Helaly M, et al. Neurolytic superior hypogastric plexus block for chronic pelvic pain associated with cancer. *Reg Anesth.* 1997;22(6):562–568.)

PART 7

INTERVENTIONAL TECHNIQUES

Interlaminar and Transforaminal Therapeutic Epidural Injections

60

QUESTIONS

1. All of the following statements are true in regard to the management of radiculopathy **EXCEPT:**
   A. Surgical care demonstrated statistically significant superiority over conservative care for the treatment of lumbar disk herniation.
   B. The natural history of discogenic radicular pain consists of slow improvement over time.
   C. Radiculopathy can be caused by impingement of a disk on the foraminal spinal nerve, spondylosis, vertebral subluxation, and infection.
   D. Radicular pain is usually caused by both pathologic compression of the spinal nerve and inflammation mediated by cytokines.
   E. All of the above are true.

2. All of the following are implicated in the pathophysiology of discogenic pain **EXCEPT:**
   A. Tumor necrosis factor-α (TNF-α) expression by the disk cells
   B. Nociceptive neural structures located in the outer third of the annulus fibrosus of the disk
   C. Nociceptive neural fibers of the disk: small unmyelinated C fibers
   D. Reduced levels of interleukin-6 (IL-6) and -8 (IL-8)
   E. All of the above are implicated.

3. Which steroid is recommended for use in cervical transforaminal epidural injections?
   A. Methylprednisolone acetate
   B. Dexamethasone
   C. Betamethasone
   D. Triamcinolone
   E. Prednisone

4. At what level should a cervical interlaminar epidural injection be performed?
   A. C4–C5
   B. C5–C6
   C. C6–C7
   D. C7–T1
   E. T1–T2

5. In relation to epidural steroid injections (ESI), what is the recommended maximum frequency to perform the procedure in the same patient?
   A. No more than 3 injections in 6 months
   B. No more than 6 injections in 6 months
   C. No more than 3 injections in 12 months
   D. Up to twice a month for 3 months until pain resolves
   E. None of the above

6. What is the most common bacteria associated with infection from epidural injections?
   A. *Streptococcus*
   B. *Staphylococcus*
   C. *Klebsiella*
   D. *Escherichia coli*
   E. *Pseudomonas*

7. Spinal cord injury resulting from ESI:
   A. Is minimized by sedating the patient to avoid unanticipated movement
   B. Most often results from direct needle trauma
   C. Can be completely avoided by use of fluoroscopy
   D. Most often results from intravascular injection
   E. Accounts for an insignificant percentage of closed claims data

8. Which of the following is considered the most proven advantage of a transforaminal approach over an interlaminar approach to the lumbar space?
A. Decreased risk of infection
B. Greater coverage of inflamed nerve roots
C. Technical ease of placement
D. Decreased risk of dural puncture
E. Decreased risk of infarction

9. When performing a transforaminal epidural, the correct arrangement of the so-called "safe triangle" includes:
A. The superior border of the pedicle, superior to the spinal nerve, and lateral to the dural sleeve
B. The inferior border of the pedicle, superior to the spinal nerve, and medial to the dural sleeve
C. The inferior border of the pedicle, superior to the spinal nerve, and lateral to the dural sleeve
D. The superior border of the lamina, posterior to the spinal cord, inferior to the spinous process
E. None of the above

10. Which of the following is true regarding intravascular injection during transforaminal epidural injection?
A. A test dose of 1 mL of normal saline is useful in identifying vascular uptake.
B. Minimizing the volume of contrast injected helps prevent injury.
C. Staying in the "safe triangle" avoids the typical location of the artery of Adamkiewicz in the inferior fifth of the foramen.
D. Digital subtraction angiography (DSA) can be used as an adjunct to detect vascular uptake.
E. It is less common during cervical spine procedures than in lumbar procedures.

11. A rare complication of cervical transforaminal epidural injection is anterior spinal artery syndrome, in which the segmental medullary arteries suffer an ischemic injury. These arteries could be branches from which of the following:
A. Vertebral artery
B. Ascending cervical artery
C. Deep cervical artery
D. All of the above
E. None of the above

12. Where is the artery of Adamkiewicz located in most of the population?
A. C5–C7
B. T1–T4
C. T4–T8
D. T8–L2
E. L2–L5

ANSWERS

1. **A.** According to data from the Spine Pain Outcomes Research Trial (SPORT), there was no statistically significant superiority of surgical discectomy over conservative care for the treatment of lumbar disk herniation.

2. **D.** Patients with disk disease have shown elevated levels of IL-6 and IL-8.

3. **B.** A nonparticulate steroid (dexamethasone) is recommended for use in cervical transforaminal epidural steroid injections, since injection of particulate steroids into arteries may cause infarctions. Dexamethasone is also recommended as the initial steroid used in a lumbar transforaminal epidural steroid injection. Particulate steroid may be considered in subsequent lumbar injections if dexamethasone does not provide sustained relief.

4. **D.** The C7–T1 level is the recommended entry site for cervical interlaminar epidural injections. At more cephalad levels, the space may be too narrow, leading to increased risk of dural sac puncture or spinal cord injury.

5. **A.** It is recommended that no more than 3 epidural steroid injections be administered in 6 months in order to minimize medication-related adverse effects.

6. **B.** Cases of abscess and meningitis associated with epidural injections were caused primarily by the *Staphylococcus* species in one case series, with a higher risk among diabetics and metastatic cancer patients. These patients typically presented within the first 2 weeks after injection with worsening back pain.

7. **B.** Catastrophic neural injury may occur as a result of direct spinal cord puncture in sedated or anesthetized patients. Fluoroscopic imaging is not necessarily protective, and closed claims data indicate a rising incidence of injuries secondary to chronic pain procedures, most of which are epidural steroid injections.

8. **D.** The classic transforaminal epidural technique uses the confines of the "safe triangle" for administration. The needle is placed lateral to the dural sleeve, decreasing the risk of dural puncture when compared with the interlaminar approach.

9. **C.** The "safe triangle" for transforaminal epidural steroid injection is a fluoroscopic region just lateral to the inferior margin of the pedicle, dorsal to the vertebral body, and cephalad to the nerve root. Because needle placement in this area avoids the nerve root, the zone was named the "safe triangle."

10. **D.** The confirmation of intravascular injection with digital subtraction angiography (DSA) has increased the detection rate of vascular puncture. Local anesthetic test dosing with 1 mL of 1%–2% lidocaine with epinephrine is also useful in detecting intravascular injection. Injection of nonionic contrast medium should demonstrate both nerve root and epidural spread. The artery of Adamkiewicz is typically found in the upper half of the foramen.

11. **D.** The segmental medullary arteries could be branches of the vertebral artery, ascending cervical artery, or deep cervical arteries.

12. **D.** In 75% of the population, the great segmental medullary artery of Adamkiewicz originates on the left side of the aorta between the T8 and L1 vertebral segments. In the remaining 25% of the population, it arises from the right side.

61 Pathogenesis, Diagnosis, and Treatment of Zygapophysial (Facet) Joint Pain

QUESTIONS

1. What is the volume capacity of a lumbar facet joint?
   A. <0.5 mL
   B. 0.5–1 mL
   C. 1–1.5 mL
   D. 1.5–2 mL
   E. 2–2.5 mL

2. A patient reports pain in her right suprascapular region and in her shoulder, but it does not extend to the mid-scapula area. The patient has concordant pain with lateral bending and rotation of her neck to the right. The rest of her examination is unremarkable. The pain is most likely referred from which structure?
   A. Right C2–3 facet joint
   B. Right shoulder joint
   C. Right C5–6 facet joint
   D. Right C6 nerve root
   E. Right T1–T2 facet joint

3. Which is the most common complication of radiofrequency denervation of the medial branch?
   A. Neuritis
   B. Spinal anesthesia
   C. Vasovagal reaction
   D. Burn
   E. Infection

4. From where does the third occipital nerve originate?
   A. C2 dorsal ramus
   B. C2 inferior branch
   C. C3 dorsal ramus
   D. C3 inferior branch
   E. Greater occipital nerve

5. Of the facet joints, which are most vertically oriented?
   A. Cervical facets
   B. Thoracic facets
   C. Lumbar facets
   D. Both cervical and thoracic facets
   E. All are oriented the same.

6. What is the most reliable method of diagnosing facet pain?
   A. Image-guided medial branch block
   B. Physical examination
   C. X-ray imaging
   D. MRI imaging
   E. Patient's history

7. Which is the most frequently implicated painful lumbar facet joint?
   A. L1–2
   B. L2–3
   C. L3–4
   D. L4–5
   E. L5–S1

8. The L4–5 facet is innervated by which nerve(s)?
   A. L3 medial branch
   B. L4 medial branch
   C. L3 and L4 medial branch
   D. L4 medial branch and L5 dorsal ramus
   E. L5 dorsal ramus

9. A patient receives an MRI that shows narrowing of the facet joint space at L4–L5 with moderate osteophyte formation and mild subarticular bone erosion at those facets bilaterally. What is the appropriate grade of degeneration corresponding to these findings?
   A. Grade 0
   B. Grade 1
   C. Grade 2
   D. Grade 3
   E. Grade 4

10. Based on clinical studies, which movement is associated with the greatest strain on the upper lumbar facet joints (L1–L2, L2–L3, L3–L4) and lower lumbar facet joints (L4–5, L5–S1) respectively?
    A. Lateral bending to the right, forward flexion
    B. Lateral bending to the left, lateral bending to the right
    C. Forward flexion, lateral bending to the right
    D. Lateral bending to the right, lateral bending to the left
    E. Lateral bending to the left, extension

11. All of the following will most likely decrease the incidence of false-positive lumbar facet blocks **EXCEPT:**
    A. Aim for a higher target on the transverse process
    B. Avoid the use of opioids or sedation
    C. Consider a single needle approach
    D. Be judicious with the use of superficial anesthesia
    E. Use comparative local anesthetic blocks

12. Which of the following factors has been associated with a positive predictor of good outcome from radiofrequency denervation of lumbar medial branch nerves?
    A. Previous back surgery
    B. Pain worsened by extension/flexion maneuvers or facet loading
    C. Lumbar paraspinal tenderness
    D. Pain from a traumatic event/motor vehicle accident
    E. Longer duration of pain

13. The medial branch innervates all of the following **EXCEPT:**
    A. Multifidus muscle
    B. Periosteum of neural arch
    C. Interspinal muscle and ligament
    D. Longissimus muscle
    E. Facet joint

14. The mamillo-accessory ligament can become calcified and be a source of nerve entrapment. This is most commonly seen at what level?
    A. C6
    B. C7
    C. L3
    D. L4
    E. L5

15. All of the following are true in regard to thoracic facet joints **EXCEPT:**
    A. These joints permit more lateral flexion compared with axial rotation.
    B. The course/location of the medial branches is consistent throughout the thoracic spine.
    C. The uppermost thoracic facet joints obtain some of their innervation from C7 and C8 medial branches.
    D. The medial branches in the midthoracic level do not run on bone.
    E. Multifidus stimulation is not reliable to confirm needle placement during radiofrequency treatment in these joints.

ANSWERS

1. **C.** The volume of a lumbar facet joint is approximately 1–1.5 mL. Cervical facet joint volume is approximately 0.5–1 mL.

2. **C.** Pain from the C5–6 facet joint is typically referred to the suprascapular region or lower part of the neck. It can also refer to the shoulder joint or midposterior neck. Pain referred from the C2–3 facet joint typically extends to the suboccipital area and the T1–2 facet joint refers to the medial border of the scapula including the lower portion and sparing the shoulder. However, it is important to note that there is considerable overlap in the referred pain regions. The patient's pain is unlikely to be caused by the C6 nerve root because of the lack of radicular symptoms down to her hand. The shoulder is an unlikely source because the examination was normal except for certain neck movements.

3. **A.** The most common complication of radiofrequency (RF) denervation of the medial branch is neuritis, but the incidence is <5%. One study showed that the administration of steroid or pentoxifylline reduced the incidence of postprocedure pain following RF denervation. Other side effects and complications include transient numbness and/or dysesthesias, burns, and thermal injury to the ventral rami.

4. **C.** The C3 dorsal ramus divides into two medial branches—the superior branch and inferior branch. The superior branch is the larger of the two and is also known as the third occipital nerve. The C2–3 facet joint is innervated mostly from the C3 dorsal ramus. The C2 dorsal ramus has a number of branches, the largest of which is the greater occipital nerve. The C2 dorsal ramus also supplies some innervation to the C2–3 facet.

5. **B.** The thoracic facets are the most vertically oriented joints with a frontal orientation. This allows for greater lateral flexion but limited axial rotation. The angle is roughly 60–70 degrees at the mid-thoracic facet joints.

6. **A.** Image-guided medial branch blocks (MBBs) or intra-articular injections of local anesthetic are the most reliable method of diagnosing facet pain. Multiple studies have shown that history, physical examination, and radiologic findings are not reliable. However, false-positive rates from 25% to 41% have been associated with diagnostic facet blocks without the use of controls. Given this finding, many view positive MBBs as more prognostic than diagnostic.

7. **E.** The most frequently implicated painful lumbar facet joint is L5–S1, followed by L4–5, then L3–4. The upper lumbar facet joints are much less likely to be the main source of axial low back pain.

8. **C.** In the lumbar spine, the facet joints are innervated by the medial branches from the posterior primary rami at the same level and the level above the facet joint. So for the L4–5 facet joint, it is innervated by the L3 and L4 medial branch nerves. Innervation of the thoracic facet joints is similar to the lumbar facet joints except that the medial branches of C7 and C8 may travel as low as T3. The innervation of the cervical facet joints is slightly more complicated. From C3–4 to C7–T1, they still receive dual innervation from the medial branches of the posterior rami at the same level and the level above. Because there are eight cervical nerve roots, the numbering is different from lumbar and thoracic facet joints. For example, the C4–5 joint is innervated by the C4 and C5 medial branch nerves.

9. **C.** Based on the findings of moderate osteophyte formation and mild subarticular bone erosions, the joint in question is best classified as grade 2. Facet joints are graded between 0 and 3 based on magnetic resonance imaging.

10. **A.** Work by Ianuzzi and colleagues showed that the greatest capsular strain in the upper lumbar facet joints was during lateral bending, usually to the right. For the lower lumbar facet joints, the greatest strain was during forward flexion. It is important to note that capsular stretch and strain can cause pain, not just loading or compression. Inflammation of the capsule can also lead to radicular symptoms because of the release of inflammatory mediators. (Ianuzzi A, Little JS, Chiu JB, et al. Human lumbar facet joint capsule strains: I. During physiological motions. *Spine J.* 2004;4(2):141–152.)

11. **A.** False-positive rates of 25%–40% have been associated with diagnostic facet blocks in the lumbar spine. There are a number of interventions that have been shown to reduce the false-positive rate and thereby improve the diagnostic ability of the block. The use of sedation and opioids has been associated with false-positive blocks because of interference with interpreting results; therefore, it is recommended to avoid sedation and opioids during the procedure. Another concern is that the local anesthetic may spread to other pain-generating structures. Studies have shown that lower volumes of anesthetic (0.5 mL for lumbar and 0.25 mL for cervical) can enhance specificity without negatively impacting sensitivity. Also, targeting *lower* on the transverse process midway between the upper border and the mamillo-accessory ligament was associated with less spread to adjacent neural structures. Other interventions include a single needle technique and/or minimizing superficial anesthetic and performing placebo-controlled or comparative local anesthetic blocks.

12. **C.** Although history, physical examination, and radiologic findings have not been shown to be reliable in the diagnosis of facet pain, in one study, paraspinal tenderness predicted successful RF denervation treatment. Factors that were associated with failed treatment included pain with hyperextension and axial rotation (i.e., facet loading), duration of pain, and previous back surgery. It is important to note that duration of pain and previous back surgery have also been associated with treatment failure for other low back pain interventions, including epidural steroid injection and surgery.

13. **D.** Along with the facet joint, the medial branch innervates the multifidus muscle, interspinal muscle and ligament, and periosteum of the neural arch. The longissimus muscle is innervated by the small intermediate branch of the posterior ramus. In the lumbar region, the lateral branch innervates the paraspinal muscles, thoracolumbar fascia, sacroiliac joint, and variable sensory fibers to the skin over the spinous processes. As a side note, since the thoracic medial branches circumvent the multifidus muscle, motor stimulation to confirm needle placement during RF treatment cannot be used reliably.

14. **E.** The mamillo-accessory ligament can become calcified, causing nerve entrapment at the L5 (20%), L4 (10%), and L3 (4%) level. It has been hypothesized that long-term benefit from the use of steroids during MBB is due to anti-inflammatory effects on the medial branch nerve trapped beneath this ligament. However, most studies have failed to corroborate these findings.

15. **B.** The vertical and frontal orientation of the thoracic facet joints allows more lateral flexion rather than axial rotation. The innervation of the facet joints is similar to the lumbar region except the medial branches of C7 and C8 may travel as low as T3. The medial branches in the mid-thoracic levels do not run on bone, but are instead suspended in the intertransverse space. They also swing laterally and circumvent the multifidus muscle. This means that motor stimulation of the multifidus muscle cannot be used reliably for needle placement during RF treatment. In addition, the superolateral corner of the transverse process may be a more accurate target point for blockade and denervation. The medial branch does become more medial at the thoracic-lumbar transition zone.

Radiofrequency Treatment

62

QUESTIONS

1. The debate about which factor during radiofrequency (RF) treatments contributed to the development of pulsed radiofrequency treatments?
   A. Current
   B. Heat
   C. Voltage
   D. Time
   E. Lesion size

2. All of the following statements regarding continuous RF treatment are true **EXCEPT:**
   A. An electrical field is created at the exposed tip of the electrode, which heats the tip and ultimately the tissues surrounding it.
   B. There is a voltage gradient between the electrode and the dispersion pad.
   C. Temperature depends on the amount of power delivered.
   D. Temperature affects lesion size.
   E. Heat is generated by friction dissipation.

3. Which of the following factors will most likely decrease the size of the lesion produced by the generator for continuous RF treatment?
   A. Increasing the power delivered
   B. Proximity to bone
   C. Proximity to blood vessels
   D. Decreased heat "washout"
   E. None of the above

4. Which of the following is used to measure continuity of the electrical circuit when performing RF ablation?
   A. Impedance monitoring
   B. Radiofrequency delivery mode
   C. Nerve stimulation
   D. Temperature monitoring
   E. Voltage monitoring

5. A 45-year-old female presents with intermittent shooting pain on the right side of her face in a V3 distribution. She reports that she is otherwise healthy. She does note that she had an episode of eye pain and vision loss in the past, which resolved. There are no neurologic deficits on examination. You make a diagnosis of trigeminal neuralgia. What is the most appropriate next step in management?
   A. MRI
   B. Diagnostic trigeminal nerve block

C. Prescription for ibuprofen
   D. Referral for desensitization therapy
   E. Radiofrequency treatment of the gasserian ganglion

6. Besides loss of facial sensation, which of the following complications of radiofrequency treatment of trigeminal neuralgia is the most common?
   A. Masseter weakness
   B. Permanent palsy of the abducens nerve
   C. Keratitis
   D. Anesthesia dolorosa
   E. Transient paralysis of cranial nerves III and IV

7. You see a 21-year-old female with episodic, one-sided headaches around her eye associated with redness, tearing, and nasal congestion. Which interventional procedure is most likely to help in the treatment of her condition?
   A. Cervical facet blocks
   B. Occipital nerve blocks
   C. Sphenopalatine ganglion radiofrequency treatment
   D. Trigeminal V3 pulsed radiofrequency treatment
   E. Gasserian ganglion block

8. During placement of the electrode for radiofrequency treatment of cluster headache, the patient experiences some paresthesia in their palate. What should you do with the needle?
   A. Keep the needle where it is
   B. Move the needle more laterally
   C. Abort the procedure
   D. Advance the needle slightly
   E. Move the needle more cephalad

9. You are performing a left C4–6 medial branch RF. While testing motor stimulation at 2 Hz, you notice that the patient's left arm starts to twitch. Which is the best course of action?
   A. Reposition the needle more anteriorly
   B. Reposition the needle more posteriorly
   C. Reposition the needle more superiorly
   D. Reposition the needle more inferiorly
   E. Leave the needle where it is

10. All of the following are potential side effects or complications of radiofrequency treatment for cervical facet pain **EXCEPT:**
    A. Dural puncture
    B. Spinal cord trauma
    C. Pneumothorax
    D. Chemical meningitis
    E. All of the above are known side effects or complications.

11. Sacroiliac joint pain is typically localized and referred to which areas, respectively?
    A. Gluteal region, posterolateral thigh
    B. Lumbar area, anterior thigh
    C. Lateral thigh, knee
    D. Gluteal region, anterior thigh
    E. Gluteal region, greater trochanter

12. Cooled RF ablation allows which of the following to be increased without causing tissue charring around the electrode?
    A. Depth
    B. Impedance
    C. Power
    D. Temperature
    E. Gauge of cannula

13. For treatment of cervical radicular pain with radiofrequency of the dorsal root ganglion, what is the most common adverse side effect?
    A. Seizure
    B. Mild burning sensation and deep neck soreness
    C. Sensory changes (hypoesthesia)
    D. Stroke
    E. Weakness

14. Why have some favored the use of cooled RF ablation for sacroiliac joint pain?
    A. Time
    B. Cost
    C. Anatomic variation of the nerves
    D. Less discomfort for the patient
    E. Ease of placement of the cannula

15. RF treatment of the dorsal root ganglion has been described for the treatment of which of the following?
    A. Facet pain
    B. Sacroiliac joint pain

C. Discogenic pain
D. Radicular pain
E. Peripheral neuropathic pain

16. During sensory stimulation for a lumbar medial branch RF ablation, at what frequency and voltage should the patient feel new pressure or tingling in the back, indicating close proximity to the medial branch nerve?
    A. 2 Hz and 0.5–1.0 V
    B. 50 Hz and 0.5–1.0 V
    C. 2 Hz and <0.5 V
    D. 50 Hz and <0.5 V
    E. 2 Hz and <1 V

17. What are the most common levels involved in cervicobrachialgia?
    A. C3 and C4
    B. C4 and C5
    C. C5 and C6
    D. C6 and C7
    E. C7 and C8

18. Which of the following is the optimum position of the RF needles outside the posterior foramen of the S1–2 levels for right lateral branch RF?
    A. Between 1:00 and 5:30
    B. Between 3:00 and 7:30
    C. Between 5:00 and 9:30
    D. Between 7:00 and 11:30
    E. Between 10:00 and 2:30

19. During pulsed RF treatment, what is the best course of action if the temperature exceeds 42°C?
    A. Change the voltage to 90 V
    B. Stop for 30 seconds, then restart
    C. Change the RF current to 250,000 Hz
    D. Change the duration of the active cycle to 40 ms
    E. Change the frequency of the active cycle to 1 Hz

20. Which of the following is **LEAST** likely to be a complication after pterygopalatine radiofrequency treatment?
    A. Dryness of the ipsilateral eye
    B. Masseter weakness
    C. Numbness of the soft palate
    D. Intravascular injection
    E. Loss of taste

ANSWERS

1. **B.** Pulsed RF treatment developed from questioning the role of heat during conventional RF treatments. For years, people thought that RF current generated heat and that the heat applied to thin nerve fibers interfered with the conduction of nociceptive stimuli. The role of heat was questioned because lesions were also successful when not performed between the nociceptive focus and the CNS. Also, RF of the dorsal root ganglion only induces transient sensory loss, but pain relief persists much longer. Finally, studies have shown no difference in outcome with two different temperatures (40°C and 67°C). Pulsed RF is based on strong, fluctuating electric fields while temperature is kept to a minimum.

2. **A.** With continuous RF treatment (as opposed to pulsed), the generator creates a voltage gradient between the electrode and the ground plate (dispersion pad). RF current creates an electric force on ions in the tissue, causing them to move back and

forth; the frictional dissipation from the movement creates heating of the tissue. The electrode is then heated by the tissue, not by the RF current itself. The lesion size depends on the temperature, and the temperature depends on the power delivered.

3. **C.** As noted in the previous question, increasing the temperature (by increasing the power delivered) will increase the size of the lesion. Heat "washout," or when heat is removed from the area by conductive loss or blood circulation, decreases the size of the lesion. When there is less heat washout, the lesion will be larger. RF lesions near bone will have less "washout," and lesions near blood vessels may have more washout.

4. **A.** A modern RF lesion generator has a number of functions, including continuous measurement of impedance, nerve stimulation, RF delivery, pulsed delivery, and monitoring of voltage, current, wattage, and temperature. The purpose of measuring impedance is to confirm the continuity of the electrical circuit.

5. **A.** Trigeminal neuralgia is characterized by brief episodes of sharp, shooting pain in one or more of the divisions of the trigeminal nerve. It is typically provoked by touch, and the patient is usually pain-free between episodes. Vascular compression of the trigeminal root likely causes the pain; however, other conditions can present with trigeminal neuralgia, including multiple sclerosis and primary brain tumors. Therefore, these conditions should be investigated or excluded, especially in younger patients or those with neurologic deficits. In this case, the patient is < 60 and may have had optic neuritis in the past, which is associated with multiple sclerosis.

6. **A.** There is very low morbidity and practically no mortality associated with radiofrequency treatment of trigeminal neuralgia. The most common side effect is loss of facial sensation and accompanying paresthesia (80%). Other complications include masseter weakness and paralysis (4.1%), anesthesia dolorosa (1%), keratitis (0.6%), and transient paralysis of cranial nerves III and IV (0.8%). Permanent palsy of cranial nerve VI is much less frequent.

7. **C.** The patient in question most likely has cluster headaches. RF treatment of the pterygopalatine (sphenopalatine) ganglion has been used to treat cluster headaches. The ganglion is a parasympathetic ganglion in the pterygopalatine fossa beneath the maxillary nerve. Afferent fibers from the nasal mucosa, soft palate, and pharynx cross the ganglion as they travel to the gasserian ganglion. The ganglion has been targeted, given the parasympathetic symptoms present with cluster headaches. RF treatment has also been used to treat atypical facial pain in the V2 distribution and posttraumatic headache. Pulsed RF treatment has been recommended, given the safety of the procedure.

8. **D.** RF treatment of the pterygopalatine (sphenopalatine) ganglion has been described for the treatment of cluster headache. The ganglion is located beneath the maxillary nerve in the pterygopalatine fossa. As the cannula is advanced into the fossa, it will contact the maxillary nerve, resulting in a paresthesia. During sensory testing, the patient may report sensations in the outside of the cheek, upper lip, or palate. The cannula is too far lateral if paresthesia occurs in the cheek or lip. The cannula should be advanced a few millimeters if the patient has a paresthesia in the palate. This is done to prevent injury to the maxillary nerve during lesioning.

9. **B.** When performing sensory testing after placement of electrodes for cervical medial branch RF, the patient should have a tingling sensation in the neck at < 0.5 V at 50 Hz. For motor testing at 2 Hz, contractions of the paraspinal muscles will be noticed. If muscle contractions are noted in the arm, the needle is too close to the exiting nerve root and should be repositioned more posteriorly.

10. **E.** Complications from cervical medial branch radiofrequency treatment are rare. If the needle is placed too anteriorly into the intervertebral foramen, puncture of the vertebral artery is possible. If the needle is too medial, intrathecal injection may occur. One observational study found the incidence of complications to be 3.9%, comparable to the lumbar area. Other complications included intravascular injection, vasovagal reactions, dural puncture, spinal cord trauma, spinal anesthesia, chemical meningitis, neural trauma, pneumothorax, and hematoma formation. Many of these complications are related to needle placement and drug administration.

11. **A.** Sacroiliac joint pain can be from sacroiliitis, infections, spondyloarthropathy, pyogenic or crystal arthropathy, fracture of the sacrum and pelvis, and diastasis. If no pathology is noted, the pain is likely from a mechanical origin and is called "sacroiliac syndrome." Pain from the sacroiliac joint is usually localized to the gluteal region (94%) and can be referred to the posterolateral thigh to the knee, sometimes in an L5 or S1 radicular pattern.

12. **C.** Cooled RF treatment has the reported advantage of creating larger lesions, which may overcome anatomic variations in the target nerves. Cooled RF involves circulating water through the device to help dissipate heat from tissues next to the electrode. This allows increased power without high impedance which could lead to tissue charring. It may be particularly helpful for RF treatments of SI joint pain given the anatomic variation of sacral lateral branches.

13. **B.** The most common side effect from radiofrequency treatment of the cervical dorsal root ganglion is a mild burning sensation in the treated dermatome and some deep neck soreness. This usually subsides within 1–3 weeks. Also, hypoesthesia may occur, but it usually

resolves within 3–4 months. Other complications are similar to those from blockade of the cervical segmental nerve, including epidural, intrathecal, or intravascular injection of local anesthetic, which can lead to local anesthetic CNS toxicity.

14. **C.** Cooled RF technology was developed to create a larger lesion size by circulating water through the device to dissipate heat from tissues surrounding the electrode. The reason for larger lesions was primarily to overcome anatomic variation of the target nerves. This approach has been favored for the treatment of sacroiliac joint pain because of the anatomic variation of the lateral branches. Placement of the cooled RF cannula is not easier than with conventional RF cannulas. Since the needle gauge is bigger for cooled RF cannulas, there may be more discomfort. Also, there is no decrease in time or cost.

15. **D.** Radiofrequency treatment of the dorsal root ganglion has been used for the treatment of cervical, thoracic, and lumbar radicular pain. Pulsed radiofrequency treatment may be helpful for peripheral neuropathies when RF lesioning is not indicated. Facet and sacroiliac joint pain have been treated with lesioning of the medial and sacral lateral branches, not the dorsal root ganglions.

16. **D.** Sensory stimulation is performed at a frequency of 50 Hz to assess proximity of the electrode to the target nerve. Stimulation is produced at 0.25 V if the needle is resting on the nerve and at 2 V if the needle is 1 cm away from the nerve. Obtaining stimulation at <0.5 V is sufficient to create a lesion that encompasses the target nerve. Motor stimulation is performed at 2 Hz and is used to check if the needle is too close to motor fibers. Since the medial branch innervates the multifidus muscle, motor stimulation may cause localized muscle contractions in the neck and back.

17. **D.** Cervicobrachialgia (cervical radicular pain) is most common at the C6 and C7 levels and to a lesser extent at C5. C4 and C8 involvement is uncommon.

18. **A.** The sacroiliac joint obtains its innervation from multiple levels, including the sacral lateral branches of S1–3. The target areas for the nerves are just lateral to the posterior foramen as the branches exit. For the S1–2 levels, the optimum position is between 1:00 and 5:30 on the right foramina and 7:00 and 11:00 on the left foramina.

19. **E.** Pulsed RF treatment is based more on the electric field effect rather than heat. Current theories of the mechanism include a neuromodulatory effect by altering synaptic transmission and transsynaptic induction of gene expression in the dorsal horn. The duty cycle of pulsed RF includes two active cycles per second of 20 ms each. The current delivered is normally at a frequency of 500,000 Hz. In some cases, the temperature at the tip of the electrode exceeds 42°C. When this happens, power output should be lowered as a precaution. Lowering the voltage (usually 45 V), decreasing the duration of the active cycle, or decreasing the frequency of the cycle results in decreased power output. It may also be best to increase the inactive time to allow more cooling rather than decrease the voltage since the electric field effect is the primary goal.

20. **B.** Complications from pterygopalatine RF treatment are rare and usually involve incorrect needle placement. Complications include intravascular injection and numbness of the soft palate, which usually resolves after 4–6 weeks. Dryness of the eye (ipsilateral) is unusual, and loss of taste is extremely rare. Masseter weakness is a potential complication of the RF treatment of the gasserian ganglion.

Sacroiliac Joint Syndrome: Sacroiliac Joint Injections and Block/Radiofrequency of the Lateral Branches

63

QUESTIONS

1. In relation to sacroiliac (SI) joint dysfunction, the following is true:
   A. The incidence of SI joint dysfunction in patients with back pain is approximately 50%–60%.
   B. SI joint dysfunction usually results in pain only above the level of L5.
   C. The presence of groin pain automatically rules out SI joint dysfunction.
   D. Radiographic testing is the gold standard to make the diagnosis.
   E. Yeoman's test appears to be a more specific and reliable maneuver than Gillet's test for SI joint dysfunction.

2. In "strip lesioning" of the SI joint, what is the recommended best distance between radiofrequency probes and duration of thermal lesion time to produce a continuous strip lesion at 90 degrees?
   A. The needle probes should be placed at 4–6 mm from each other along the sides of the foramen and lesion duration should be 120–150 seconds.
   B. The needle probes should be placed at 6–8 mm from each other along the sides of the foramen and lesion duration should be 60–90 seconds.
   C. The needle probes should be placed at 8–10 mm from each other along the sides of the foramen and lesion duration should be 90–120 seconds.
   D. The needle probes should be placed at 10–12 mm from each other along the sides of the foramen and lesion duration should be 120–150 seconds.
   E. The needle probes should be placed at 4–6 mm from each other along the sides of the foramen and lesion duration should be 60–90 seconds.

3. Which of the following about SI joint radiofrequency ablation (RFA) is true?
   A. Bipolar strip lesioning is an alternative to making several unipolar lesions with thermal RF needles, as the burn area with unipolar thermal RF lesioning is small.
   B. Bipolar strip lesioning is more effective than water-cooled RF for lateral sacral branch neurolysis.
   C. Targeting the ventral innervation of the SI joint produces more effective pain relief compared to targeting the dorsal innervation.
   D. Relief obtained from SI joint injection with local anesthetic and steroid is more prolonged than by thermal RF lesioning of the SI joint or the lateral branches of the primary ramus of the L5–S3 nerves.
   E. All of the above

4. Where is the typical location of SI joint pain?
   A. Dorsal foot
   B. Groin
   C. Above buttocks
   D. Medial ankle
   E. Contralateral hip

5. Which of the following is true regarding SI joint injection?
   A. There is often a change in resistance noted when the capsule is entered.
   B. Imaging guidance is optional because of ease of entering the joint blindly.
   C. The medial line on anteroposterior (AP) imaging of the SI joint under fluoroscopy typically correlates with the ventral aspect of the joint space.
   D. Given the large size of the joint, it is recommended to use injectate volumes between 3 and 4 mL.
   E. All of the above

6. In a normal Gillet's test, when the patient maximally flexes the hip, the posterior superior iliac spine (PSIS):
   A. Remains at the level of the S2 spinous process
   B. Moves superior to the S2 spinous process
   C. Moves inferior to the S2 spinous process
   D. Moves laterally to the S2 spinous process
   E. Remains at the level of the S1 spinous process

7. What are the ligaments that attach near the sacral foramina?
   A. Sacrospinous ligaments
   B. Ischiofemoral ligaments
   C. Sacrococcygeal ligaments
   D. Posterior sacroiliac ligaments
   E. Supraspinous ligaments

8. To perform a diagnostic block of the lateral branches of the sacral nerves, the needle should be advanced approximately 5 mm laterally to which position on the R and L foramen, respectively?
   A. 1:00 and 4:00 o'clock, 6:00 and 9:00 o'clock
   B. 2:00 and 5:00 o'clock, 7:00 and 10:00 o'clock
   C. 12:00 and 3:00 o'clock, 8:00 and 1:00 o'clock
   D. 11:00 and 2:00 o'clock, 9:00 and 3:00 o'clock
   E. 1:00 and 4:00 o'clock, 7:00 and 10:00 o'clock

9. Which of the following is the most sensitive indicator of SI joint dysfunction?
   A. Positive Gaenslen's test
   B. Abnormal appearance on X-ray examination
   C. PSIS pain
   D. Positive straight leg raise
   E. Femoral nerve stretch

10. Which of the following is the **LEAST** diagnostic of SI joint disease?
    A. Pain while sitting and driving, but relieved while standing and walking
    B. Pain over the sacral sulcus
    C. X-ray examination of SI joint
    D. Diagnostic local anesthetic block
    E. SI joint pain and pain into groin

11. All of the following anatomic considerations about the SI joint are true **EXCEPT:**
    A. The function of the joint is to transmit or dissipate the loading of the trunk to the lower extremities.
    B. The irregular contour of the joint increases the joint's stability.
    C. The posterior joint innervation is derived from primarily the dorsal ramus of L5 and lateral branches of S1–3.
    D. Blood supply is derived from the median sacral artery and lateral sacral branches from the internal iliac artery.
    E. It is a pseudojoint because of its lack of synovial fluid and joint capsule.

ANSWERS

1. **E.** The incidence of SI joint dysfunction is approximately 15%–30%. Two distinguishing features include presence of groin pain and absence of pain above the level L5. Yeoman's test stretches the femoral nerve and extends the lumbar spine, but appears to be a more specific and reliable maneuver for SI joint dysfunction.

2. **A.** Pino and colleagues studied the shortest distance needed to create a strip lesion between two needles. Continuous strip lesions were produced when probes were placed less than 6 mm apart for 120-150 seconds. (Pino CA, Hoeft MA, Hofsess C, et al. Morphologic analysis of bipolar radiofrequency lesions: implications for treatment of the sacroiliac joint. *Reg Anesth Pain Med.* 2005;30(4):335-338.)

3. **A.** Bipolar strip lesion technique is an alternative method to conventional unipolar lesions for denervating the posterior SI joint, because the burn area with unipolar probes directed to the lateral branches is small.

4. **B.** SI joint pain will typically present in the groin and there is an absence of pain above the L5 level. Pain can be felt in the superior medial quadrant of the buttock, the lateral buttock, inferior to the PSIS, upper lateral thigh, and greater trochanter. Less commonly, it can refer to the posterior thigh and below the knee.

5. **A.** There is often a subtle change in resistance felt when entering the joint capsule. Imaging is recommended, as blind injections can result in incorrect needle placement. The medial line on AP fluoroscopic imaging is typically the posterior joint space. The joint will typically not accommodate more volume than 2.5 mL.

6. **C.** In a normal Gillet's test, the PSIS moves inferior to the second sacral spinous process with hip flexion. In an abnormal test, suggesting SI joint dysfunction, the PSIS will remain at the level of the S2 spinous process or move superior.

7. **D.** The anterior sacroiliac ligament traverses the ilium to the sacrum. The posterior sacroiliac ligament traverses the posterior iliac ridge to the sacrum and attaches near the foramina. The interosseous ligament provides stability to the joint. The sacrospinous ligaments are distal to the foramen. The ischiofemoral ligaments are lateral structures attaching to the femur. The sacrococcygeal ligaments are distal structures attaching the sacrum to the coccyx.

8. **B.** Relative to the lateral border of the right foramen, target needle placement is the 2:00 and 5:00 position. Relative to the lateral border of the left foramen, target needle placement is the 7:00 and 10:00 position.

9. **C.** Pain on palpation of the SI joint or the sacral sulcus, buttock pain, and the patient pointing to pain over the PSIS are more sensitive for SI joint pathology than the other tests listed.

10. **C.** Radiographic evaluation rarely aids in diagnosis of SI joint dysfunction.

11. **E.** The SI joint is a true diarthrodial joint, which contains synovial fluid and a joint capsule. The cartilaginous surface allows for motion to occur.

Myofascial Injections: Trigger Point, Piriformis, Iliopsoas, and Scalene Injections

64

QUESTIONS

1. All of the following are true about myofascial trigger points **EXCEPT:**
   A. The muscles most commonly involved are the trapezius, splenii, cervical and lumbar paraspinals, and quadratus lumborum.
   B. Palpation of trigger points produces characteristic nondermatomal referral patterns.
   C. Trigger points only produce pain when palpated.
   D. Alteration in blood flow is thought to occur at trigger points.
   E. Tizanidine has shown efficacy in the treatment of myofascial pain.

2. When you perform a trigger point injection of the trapezius muscle using a 25-gauge, 1.5-inch needle in a 50-kg patient with myofascial pain, the patient begins to cough. You should be most concerned about which of the following?
   A. Hematoma
   B. Infection
   C. Pneumothorax
   D. Pleural effusion
   E. Pulmonary embolus

3. Which of the following is true regarding trigger point injections?
   A. Trigger point injections with local anesthetic are more effective than dry needling.
   B. Under ultrasound, trigger points appear as well-defined, circumscribed, hyperechoic regions.
   C. Trigger point injections are thought to be more effective when a muscle twitch response is elicited with needle penetration of the trigger point.
   D. Patients with chronic widespread myofascial pain are more likely to respond to trigger point injection than patients with focal myofascial pain.
   E. Stretching and strengthening of muscle through physical therapy provides no additional benefit to trigger point injections for myofascial pain.

4. All of the following are benefits of ultrasound-guided trigger point injections **EXCEPT:**
   A. Visualization of the focal trigger point in the muscle
   B. Assurance of needle penetration of the myofascial trigger point rather than adipose tissue
   C. Visualization of the focal muscle twitch response

D. Avoidance of neurovascular structures
E. Randomized control trial (RCT) evidence of improved efficacy relative to blind trigger point injection

5. What percentage of patients have aberrant piriformis muscle anatomy such that the sciatic nerve passes either through or posterior to the piriformis muscle?
   A. 0.1%–1%
   B. 1%–8%
   C. 12%–21%
   D. 30%–40%
   E. 42%–56%

6. When performing an ultrasound-guided piriformis injection at the greater sciatic notch, which is the correct order of anatomic structures (superficial to deep), assuming typical sciatic nerve location?
   A. Piriformis muscle, gluteus maximus muscle, sciatic nerve
   B. Gluteus maximus muscle, sciatic nerve, piriformis muscle
   C. Sciatic nerve, piriformis muscle, gluteus maximus muscle
   D. Gluteus maximus muscle, piriformis muscle, sciatic nerve
   E. Piriformis muscle, sciatic nerve, gluteus maximus muscle

7. In a prone patient undergoing a buttock injection under ultrasound, flexing the knee to 90 degrees followed by internal and external rotation of the hip promotes visualization of which sliding muscular structure?
   A. Gluteus maximus
   B. Piriformis
   C. Ischiococcygeus
   D. Puborectalis
   E. Quadratus femoris

8. All of the following are provocative physical examination tests for iliopsoas muscle pathology **EXCEPT:**
   A. Pain on palpation of the iliopsoas tendon while flexing the hip against resistance
   B. Supine patient with inability to extend the affected hip completely with the contralateral hip fully flexed

C. Prone patient who experiences pain posteriorly with passive extension of the affected hip
D. Supine patient who experiences anterior pain with passive extension of the affected hip hanging off the examination table while the contralateral hip is flexed
E. Supine patient who experiences anterior pain with flexion, abduction, and external rotation of the affected hip

9. "A supine patient with inability to extend the affected hip completely with the contralateral hip fully flexed" describes which of the following tests?
A. Yeoman's test
B. Patrick's test
C. Thomas's test
D. Gaenslen's test
E. Snapping hip test

10. All of the following are considered reasonable treatments of iliopsoas syndrome **EXCEPT:**
A. Botox injection of the iliopsoas muscle
B. Local anesthetic with steroid injection of the iliopsoas muscle
C. Stretching and strengthening exercises of the iliopsoas muscle
D. Dry needling of the iliopsoas muscle
E. Radiofrequency ablation (RFA) of the iliopsoas muscle

11. The psoas muscle originates from which of the following anatomic structures?
A. Transverse processes of L1–5
B. All of the lumbar disks except L5–S1
C. Lateral surfaces of the T12–L4 vertebral bodies
D. A and C
E. All of the above

12. Which is the most common form of thoracic outlet syndrome?
A. Neurogenic
B. Arterial
C. Venous
D. Lymphatic
E. A and B have equal prevalence and are both the most common.

13. Neurogenic thoracic outlet syndrome can be caused by which of the following?
A. Trauma from whiplash-induced injuries
B. Scalene muscle anomalies
C. Cervical rib
D. Tumor metastases
E. All of the above

14. While scanning the patient's neck with ultrasound in preparation for a scalene muscle injection for neurogenic thoracic outlet syndrome, you notice the roots of the brachial plexus passing through the middle scalene muscle. What is the best course of action?
A. Abort the injection
B. Inject local anesthetic into both the middle and anterior scalene muscles, as planned
C. Inject local anesthetic into only the anterior scalene muscle
D. Target the brachial plexus in the interscalene groove in addition to the middle scalene muscle
E. Target the brachial plexus in the interscalene groove only

15. Patients with neurogenic thoracic outlet syndrome often present with paresthesias in which nerve distribution?
A. Ulnar nerve
B. Median nerve
C. Radial nerve
D. Musculocutaneous nerve
E. Axillary nerve

ANSWERS

1. **C.** There are two types of trigger points. Active trigger points produce spontaneous pain without stimulation as well as pain on palpation; latent trigger points only produce pain on palpation.

2. **C.** Performing trigger point injections in a thin, 50-kg patient in the upper thoracic region necessitates concern for pneumothorax, which can be indicated by coughing from the patient.

3. **C.** Trigger point injections (TPIs) are thought to be equally efficacious to dry needling, although the latter is often more painful. Ultrasound depicts trigger points as hypoechoic (dark) focal regions rather than hyperechoic. Patients with focal myofascial pain are thought to be greater responders to TPIs. Physical therapy is helpful in addition to TPIs for myofascial pain.

4. **E.** All of the points are theoretically true for ultrasound-guided TPIs; no RCT, however, has shown superiority of ultrasound guidance vs. blind TPI.

5. **C.** In 12%–21% of the population, the sciatic nerve either divides through or passes posterior to the piriformis muscle with resultant risk for piriformis syndrome.

6. **D.** The correct order, from superficial to deep, is (1) the gluteus maximus muscle, (2) piriformis muscle, and (3) sciatic nerve, assuming normal sciatic nerve location.

7. **B.** Internal and external rotation of the hip in a prone position with flexed knee promotes visualization of the piriformis muscle, which will slide over the ischium while the gluteus maximus muscle remains immobile.

8. **C.** This is a description of Yeoman's test. When pain is felt posteriorly, it is indicative of sacroiliac joint pathology. When pain is felt anteriorly, it is suggestive of iliopsoas pathology.

9. **C.** This is a description of Thomas's test for a tight, painful iliopsoas hip flexor muscle.

10. **E.** All are correct and reasonable treatments for iliopsoas syndrome except RFA of the iliopsoas muscle.

11. **E.** All of the listed structures are anatomic origins of the psoas muscle.

12. **A.** The most common type of thoracic outlet syndrome is the neurogenic form, which accounts for 95% of all cases, and results from compression of the brachial plexus between the anterior and middle scalene muscles and the first rib.

13. **E.** All of the listed etiologies contribute to neurogenic thoracic outlet syndrome.

14. **C.** Many clinicians inject only the anterior scalene muscle, with excellent though temporary relief of thoracic outlet syndrome. Injecting the middle scalene muscle in addition will more likely result in brachial plexus neural blockade in this instance, which is unnecessary for a therapeutic block and will result in weakness and numbness of the ipsilateral arm, necessitating an arm sling for protection.

15. **A.** Ulnar nerve paresthesias are common with neurogenic thoracic outlet syndrome.

65 Lumbar Discogenic Pain and Diskography

QUESTIONS

1. In patients with chronic low back pain who have not returned to work, which of the following are the correct lifetime return-to-work rates if the patient has not worked for 6 months, 12 months, and 2 years, respectively?
   A. 50%, 25%, 5%
   B. 25%, 5%, 1%
   C. 60%, 40%, 20%
   D. 75%, 50%, 25%
   E. 10%, 5%, 1%

2. For the interpretation of provocation diskography using manometry, which of the following denotes a chemically sensitive disk?
   A. Concordant pain noted at >15 psi above opening pressure
   B. Concordant pain noted at <15 psi above opening pressure
   C. Concordant pain noted at <30 psi above opening pressure
   D. Concordant pain noted at 15–50 psi above opening pressure
   E. Concordant pain noted at 50–100 psi above opening pressure

3. What can be concluded about concordant pain provocation >50 psi above opening pressure?
   A. The response cannot be considered clinically significant.
   B. This is a chemically sensitive disk.
   C. This is a mechanically sensitive disk.
   D. This is an indeterminate disk.
   E. Both A and D

4. All of the following are causes of false–positive provocation diskography **EXCEPT:**
   A. Needle placement in the annulus
   B. Needle placement too close to the vertebral endplate
   C. Pressurizing the disk too rapidly
   D. Diffuse contrast extravasation and underpressurization
   E. Undersedation of the patient

5. Which of the following is true regarding Modic changes of the endplates?
   A. Type I changes are hypointense on T1, hyperintense on T2, and signify fatty degeneration.
   B. Type I changes are hypointense on T1, hyperintense on T2, and signify edema.
   C. Type II changes are hyperintense on T1, hypointense on T2, and signify edema.
   D. Type III changes are hyperintense on both T1 and T2, and signify bony sclerosis.
   E. Type II changes are hypointense on both T1 and T2, and signify fatty degeneration.

6. What is the most sensitive indicator of diskitis?
   A. Elevated erythrocyte sedimentation rate (ESR) and C-reactive protein (CRP)
   B. Low back pain
   C. Fever
   D. Elevated white blood count (WBC)
   E. Neurologic changes on examination

7. The referral pattern from L3–4 disk provocation often radiates from the low back into which distal location?
   A. Anterior thigh
   B. Posterior thigh
   C. Dorsal foot
   D. Plantar foot
   E. Lateral foot

8. What is thought to be the most common etiology of chronic axial low back pain in young and middle-aged individuals?
   A. Myofascial pain
   B. Discogenic pain
   C. Facetogenic pain
   D. Sacroiliac joint pain
   E. Fibromyalgia

9. The annulus fibrosus (AF) is weakest in which anatomic region?
   A. Lateral
   B. Anterior
   C. Anterolateral
   D. Posterior
   E. A and D

10. What is the earliest period of life at which histologic studies have revealed that a reduction in blood flow to the intervertebral disk leads to diminished nutritional supply to the endplate resulting in tissue breakdown within the disk?
    A. Newborn period
    B. First decade
    C. Second decade
    D. Fifth decade
    E. Sixth decade

11. Which of the following statements about discogenic pain or diskography is true?
    A. The results are conflicting regarding whether preoperative diskography improves fusion outcomes in patients with discogenic low back pain.
    B. Detection of a high intensity zone (HIZ) on MRI is both sensitive and specific for discogenic low back pain.
    C. Diskography has not been associated with acceleration of disk degeneration.
    D. Intradiskal injection of cefazolin mixed with contrast is contraindicated during diskography.
    E. Modic type I changes are unlikely to transition to type II changes over time.

12. Carragee and colleagues' landmark prospective study evaluating potential long-term disk effects postdiskography revealed which of the following? (Carragee EJ, Don AS, Hurwitz EL. 2009 ISSLS Prize Winner: Does discography cause accelerated progression of degeneration changes in the lumbar disc: a ten-year matched cohort study. *Spine* 2009;34(21):2338-2345)
    A. Disks that had undergone diskographic evaluation demonstrated equal progression of degeneration relative to noninjected disks.
    B. New disk herniations were disproportionately found on the side of the annular puncture.
    C. Disk height was overall unchanged between the diskography and control groups.
    D. New disk herniations were disproportionately found on the side contralateral to the annular puncture.
    E. Over the 2-year study period, no changes were noted.

13. Which of the following is correct in regard to performing diskography?
    A. The disk level considered most likely to produce intense pain should be injected last.

    B. Generous use of sedation is encouraged secondary to significant pain associated with disk stimulation.
    C. Ionic dye is used to minimize the risk of allergic reactions.
    D. Intradiskal gadolinium is contraindicated in iodine-allergic patients.
    E. The L5–S1 disk is the easiest lumbar disk level to access for diskography.

14. All of the following are absolute contraindications to performing diskography **EXCEPT:**
    A. Inability of the patient to report pain response
    B. Localized infection
    C. Untreated coagulopathy
    D. Pregnancy
    E. Iodinated contrast allergy

15. In Fig. 65.1 depicting innervation of the intervertebral disk (ID) and vertebral body (VB), which structure is represented by number 6?
    A. Sympathetic trunk
    B. Sinuvertebral nerve
    C. Anterior plexus
    D. Posterior plexus
    E. Ventral ramus

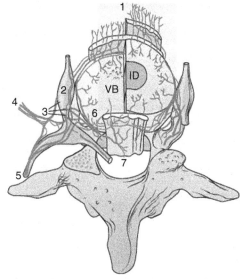

Fig. 65.1   Reprinted from Benzon H, Rathmell J. *Practical Management of Pain.* 5th ed. Philadelphia, PA: Elsevier Mosby; 2014:887.

ANSWERS

1. **A.** Low back pain patients who have not worked for 6 months have a 50% lifetime return-to-work rate; 12 months out of work translates to a 25% return-to-work rate; 2 years out of work has a much lower 5% lifetime rate of return to work. These statistics support encouraging early return to work to prevent disability.

2. **B.** A chemically sensitive disk on provocation diskography is defined as generation of concordant pain at low pressures (<15 psi) above opening pressure.

3. **E.** If concordant pain is noted at >50 psi above opening pressure, the response is not considered clinically significant and the disk is denoted indeterminate.

4. **D.** All of the choices can result in a false–positive result except diffuse contrast extravasation and underpressurization, which can result in a false-negative result.

5. **B.** The true statement relates to type I Modic endplate changes, which are characteristically hypointense on T1, hyperintense on T2, and signify edema secondary to disruption and fissuring of the endplate.

6. **A.** An elevated ESR and CRP are the most sensitive indicators of postdiskography diskitis, but elevation does not usually occur until 3 weeks postprocedurally. If elevated, an MRI or bone scan is necessary to rule out diskitis.

7. **A.** L3–4 positive diskograms frequently result in lumbar pain referring into the anterior thigh and anterior leg. In contrast, for L4–5 diskograms, equivalent anterior and posterior thigh pain referral is often noted. For L5–S1 disks, posterior thigh referral is much more common.

8. **B.** Discogenic pain appears to be the major source of pain in more than one-third of patients with chronic axial low back pain utilizing MRI and diskography, with greater prevalence in young and middle-aged individuals. Facet joint pain prevalence increases in the elderly population.

9. **D.** The AF comprises type I collagen arranged in concentric lamellae. The AF is thickest and strongest in the anterior and lateral regions, but it tends to be weaker posteriorly, where most disk herniations occur.

10. **C.** As early as the second decade of life, there is demonstrable reduction in blood flow and nutritional supply to the endplate, causing tissue breakdown within the nucleus pulposus and thereafter in the vertebral endplates.

11. **A.** There is no clear consensus on whether diskography improves surgical results for discogenic pain. Detection of HIZ is thought to be specific but relatively insensitive for discogenic low back pain. Diskography has been associated with accelerated disk degeneration. Intradiskal cefazolin is one strategy for reducing periprocedural risk of diskitis following diskography. Type I Modic changes tend to convert to type II changes over time.

12. **B.** This long-term 7- to 10-year prospective study revealed a disproportionate number of disk herniations on the side of disk puncture as well as more disk herniations of the postdiskography disks.

13. **A.** The disk deemed most likely to produce intense pain should be injected last, because once severe pain is produced, the patient may be less likely to tolerate or judge subsequent injections. Excessive sedation is discouraged to avoid a false–negative response. Nonionic dye minimizes the risk of allergic reactions. Gadolinium can be used for disk pressurization in patients with known prior contrast reactions. The L5–S1 level is the most challenging disk level secondary to presence of the iliac crests.

14. **E.** Iodinated contrast allergy is not a contraindication because gadolinium can be utilized instead of iodinated contrast for diskography. All of the other answer choices listed are contraindications to diskography.

15. **B.** The sinuvertebral nerve is depicted by number 6 and innervates the posterolateral margin of the intervertebral disk.

Intradiskal Procedures for the Treatment of Discogenic Lower Back and Leg Pain

66

QUESTIONS

1. Nociceptors are normally limited to which portion of the annulus fibrosis?
   A. Outer 1/3
   B. Outer 1/2
   C. Outer 2/3
   D. Inner 1/3
   E. Inner 1/2

2. All of these patients have a lower chance of treatment success with intradiscal electrothermal therapy (IDET) **EXCEPT:**
   A. Patients with multilevel disk degeneration on MRI
   B. Overweight patients
   C. Patients receiving Workers' Compensation benefits
   D. Patients undergoing provocative diskography that replicates concordant pain at low disk pressures <50 psi
   E. Patients with axial low back pain that improves with prolonged sitting and Valsalva maneuver

3. Which of the following intradiskal procedures utilizes bipolar cooled radiofrequency electrodes?
   A. Coblation nucleoplasty
   B. Dekompressor percutaneous disk decompression
   C. Intradiskal biacuplasty
   D. Nucleotome disk treatment
   E. Percutaneous laser disk decompression

4. All of the following statements are true regarding percutaneous disk decompression **EXCEPT:**
   A. Applying heat through radiofrequency within the nucleus can cause a decrease in intradiskal pressure and retraction of the herniation away from a compressed nerve root.
   B. Patients with high-grade (Dallas 5) fissures are optimal candidates for this procedure.
   C. The procedure is for patients with predominantly radicular leg pain.

D. Patients considered for this procedure should have a contained disk herniation with intact annular wall.
E. Multiple observational and prospective studies have shown an improvement in functional capacity using coblation nucleoplasty.

5. What is the temperature and heat time used for intradiskal biacuplasty?
   A. 45°C for 5 minutes
   B. 500°C for 15 minutes
   C. 70°C for 10 minutes
   D. 80°C for 90 seconds
   E. 80°C for 15 minutes

6. The extent of tissue damage with radiofrequency (RF) application depends on multiple factors including:
   A. Temperature
   B. Electrode thickness
   C. Duration of heating
   D. A and B
   E. All of the above

7. The incidence of disk herniation following percutaneous annuloplasty could be as high as:
   A. 0.3%
   B. 3%
   C. 10%
   D. 25%
   E. 33%

8. Which of the following terms is defined by the fact that the greatest distance in any plane between the edges of disk material beyond the disk space is less than the distance between the edges of the disk base in the same plane?
   A. Protrusion
   B. Extrusion

C. Sequestration
D. Bulge
E. Subarticular stenosis

9. Which of the percutaneous disk treatments is intended for discogenic low back pain verified by diskography and involves focal heating of the posterior annulus via careful advancement of an elongated small-diameter resistive coil?
   A. Intradiskal biacuplasty
   B. Intradiskal electrothermal therapy

C. Coblation nucleoplasty
D. Laser disk decompression
E. Percutaneous disc Dekompressor

10. The following complications have been reported after the IDET procedure:
    A. Diskitis
    B. Catheter breakage
    C. Vertebral osteonecrosis
    D. Cauda equine syndrome
    E. All of the above

ANSWERS

1. **A.** Nociceptors (C and A-delta fibers) are normally located in the outer 1/3 of the annulus. They penetrate further into the disk with greater degeneration, as in fissures.

2. **D.** The ideal patient for IDET consideration has persistent discogenic low back pain that typically worsens with sitting and Valsalva maneuver, concordant pain on provocative diskography at low disk pressures <50 psi, one degenerated disk on MRI, normal BMI, and is not receiving Workers' Compensation benefits.

3. **C.** Intradiskal biacuplasty uses bipolar cooled radiofrequency electrodes spaced <3 cm apart within the posterior annulus of the diseased lumbar disk; heat is distributed to the posterior annulus.

4. **B.** Retraction of the disk herniation away from the compressed nerve may not be possible if the disk contains a high-grade (Dallas 5) fissure or if the elasticity of the disk is not preserved.

5. **B.** Intradiskal biacuplasty utilizes bilateral percutaneously placed cooled electrodes whereby the temperature increases gradually to 50°C with an overall heating time of 15 minutes.

6. **E.** During the application of RF, alternating flow of electrical current produces thermal injury that depends on multiple factors including temperature, electrode thickness, and duration of heating.

7. **A.** Disk herniation following annuloplasty can be as high as 0.3% and is thought to be secondary to thermally mediated loss of tensile strength of the annular collagen fibers.

8. **A.** A protrusion is defined by the fact that the greatest distance in any plane between the edges of disk material *beyond the disk space* is <u>less than</u> the distance between the edges of the disk *base* in the same plane. In contrast, an extrusion is present if the diameter of the herniated disc material is greater than the base in the same plane.

9. **B.** This description applies to IDET, during which a resistive coil is carefully advanced percutaneously along the posterior annulus to focally heat disk nociceptors.

10. **E.** All of these rare complications have been reported following IDET.

Minimally Invasive Procedures for Vertebral Compression Fractures

67

1. A new patient presents with chronic back pain with focal tenderness. They show you a recent CT scan of their lumbar spine, indicating a vertebral fracture. What is the most appropriate course of action?
   A. Continue medication therapy
   B. Order an MRI of the lumbar spine
   C. Refer the patient to physical therapy
   D. Schedule the patient for vertebral augmentation
   E. Refer the patient to a neurosurgeon

2. What is the main advantage of the bipedicular approach in vertebral augmentation?
   A. Decreased lateral to medial angulation
   B. Decreased risk of cement extravasation
   C. Improved pain relief
   D. Decreased risk of fracture from hemivertebral fill
   E. Decreased risk of infarction

3. You perform a vertebroplasty at the L4 level on a patient with an osteoporotic compression fracture. They report pain in the right leg following the procedure and no weakness or sensory abnormalities are evident. An MRI reveals cement extravasation into a foraminal vein near the L4 nerve root. What is the next most appropriate step?
   A. Emergent neurosurgical consultation
   B. Electromyography to evaluate for radiculopathy
   C. Oral steroid prescription
   D. Right L4–5 transforaminal epidural
   E. C or D

4. A 75-year-old female patient sustains a T4 vertebral body fracture while trying to lift weights at the gym. She is discovered to be osteoporotic and her vertebral height loss is > 75% of her baseline. On MRI, she has retropulsion of fracture fragments and a physical examination reveals she has myelopathic features. She has tried conservative treatment but has not had any benefit in terms of pain control. She is worried that her sedentary situation is going to "slow her down." She is still in a great deal of pain. Which of the following is the most appropriate next step in her management?
   A. Recommend performing a vertebroplasty, given the potential for benefit of the procedure
   B. Recommend prolonged strict bed rest

C. Continue with conservative treatment, given the presence of at least one absolute contraindication to vertebroplasty
D. Recommend aggressive treatment for osteoporosis and wait until a dual energy X-ray absorptiometry (DEXA) scan shows signs of improvement, then perform a vertebroplasty

5. What is the most important aspect of needle placement in vertebral augmentation procedures?
   A. Keep the needle trajectory medial to the medial cortex and superior to the inferior cortex of the pedicle
   B. Keep the needle trajectory lateral to the medial cortex and superior to the inferior cortex of the pedicle
   C. Keep the needle trajectory lateral to the medial cortex and inferior to the inferior cortex of the pedicle
   D. Keep the needle trajectory through the midline of the vertebral body
   E. Keep the needle trajectory anterior to the vertebral column

6. When performing a vertebroplasty, what is the recommended maximum number of level(s) to perform per session?
   A. A single level
   B. No more than three levels per session
   C. A maximum of four levels if the patient has no mass with potential for posterior displacement
   D. As many levels as needed to minimize the risk of anesthesia from repeated sessions
   E. None of the above

7. During a vertebroplasty, your patient suddenly has a significant reduction in blood pressure and oxygen saturation. Which of the following is a potential cause for this?
   A. Allergic reaction to cement
   B. Pulmonary embolism from fat or cement
   C. Depressed myocardial function
   D. All of the above
   E. None of the above

8. Which of the following is associated with a unipedicular approach to vertebroplasty?
   A. Higher risk of cement leakage
   B. Better pain relief

C. Decrease in procedure time
D. Less risk of vessel or nerve damage
E. Worsening fracture

9. What is the recommended imaging study to determine whether a vertebral fracture is acute or chronic?
A. T1-weighted MRI
B. CT scan
C. MRI with STIR
D. Nuclear scintigraphy bone scan
E. DEXA scan

10. Which of the following is an advantage of the parapedicular approach over the transpedicular approach to vertebroplasty?
A. Less cement leakage
B. More medial tip placement

C. Better pain relief
D. Less injury to nearby structures
E. All of the above

11. What is the recommended volume of cement that should be injected at each vertebroplasty level?
A. 0.5 mL
B. 1 mL
C. 2 mL
D. 5 mL
E. There is no consensus on the volume of cement that should be injected.

ANSWERS

1. **B.** In this setting, an MRI with STIR or T2-weighted sequences with fat saturation should be obtained to identify marrow edema, which distinguishes acute from chronic fractures. This should be done as part of the preprocedure evaluation for vertebral augmentation.

2. **A.** The major advantage of a bipedicular approach in vertebral augmentation is that access is typically transpedicular with a less aggressive lateral to medial approach. This may result in less paravertebral vessel and nerve injury as well as a potential biomechanical advantage for bilateral delivery of cement.

3. **E.** Extraosseous passage of cement is an important source of complications during vertebral augmentation. Although most cases are asymptomatic, even small amounts of PMMA cement adjacent to a nerve root within the foraminal veins can produce radicular pain. This pain can be treated with a nerve root block or systemic steroids. Surgical decompression becomes necessary only in the setting of frank root compression, cord compression, or cauda equina syndrome.

4. **C.** This patient has fracture retropulsion with evidence of myelopathy, which is an absolute contraindication to vertebroplasty. She also has two relative contraindications to vertebroplasty (loss of vertebral body height > 75% and fracture above T5). Thus, conservative therapy should be continued with this patient. Caution must be used with prolonged strict bed rest because it can lead to loss of bone mass and muscle strength, decubitus ulceration, and venous thromboembolism.

5. **B.** The most important aspect of needle placement is to keep the needle trajectory lateral to the medial cortex and superior to the inferior cortex of the pedicle. This prevents entry of the needle into the spinal canal or neural foramen.

6. **B.** A patient scheduled for vertebral augmentation may have multiple fractures that require treatment. However, treating an excessive number of levels in a single session has multiple associated risks. Elderly patients might find it difficult to lie prone for the duration of time required. Patient discomfort and potential fat embolization are other issues. Even though there is no established guideline, a good rule of thumb is to treat a maximum of three levels per session.

7. **D.** Potential complications of vertebral augmentation that may result in hemodynamic changes include pulmonary embolism secondary to cement or fat, depressed myocardial function secondary to free methyl methacrylate monomer or fat emboli, or anaphylaxis to the cement.

8. **C.** The advantages of a unipedicular approach include a decrease in procedure time and elimination of the risk associated with the placement of a second needle. A unipedicular approach is also associated with lower rates of cement leakage.

9. **C.** MRI with STIR or T2-weighted sequences with fat saturation should be obtained in all patients, unless contraindicated. These sequences identify marrow edema, which distinguishes acute from chronic fractures.

10. **B.** In the parapedicular approach, the needle is directed along the lateral surface of the pedicle, which can allow for a more medial tip placement when compared with a transpedicular approach.

11. **E.** There is no consensus on the amount of cement that should be injected. Studies have not shown an association between the volume of cement injected and the clinical outcomes of pain and medication use. The volume used is at the discretion of the physician.

Biopsychosocial Prescreening for Spinal Cord and Peripheral Nerve Stimulation Devices

68

QUESTIONS

1. Conditions that are commonly treated with spinal cord stimulation (SCS) include all of the following **EXCEPT**:
   A. Failed back surgery syndrome
   B. Peripheral vascular disease
   C. Neuropathic pain
   D. Multiple sclerosis
   E. Acute vertebral fracture

2. Which of the following scales in the Minnesota Multiphasic Personality Inventory-2 (MMPI-2) is associated with a negative influence on surgical clinical outcomes?
   A. Scales 1 and 3: pain sensitivity
   B. Scale 2: depression
   C. Scale 4: anger
   D. Scale 7: anxiety
   E. All of the above

3. Which of the following questionnaires is the most commonly used as a personality assessment for patients with chronic pain?
   A. Beck Depression Inventory
   B. Medical Outcomes Survey 36-Item Short Form Health Survey
   C. Million Visual Analog Scale (MVAS)
   D. MMPI-2
   E. Oswestry Disability Questionnaire

4. All of the following are considered psychosocial risk factors for failure of a spinal cord stimulator to control pain **EXCEPT**:
   A. Chronic or reactive depression
   B. Pain sensitivity
   C. Job dissatisfaction
   D. Education level
   E. Substance abuse

5. Which of the following pain conditions would least likely be controlled with a spinal cord stimulator?
   A. Complex regional pain syndrome
   B. Failed back surgery syndrome
   C. Multiple sclerosis
   D. Neuropathic pain
   E. Occipital neuralgia

6. All of the following are medical risk factors for poor outcomes after spinal cord stimulator placement **EXCEPT**:
   A. Obesity
   B. Tobacco use
   C. Pending litigation
   D. Old age
   E. Multiple positive Waddell's signs

7. If a patient's self-reported pain is higher than expected based on objective physical findings, which scale would help determine a potential contributory psychological component?
   A. MVAS
   B. Visual Analog Scale
   C. MMPI-2
   D. Pain Medication Questionnaire
   E. Wong-Baker Scale

8. On the MVAS, moderately disabling pain is indicated by a score of:
   A. 0–19
   B. 20–39
   C. 40–84
   D. 85–90
   E. 91–100

9. A general survey of pain symptoms is a necessary starting point for any pretreatment evaluation in a pain program. A general intake assessment should include which of the following?
   A. Survey of pain symptoms
   B. Demographic information
   C. Date of onset and pertinent details of the pain condition
   D. Prior treatments or surgeries
   E. All of the above

10. All of the following are examples of assessment tools that have been utilized for prescreening for SCS **EXCEPT**:
    A. MVAS
    B. Oswestry Disability Questionnaire
    C. Pain Medication Questionnaire
    D. Beck Depression Inventory
    E. DOLOPLUS-2

ANSWERS

1. **E.** SCS has been successfully used for the management of various forms of chronic pain including failed back surgery syndrome, neuropathic pain, peripheral vascular disease, multiple sclerosis, and complex regional pain syndrome. This is in contrast to acute vertebral fracture, which can be treated with vertebroplasty, not SCS.

2. **E.** MMPI-2 has been validated as a predictor of outcomes for spine surgery candidates. Scale elevations on the MMPI-2 associated with pain sensitivity (scales 1 and 3), depression (scale 2), anger (scale 4), and anxiety (scale 7) were the most noteworthy factors negatively influencing outcomes.

3. **D.** The MMPI-2 has been extensively used in chronic pain research. It is a 567-item, self-report measure of personality functioning and psychiatric symptoms. It is the most commonly used personality assessment for patients with chronic pain. Findings can assist with the identification of psychopathology, personality and behavioral characteristics, treatment planning, and prediction of outcomes.

4. **D.** Schocket and colleagues used both psychosocial as well as medical risk factors to select suitable surgical candidates. Education level was not included in this algorithm. (Schocket KG, Gatchel RJ, Stowell AW, et al. A demonstration of a presurgical behavioral medicine evaluation for categorizing patients for implantable therapies: a preliminary study. *Neuromodulation* 2008;11(4):237-248.)

5. **E.** Peripheral nerve stimulation (PNS) techniques are better suited for treating pain in a nerve region that is not easily accessible by SCS. Nerve regions that are more easily accessed by PNS include the occipital nerve, trigeminal nerve, and subcutaneous peripheral nerves, making PNS the preferred procedure for pain syndromes in these areas.

6. **D.** Schocket and colleagues used both psychosocial and medical risk factors to select suitable surgical candidates. Old age has not been specified as a medical risk factor. (Schocket KG, Gatchel RJ, Stowell AW, et al. A demonstration of a presurgical behavioral medicine evaluation for categorizing patients for implantable therapies: a preliminary study. *Neuromodulation* 2008;11(4):237–248.)

7. **A.** The MVAS consists of 15 self-reported items specific to perceived pain and disability. The MVAS is especially helpful for discrepancies, such as when self-reported pain is higher than expected based on objective findings, and suggests a contributing psychological component.

8. **C.** The MVAS is a 15-item questionnaire about disability and pain intensity in patients with low back pain. It is scored on a 100-mm visual analog scale (VAS). Scores of 40–84 indicate "moderately disabling" pain.

9. **E.** The general intake assessment should include a survey of pain symptoms along with other pertinent information such as demographics, date of onset, details of the pain condition, prior treatments or surgeries, employment status, education level, disability payment status, Workers' Compensation status, health care utilization, and other comorbid chronic health problems. These are reflected in the various assessment tools for prescreening.

10. **E.** Standardized self-reported instruments to evaluate the patient's pain intensity, functional abilities, beliefs and expectations, and emotional distress are available and can be administered by the physician to assist in treatment planning. The MVAS, Oswestry Disability Questionnaire, Pain Medication Questionnaire, and Beck Depression Inventory are all examples of validated instruments. DOLOPLUS-2 is used for pain assessment in cognitively impaired patients, not for SCS prescreening.

Spinal Cord and Peripheral Nerve Stimulation

69

QUESTIONS

1. Which of the following is most likely correlated with a positive response to spinal cord stimulation (SCS) in patients with complex regional pain syndrome (CRPS)?
   A. Mechanical allodynia of the affected limb
   B. Age above 50 years
   C. Age below 50 years
   D. SCS treatment initiated within 1 year of symptom initiation
   E. Positive response to sympathetic block of affected limb

2. All of the following are true regarding the sterile setup for both SCS trials and permanent implant **EXCEPT**:
   A. Physicians should perform a surgical scrub prior to placement of both SCS trial and permanent leads.
   B. Patients should undertake a preprocedure chlorhexidine shower for both SCS trial and permanent leads.
   C. Preoperative antibiotics for coverage of skin flora (cefazolin or clindamycin) should be given for both SCS trial and permanent lead placement.
   D. Sterile covering for the fluoroscopic machine should be used with both SCS trial and permanent lead placement.
   E. Full surgical drape should be used for both SCS trial and permanent lead placement.

3. What is a disadvantage of using a permanent lead in a stimulator trial?
   A. Propensity to implant regardless of outcome
   B. Extra cost of a new electrode
   C. Increased infection risk
   D. Higher incidence of lead migration after implantation
   E. All of the above

4. Spinal cord stimulation acting on the dorsal horn may provide analgesia through which of the following mechanisms?
   A. Decreasing gamma-aminobutyric acid
   B. Increasing aspartate
   C. Increasing glutamate
   D. Increasing serotonin
   E. Increasing substance P

5. Which of the following psychological comorbidities or constructs has been demonstrated to be detrimental to a positive SCS outcome in patients with CRPS?
   A. Anxiety
   B. Somatization
   C. Catastrophizing
   D. A and B
   E. All of the above

6. A patient with an implanted SCS loses pain coverage. The patient regains analgesia by increasing the voltage supplied by the generator. Which parameter has been adjusted?
   A. Amplitude
   B. Electrode selection
   C. Frequency
   D. Pulse width
   E. Rate

7. Which of the following patients is the best candidate for SCS therapy?
   A. A 24-year-old female with a history of CRPS of the right arm and comorbid schizophrenia, anxiety, and fibromyalgia
   B. A 65-year-old male with a 3-month history of axial low back pain after lumbar laminectomy and fusion
   C. A 45-year-old male with peripheral vascular disease who is homeless and has a history of PTSD
   D. A 70-year-old female with a 20-year history of radicular pain after two lumbar surgeries
   E. A 55-year-old male with failed back surgery syndrome following a Workers' Compensation injury

8. Which of the following interventions may be beneficial in decreasing the incidence of postimplantation complications?
   A. Incorporation of a strain relief loop during implantation
   B. Early physical therapy
   C. Preimplantation course of oral antibiotics
   D. Avoid burying the anchor through the deep fascia
   E. None of the above

9. What is the most common complication of SCS?
   A. Lead migration
   B. Infection
   C. Postdural puncture headache
   D. Peripheral nerve injury
   E. Paraplegia

10. Which of the following statements is true regarding spinal cord stimulation for peripheral ischemia and angina?
    A. Microvascular perfusion is probably improved after SCS therapy.
    B. There is no demonstrated relationship between pain relief and limb survival.
    C. There are no blinded, randomized controlled trials for SCS therapy in angina.
    D. SCS has been shown to have similar efficacy to coronary bypass surgery in treating refractory angina but with lower acute morbidity and mortality rates.
    E. All of the above

11. Which of the following statements is true regarding programming in SCS?
    A. Amplitude is the intensity or strength of stimulation measured in kW.
    B. Pulse width is measured in Hz. The smaller the pulse width, the broader the coverage.
    C. There are four parameters in neurostimulation: amplitude, pulse width, rate, and intensity.
    D. At a lower rate, the patient feels more of a buzz, whereas at higher rates, the feeling is more of a thump.
    E. The primary target is at the cathode (–); electrons flow from the cathode (–) to the anode (+).

12. Based on the image provided (Fig. 69.1), which of the following can be most confidently inferred?
    A. The leads are located in the anterior epidural space.
    B. The leads are located in the posterior epidural space.
    C. The patient is receiving therapy for refractory angina.
    D. The patient is receiving therapy for failed back surgery syndrome.
    E. The leads are located at T4.

13. All the following have Level A recommendations with regard to placement of a SCS **EXCEPT**:
    A. Failed back surgery syndrome
    B. CRPS
    C. Peripheral ischemia
    D. Angina pectoris
    E. None of the above: all have Level A recommendation.

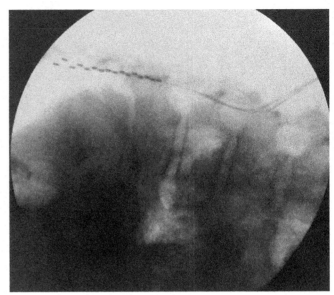

Fig. 69.1   Courtesy Anna Woodbury, MD.

14. Which of the following statements is true regarding SCS?
    A. The mechanism of action for SCS is completely understood and well defined.
    B. To be effective, SCS should be applied continuously or in cycles at least 20 minutes before the onset of analgesia.
    C. Analgesia develops quickly and usually dissipates immediately after cessation of stimulation.
    D. There is no evidence for clinical effectiveness of SCS in treating occipital neuralgia.
    E. Paddle leads are superior to percutaneous leads in terms of improved efficacy and reduced complication rates.

15. When analyzing SCS trial to permanent ratios, what is generally considered an acceptable level of progression to implant?
    A. 25%
    B. 35%
    C. 50%
    D. 55 %
    E. 75%

ANSWERS

1. **E.** In studies of CRPS treated with SCS, mechanical allodynia was negatively correlated with SCS success, while patient age, sex, duration, and pain intensity had no impact. Response to sympathetic blockade of the affected limb may positively correlate with outcomes in SCS therapy. Psychological testing is also an important predictor of outcomes for SCS.

2. **C.** Preoperative antibiotic coverage for skin flora is indicated for permanent SCS implantation, but not for placement of trial leads.

3. **C.** A lead should not be permanently implanted if there is insufficient relief with the trial, regardless of the trial method. The permanent lead trial saves the cost of a new electrode at implant and ensures that the implanted lead position matches the trial lead position. However, there is an increased infection risk related to the percutaneous temporary extension that would be used for the permanent lead trial. The percutaneous lead trial avoids two trips to the operating room, avoids an incision and related pain for the trial, and avoids the risk of infection associated with a percutaneous temporary extension.

4. **D.** SCS may alter local neurochemistry at the dorsal horn and produce analgesia by decreasing excitability of the wide dynamic range neuron through increasing serotonin and gamma-aminobutyric acid (GABA) while suppressing glutamate, aspartate, and other excitatory mediators.

5. **D.** Although depression, anxiety, poor coping skills, and somatization are predictors of poor outcomes with SCS, catastrophizing was not found to be detrimental to a positive SCS outcome in patients with CRPS.

6. **A.** Amplitude, pulse width, rate, and electrode selection are adjustable parameters in SCS programming. Amplitude, measured in volts, is the strength or intensity of stimulation.

7. **D.** Patients must be carefully selected both on the basis of their pathology and their comorbid conditions. In the United States, SCS is most commonly used to treat radicular symptoms following failed back surgery syndrome (FBSS); it has high-level evidence for this indication. Psychiatric and psychological factors such as anxiety, depression, and a poor social network may lead to poor outcomes with SCS. Workers' Compensation patients tend to perform poorly with SCS as well as other therapies. Thus, the 70-year-old female with FBSS and radicular symptoms is the best candidate for SCS of the patients presented.

8. **A.** To decrease lead migration and breakage, a strain relief loop is recommended between the anchor, which should be pushed through deep fascia, and the implantable pulse generator (IPG).

9. **A.** Lead migration and breakage remain the most common complications of spinal cord stimulation. Breakage occurs almost twice as often with paddle leads as compared with percutaneous leads. Both of these complications result in the need for revision or replacement.

10. **E.** SCS therapy is thought to improve microvascular perfusion and oxygen supply in angina and peripheral vascular disease, although there is no association between pain relief and limb salvage and no correlation with decreased amputation. Although randomized controlled trials have been performed, blinding has been difficult because of SCS-related chest paresthesias. SCS with leads placed at the T1–2 level, just left of midline, has been shown to have similar efficacy as coronary bypass surgery for refractory angina with lower short-term morbidity and mortality.

11. **E.** Amplitude is measured in volts. Pulse width is measured in microseconds. Increasing pulse width can broaden coverage of the painful area. The four parameters include electrode selection (amplitude sets the intensity of stimulation, thus these are essentially the same thing). At higher rates, a buzzing is felt, whereas at lower rates, a thump is felt.

12. **B.** The leads are located in the posterior epidural space, in the posterior aspect of the visualized neural foramina. If they were located in the anterior epidural space, the patient would experience abdominal or potentially chest wall stimulation, depending on the level. This particular patient was receiving SCS therapy for CRPS, although this would not be evident from visualization of this image alone.

13. **B.** SCS therapy in CRPS retains a Level B recommendation, despite its common usage for this indication.

14. **B.** It is true that, to be effective, spinal cord stimulation should be applied continuously or in cycles at least 20 minutes before the onset of analgesia. The mechanism of action for SCS is still not fully understood. Analgesia develops slowly and usually lasts for hours even after cessation of stimulation. There is evidence for efficacy in occipital neuralgia. The role of percutaneous versus paddle leads is still debatable.

15. **E.** The cost of SCS therapy is high and poor selection of patients leads to lower trial to permanent ratios that impose costs to both the system and to the patient. A recommended trial to permanent ratio should be around 75%. Physicians should reevaluate their practice in terms of patient selection and SCS trial technique if their ratios are <50%.

70 Intrathecal Drug Delivery: Patient Selection, Trialing, and Implantation

QUESTIONS

1. Implantable intrathecal infusion pumps are generally recommended for patients with greater than _____ of life expectancy but can be considered in patients with a life expectancy as low as _____.
   A. 12 months, 6 months
   B. 24 months, 12 months
   C. 6 months, 2 months
   D. 9 months, 6 months
   E. 3 months, 1 month

2. All of the following are additional practices that can reduce the risk of infection during the placement of an intrathecal pump **EXCEPT**:
   A. Soaking the pump in a mixture of saline-povidone-iodine solution
   B. Packing the wound with povidone-iodine soaked sponges for a few months
   C. Regloving after the surgical dissection is complete and before handling the pump
   D. Shaving the site before surgery
   E. Double gloving to reduce infection risks associated with glove puncture

3. After placing the catheter for an intrathecal pump, you meet slight resistance when attempting to withdraw the catheter through the needle. What is the most appropriate next step?
   A. Gently rotate the catheter and reattempt
   B. Gently use more force to withdraw the catheter
   C. Turn the bevel of the needle and reattempt
   D. Abort the procedure
   E. Remove the needle and catheter together and restart needle placement

4. All of the following are FDA-approved for use in the SynchroMed II **EXCEPT**:
   A. Baclofen
   B. Morphine
   C. Hydromorphone
   D. Ziconotide
   E. None of the above

5. The most common catheter-related complication is:
   A. Puncture
   B. Disconnection

C. Migration
D. Fracture
E. Dislodgment

6. The most common medication involved in granuloma formation is:
   A. Hydromorphone
   B. Fentanyl
   C. Morphine
   D. Baclofen
   E. Ziconotide

7. A 57-year-old patient with metastatic prostate cancer develops intractable pain and has a life expectancy of 9 months. You deem them a candidate for implantation of a Medtronic SynchroMed II intrathecal pump. Which of the following is true regarding this intrathecal drug delivery system?
   A. It is FDA approved for morphine only.
   B. It has a battery life of 10 years.
   C. It uses a ceramic drive flow valve system to maintain the infusion rate.
   D. It allows patient-controlled intrathecal bolus dosing via a remote control device.
   E. It has a negative-pressure reservoir to improve safety with pump refills.

8. All of the following constitute absolute contraindications to implantation of an intrathecal drug delivery system **EXCEPT**:
   A. Uncontrolled depression
   B. Active psychosis
   C. Active infection
   D. Unstable pathologic fractures
   E. Severe cognitive deficit

9. A patient with an intrathecal drug delivery system who you have been following for over one year suddenly complains of worsening pain. Which of the following catheter-related problems is most likely?
   A. Disconnection
   B. Dislodgment
   C. Fracture
   D. Migration
   E. Puncture

ANSWERS

1. **C.** The general recommendation is that implanted pumps be used only in patients with a life expectancy greater than 6 months. However, pumps can improve the quality of life in patients with life expectancy as low as 2 months. Patients with lower life expectancy should undergo very stringent selection criteria, and costs and benefits must be appropriately weighed.

2. **D.** Shaving can increase the risk of infection, because it has been shown to cause microtrauma of the skin. The other choices describe practices that reduce the risk of contamination and infection.

3. **E.** The needle and catheter should be removed together and the process restarted if even the slightest resistance is noticed.

4. **C.** The SynchroMed II is FDA approved for use with baclofen, morphine, and ziconotide. The Prometra is a device that only comes with a 20-mL reservoir and is FDA approved for morphine.

5. **C.** The most common complications after the intrathecal drug delivery system are catheter related. Follet and Naumann found a catheter-related complication rate of 18.6% in a prospective study. Among these problems, catheter migration, which can occur from improper anchoring to fascia, is the most common. (Follett KA, Naumann CP. A prospective study of catheter-related complications of intrathecal drug delivery systems. *J Pain Symptom Manage.* 2000;19(3);209-215)

6. **C.** High doses and concentration infusions of opioids (except fentanyl) can lead to granuloma formation, with the most commonly implicated drug being morphine.

7. **D.** The Medronic SynchroMed II has a pump life of 7 years. Prometra is a pump with a 10-year battery life. SynchroMed II uses a peristaltic roller system to move the drug and is FDA approved for not only morphine but also ziconotide and baclofen. It requires positive pressure for pump refills, as opposed to the Medallion, which uses negative pressure to improve the safety of refill injections. Hence, the only true statement is that regarding bolus dosing.

8. **D.** The presence of uncontrolled depression (particularly with suicidal or homicidal ideation), active psychosis, severe cognitive deficits, and drug abuse are absolute contraindications to implantation, as are active bacterial or fungal infectious processes. Pathologic fractures are not a contraindication to implantation.

9. **D.** Catheter failures can present with inadequate analgesia, CSF leaks, or withdrawal, and are caused by catheter fracture, puncture, disconnection, migration, or dislodgment from the intrathecal space. Catheter migration is the most common of these complications.

71 Joint Injections

QUESTIONS

1. Which of the following is the most myotoxic local anesthetic?
   A. Bupivacaine
   B. Lidocaine
   C. Ropivacaine
   D. Prilocaine
   E. Mepivacaine

2. Ultrasound-guided joint injections have been shown to have which of the following advantages relative to blind joint injections?
   A. Reduction in procedural pain
   B. Reduced pain scores at 2 weeks postinjection
   C. Improved detection of joint effusion
   D. Increased aspirated joint fluid volume
   E. All of the above

3. How long does acute hyperglycemia typically last in a diabetic patient following corticosteroid injection?
   A. 2–3 days
   B. 7–10 days
   C. 14–17 days
   D. 21–23 days
   E. 30–35 days

4. Which of the following is the least soluble corticosteroid?
   A. Triamcinolone hexacetonide
   B. Triamcinolone acetonide
   C. Methylprednisolone
   D. Dexamethasone
   E. Betamethasone acetate

5. Which of the following has the most anti-inflammatory potency of the listed corticosteroids?
   A. Hydrocortisone
   B. Methylprednisolone
   C. Triamcinolone acetonide
   D. Triamcinolone hexacetonide
   E. Betamethasone

6. All of the following are absolute contraindications to intra-articular joint injection with corticosteroids **EXCEPT:**
   A. Overlying skin infection
   B. Suspected bacteremia
   C. Severely compromised immune status
   D. Joint prosthesis
   E. Suspected infectious arthritis

7. A patient receives a subdeltoid subacromial bursa injection and subsequently develops hives, pruritus, and audible wheezing. Which of the following local anesthetics was most likely injected?
   A. Lidocaine
   B. Bupivacaine
   C. Ropivacaine
   D. Chloroprocaine
   E. Mepivacaine

8. Which joint is most likely to develop avascular necrosis after repeat intra-articular injections?
   A. Knee
   B. Shoulder
   C. Elbow
   D. Hip
   E. Ankle

9. All of the following statements are true regarding local anesthetics **EXCEPT:**
   A. They bind reversibly to sodium channels on neural cell membranes and thereby block nerve conduction.
   B. They have a transient anti-inflammatory effect and inhibit several leukocyte functions.
   C. Local anesthetics induce myonecrosis through degeneration of the sarcoplasmic reticulum and muscle mitochondria.
   D. Chondrolysis is found to occur less frequently with continuous intra-articular local anesthetic infusion relative to single articular injections.
   E. Chondrotoxicity increases with higher concentration of local anesthetic.

10. During the treatment of cardiac arrest from suspected local anesthetic systemic toxicity (LAST), the recommended initial bolus dose and continuous infusion rate for lipid emulsion (20%) therapy is:
    A. 1.0 mL/kg and 0.25 mL/kg/min respectively
    B. 1.0 mL/kg and 0.50 mL/kg/min respectively
    C. 1.5 mL/kg and 0.25 mL/kg/min respectively
    D. 1.5 mL/kg and 0.50 mL/kg/min respectively
    E. 2.0 mL/kg and 0.25 mL/kg/min respectively

11. Which of the following drugs should be avoided during pharmacologic treatment of LAST?
    A. Epinephrine
    B. Propofol
    C. Vasopressin
    D. A and B
    E. B and C

12. Which of the following conditions increases the likelihood of local anesthetic systemic toxicity?
    A. Advanced age
    B. Ischemic heart disease
    C. Cirrhosis
    D. Metabolic or respiratory acidosis
    E. All of the above

13. A 63-year-old male with no significant past medical history receives a corticosteroid injection for knee osteoarthritis. Five hours after the injection, he calls the clinic to report increased pain in his knee. What is the most likely etiology?
    A. Hematoma
    B. Septic arthritis
    C. Steroid flare
    D. Avascular necrosis
    E. Tendon rupture

14. Cross-linking of hyaluronic acid is thought to confer which of the following?
    A. Increased molecular weight to more closely resemble native synovial fluid
    B. Prolongation of intra-articular half-life
    C. Increased risk of immune reaction and pseudosepsis
    D. A and B
    E. All of the above

15. The majority of available evidence supporting glenohumeral joint injection is for which clinical indication?
    A. Adhesive capsulitis
    B. Subacromial bursitis
    C. Impingement
    D. Glenohumeral arthritis
    E. Supraspinatus tendinopathy

ANSWERS

1. **A.** Bupivacaine is the most myotoxic local anesthetic, although myotoxicity is typically not clinically relevant because muscle regenerates.

2. **E.** Sonographic needle guidance is found to be statistically superior to blind palpation-guided injections in multiple areas: reduced procedural pain, reduced absolute pain scores at 2 weeks postinjection, increase in responder rate, improved detection of joint effusion, and increased aspirated fluid volume from the joint.

3. **A.** Hyperglycemia in diabetic patients with appropriate glucose control typically persists for 2–3 days post-steroid injection with peak glucose levels generally reaching about 300 mg/dL.

4. **A.** Corticosteroid solubility may influence duration of action, although data are conflicting. Triamcinolone hexacetonide is the most insoluble (least soluble) injectable corticosteroid.

5. **E.** Hydrocortisone is the relative baseline with an anti-inflammatory potency of 1. The potency of betamethasone is 25; the potency of methylprednisolone acetate, triamcinolone acetonide, and triamcinolone hexacetonide are all 5. Therefore, betamethasone is the most potent.

6. **D.** Absolute contraindications for intra-articular joint steroid injections include overlying skin infection, fracture site, severely compromised immune status, suspected bacteremia, or suspected septic arthritis. Relative contraindications include coagulopathy, joint prosthesis, poorly controlled diabetes mellitus, and previous lack of efficacy.

- 7. **D.** Pruritic rash, hives, and bronchospasm postinjection are indicative of allergic reaction, which is more common with amino-ester local anesthetics (only one "i" in the spelling) relative to amino-amides (two "i's" in the spelling). The ester class (including chloroprocaine) results in production of para-aminobenzoic acid (PABA) metabolites, which are more prone to allergy. The other listed local anesthetics are all amides.

8. **D.** Avascular necrosis is reported most commonly of the hip joint, occurring more commonly after multiple joint steroid injections and in patients who are concurrently taking oral corticosteroids.

9. **D.** Chondrolysis has been *most* reported after *continuous* intraarticular infusion to manage postoperative pain rather than single injections. The other choices are all true.

10. **C.** Lipid emulsion (20%) therapy for LAST is initiated on the basis of clinical judgment, severity, and rate of progression of LAST. Initially, bolus 1.5 mL/kg lean body mass IV over 1 minute, then start a continuous infusion of 0.25 mL/kg/min. Repeat the bolus once or twice for persistent cardiovascular collapse. Double the infusion rate to 0.5 mL/kg/min if blood pressure remains low. Continue the infusion for at least 10 minutes after attaining circulatory stability. The recommended upper dosing limit is approximately 10 mL/kg lipid emulsion over the first 30 minutes.

11. **E.** Because propofol may result in hypotension, it should be avoided in patients with cardiovascular instability. Benzodiazepines are the preferred antiepileptic medication. Vasopressin should also

be avoided for local anesthetic toxicity treatment. Epinephrine is indicated in smaller doses (< 1 μg/kg) for treating associated hypotension.

12. **E.** Factors that can increase the likelihood of LAST include advanced age, heart failure, ischemic heart disease, conduction abnormalities, liver disease, and metabolic or respiratory acidosis.

13. **C.** Steroid injections are commonly associated with a postinjection flare in pain with a prevalence of 2%–25%, typically presenting within a few hours of injection and resolving within 1–3 days. The other listed complications are much less likely.

14. **E.** Chemically modified cross-linked hyaluronic acid (HA) such as Synvisc or Synvisc-One is thought to increase the molecular weight of the HA to resemble native synovial fluid more closely and to lengthen intra-articular half-life, although there is no conclusive evidence that efficacy is improved with cross-linking. Because cross-linked HA molecules are larger and more complex, they may activate the immune system inflammatory response more readily.

15. **A.** The majority of available evidence for therapeutic glenohumeral joint injection supports its use for adhesive capsulitis (frozen shoulder). These injections provide improved range of motion and reduced pain from 6–16 weeks.

Radiation Safety and Radiographic Contrast Agents in Pain Medicine

72

QUESTIONS

1. Hyperosmolar reactions from contrast media include all of the following **EXCEPT:**
   A. Hemolysis
   B. Endothelial damage
   C. Vasodilation
   D. Increased cardiac contractility
   E. Hypervolemia

2. A patient scheduled for a lumbar interlaminar epidural steroid injection using low-osmolar, nonionic radiographic contrast media tells you he has a shellfish allergy. Which of the following is the best response?
   A. Pretreat with a corticosteroid
   B. Iodinated radiographic contrast media is contraindicated.
   C. The risk of reaction for this patient is similar to those who have asthma or other food allergies.
   D. Pretreat with diphenhydramine
   E. Gadolinium-based contrast should be used.

3. What is vignetting?
   A. Splaying outward of objects toward the periphery of the image
   B. Decreasing the size of the image by using shutters
   C. Having less sharpness at the periphery because of a decrease in brightness
   D. Increasing kVp (kilovoltage peak energy levels) by using manual mode instead of automatic brightness control
   E. Using pulsed mode during live fluoroscopy

4. In which of the following situations is gadolinium-based contrast contraindicated?
   A. Shellfish allergy
   B. Liver disease
   C. Congestive heart failure
   D. Chronic kidney disease stage 4–5 (GFR $< 30\,mL/min/1.72\,m^2$)
   E. None of the above

5. What is the function of the collimator?
   A. Changes the ionizing radiation power of the X-ray beam
   B. Changes the size or shape of the X-ray beam
   C. Changes the axis of the X-ray beam
   D. Intensifies the image
   E. Converts X-rays to visible light

6. The clarity of small structures, or image detail, can be improved by all of the following **EXCEPT:**
   A. Increasing kVp
   B. Reducing the distance between the patient and the image intensifier
   C. Using collimation to limit the field of exposure to only those structures of interest
   D. Placing the structure of interest in the center of the image
   E. All of the above

7. What is the minimum radiation dose that will produce erythema (in rad)?
   A. 100
   B. 200
   C. 300
   D. 500
   E. 700

8. The relationship between the radiation source and radiation exposure is best expressed by which of the following (where d is the distance from the radiation source)?
   A. d^2
   B. $1/d^2$
   C. $1/d^3$
   D. d^3
   E. $1/\sqrt{d}$

9. Which of the following produces more X-rays when applied to the X-ray tube?
   A. Increased voltage
   B. Decreased voltage
   C. Increased current
   D. Decreased current
   E. Both increased voltage and increased current

10. When compared with a chest X-ray examination, the approximate radiation dosage of a lumbar transforaminal or facet injection using intermittent fluoroscopy is:
    A. 10× more
    B. 10× less
    C. The same
    D. 100× less
    E. 100× more

11. The following are techniques that can be used to minimize radiation exposure to patients **EXCEPT:**
    A. Shielding
    B. Increasing kVp while minimizing mA
    C. Utilizing pulsed mode
    D. Using collimation
    E. Positioning the image intensifier as far from the patient as possible

12. The following are techniques that can be used to minimize radiation exposure to the practitioner **EXCEPT:**
    A. Shielding of all personnel in the fluoroscopy suite
    B. Using an intravenous extension tube during periods of continuous or live fluoroscopy
    C. When in lateral position, standing on the side of the table of the image intensifier
    D. Having the X-ray tube above the table
    E. Having only the personnel needed to conduct the procedure in the fluoroscopy suite

13. Which of the following techniques for minimizing radiation exposure is least helpful in fluoroscopy units with automatic brightness control?
    A. Collimation
    B. Using leaded gloves
    C. Using leaded eyewear
    D. Using an intravenous extension tube during periods of continuous or live fluoroscopy
    E. Positioning image intensifier as close to the patient as possible, without including unnecessary structures in the field of view

14. The only nonionic monomers approved for intrathecal use are:
    A. Iohexol and iopamidol
    B. Iohexol and ioversol
    C. Iodixanol and iopamidol
    D. Iodixanol and ioversol
    E. Iopamidol and ioversol

15. Which of the following is least likely to increase the risk of severe adverse drug reactions to intravenous injection of low-osmolar, nonionic radiographic contrast media?
    A. Diabetes mellitus
    B. Advanced heart disease
    C. Asthma
    D. Liver disease
    E. History of allergies

ANSWERS

1. **D.** Hyperosmolar reactions are a subgroup of nonidiosyncratic anaphylactoid reactions from iodinated contrast agents. Reactions include hemolysis, endothelial damage (capillary leakage and edema), vasodilation, hypervolemia, and direct cardiac depression. Fortunately, these reactions are exceedingly rare with the use of low-osmolar, nonionic agents and also when receiving small volumes for needle localization during image-guided pain treatments.

2. **C.** In patients with a seafood or shellfish allergy, the risk of an idiosyncratic anaphylactoid reaction to radiographic contrast media (RCM) is similar to those with other food allergies or asthma. It is not a contraindication to the use of RCM. Unfortunately, there is no known premedication regimen that reliably eliminates the risk of severe reactions to RCM. Corticosteroids and antihistamines have been suggested and proven to reduce the incidence of adverse reactions in patients with a history of previous reaction to high-osmolar contrast agents. It is less clear if prophylaxis is needed when using low-osmolar, nonionic agents. Gadolinium, often used with magnetic resonance imaging, can be used instead, but the radiopacity is less than that of iodinated contrast agents. Also, some have advocated avoiding radiographic contrast altogether in patients at elevated risk of adverse reactions if it is not required to carry out the procedure safely.

3. **C.** Vignetting is a phenomenon seen with fluoroscopic images where there is less sharpness at the periphery due to a fall-off of brightness and spatial resolution. By placing the structure of interest in the center of the image, maximum image detail can be obtained. Another phenomenon, pincushion distortion, results in a splaying outward of objects toward the periphery. This is because X-rays are emitted from a spherical surface but detected on a flat surface. Electronic flat plate detectors that replace conventional image intensifiers can eliminate both vignetting and pincushion distortion. Decreasing the size of the image by using shutters is called collimation.

4. **D.** Gadolinium-based contrast is contraindicated in patients with GFR $< 30 \, \text{mL/min}/1.72 \, \text{m}^2$. Caution is also advised in patients with moderately reduced kidney function (30–60 mL/min). Gadolinium-based contrast is an alternative in patients with risk factors for adverse reactions from iodinated contrast.

5. **B.** Collimators, both linear and circular (or iris), are used to adjust the size and shape of the X-ray beam after exiting the X-ray tube and before entering the patient. Linear collimation is useful in imaging long, thin structures such as the spine, whereas iris collimation is helpful for small, circular areas. They both can exclude areas of greatly varying radiodensity and improve image quality.

6. **A.** Reducing the distance between the patient and the image intensifier, using collimation, and placing the structure of interest in the center of the image are all techniques that should be used to maximize image detail. Increasing kVp produces X-rays of higher energy, which improves penetration (useful for obese patients). However, the resulting image is brighter with less contrast between different tissues, thereby reducing image detail.

7. **D.** Erythema results at a minimum radiation dose of 500 rad. Cataract formation occurs at 200 rad.

8. **B.** Radiation exposure is inversely proportional to the square of the distance from the radiation source. One of the most important actions that can minimize exposure is standing as far from the X-ray tube as practical.

9. **C.** Increased current (mA) applied to the X-ray tube will produce more X-rays. Also, lengthening the exposure time will increase the number of X-rays. Increased voltage (kVp) results in X-rays at a higher energy level. In general, it is best to use a high kVp and low mA to optimize image quality while minimizing radiation exposure.

10. **B.** A chest X-ray image produces a dose of approximately 0.1 mSv or 10 mrem. Using intermittent fluoroscopy for a procedure such as a lumbar transforaminal epidural steroid injection or facet injection produces about 0.007–0.003 mSv or 0.7–3 mrem. However, the use of high-dose continuous fluoroscopy and digital subtraction can lead to markedly higher doses.

11. **E.** To minimize radiation exposure to a patient, the X-ray tube should be as far from the patient as possible, without including unnecessary structures in the field of view. Positioning the image intensifier far from the patient will lead to the X-ray tube being close to the patient, which would cause the small area of skin near the X-ray tube to be exposed to a much higher dose. Shielding can be used to protect the gonads (or in rare cases, the fetus), but must be placed on the table underneath the patient to block the X-ray beam before penetrating the patient. They are not often used during image-guided injections of the lumbosacral spine.

12. **D.** Radiation exposure to the practitioner (and the patient) is significantly increased by inverting the C-arm so that the X-ray tube is above the table. This practice has been used to increase the C-arm's range of lateral movement. In lateral position, stand completely away from the table behind the X-ray tube or move to the side of the table opposite the X-ray tube. The other choices are additional methods for minimizing practitioner exposure.

13. **B.** When using automatic brightness control (ABC), the unit will increase output to compensate for radiodense areas created by leaded gloves, thus negating the protective effect. All other options are still useful with ABC, as explained in previous questions.

14. **A.** Iohexol and iopamidol are the only nonionic monomers approved for intrathecal use. Ionic agents should be avoided if there is a possibility of inadvertent intrathecal injection.

15. **D.** Liver disease does not appear to significantly increase the risk of adverse reactions to intravenous contrast. There is an eightfold risk increase in patients with asthma, a sixfold increase in patients with a previous reaction, a fourfold increase in allergic and atopic patients, and a threefold increase in patients with advanced heart disease.

The Management of Pain from Sickle Cell Disease

73

QUESTIONS

1. All of the following pain syndromes, distinct from vaso-occlusive episodes, are commonly seen in sickle cell disease **EXCEPT:**
   A. Avascular necrosis
   B. Osteomyelitis
   C. Leg ulcers
   D. Headaches
   E. Tendonitis

2. Sickle hemoglobin has a single mutation that results in the replacement of:
   A. Glycine with arginine
   B. Arginine with glycine
   C. Glutamine with valine
   D. Valine with glutamine
   E. Valine with glycine

3. Which of the following is recommended as initial therapy at the onset of typical vaso-occlusive pain?
   A. Topical lidocaine
   B. Acetaminophen
   C. Codeine

D. Oxycodone
E. Morphine

4. A 35-year-old female with sickle cell disease develops a severe headache preceded by a visual aura and associated with photophobia and nausea. All of the following are indicated for the treatment of this headache **EXCEPT:**
   A. Sumatriptan
   B. Acetaminophen
   C. Naproxen
   D. Topamax
   E. Magnesium

5. Which of the following have been associated with significant pharmacogenetic issues specifically in patients with sickle cell disease?
   A. Acetaminophen
   B. Codeine
   C. Oxycodone
   D. Morphine
   E. B and D

ANSWERS

1. **E.** Typical vaso-occlusive pain develops from hypoxia and reperfusion injury; however, there are a number of other pain syndromes distinct from vaso-occlusive episodes. These conditions need to be considered when evaluating pain in a patient with sickle cell disease and include acute splenic sequestration, splenic infarction, acute bone infarction, avascular necrosis, osteomyelitis, acute cholelithiasis, leg ulcers, and headache. Tendonitis

is not a common pain syndrome seen in sickle cell disease.

2. **C.** Sickle hemoglobin has a single mutation resulting in the replacement of glutamine with valine at the sixth amino acid position in the beta-globin subunit. With deoxygenation, sickle hemoglobin polymerizes, which physically deforms the red blood cells and leads to obstruction of blood flow.

3. **B.** Low-potency analgesics, which include acetaminophen and ibuprofen, are recommended as initial therapy for vaso-occlusive pain. For more severe pain, oral opioids such as hydrocodone and oxycodone preparations can be used. Topical lidocaine may be used as an adjuvant therapy, but it is not recommended as initial, sole therapy. Morphine would normally be reserved for the acute care or inpatient setting. Long-acting oral morphine would be a treatment option for chronic pain in sickle cell disease.

4. **A.** The patient is probably experiencing a migraine headache, which is a common pain syndrome in sickle cell disease. All of the choices are proven therapies for migraine headaches; however, triptans are contraindicated in sickle cell disease because of cardiovascular concerns.

5. **E.** Both codeine and morphine have been associated with pharmacogenetic issues that affect their use, especially in patients with sickle cell disease. Genetic variability of cytochrome P450-2D6, which metabolizes codeine into morphine, leads to differing levels of metabolism of codeine. On the two extremes are ultra-rapid and poor metabolizers, which cause excessive toxicity or inadequate efficacy, respectively. There is also variability in hepatic and renal clearance of morphine in this population. Dose amounts and frequency may need to be individualized.

QUESTIONS

1. Which type of burn is best characterized by blisters, pink and wet in appearance, and is painful to touch?
   A. First-degree burn
   B. Deep partial-thickness burn
   C. Third-degree burn
   D. Superficial partial-thickness burn
   E. Full-thickness burn

2. Given the properties of fentanyl, it is most useful for the treatment of which type of burn pain?
   A. Rest pain
   B. Breakthrough pain
   C. Procedural pain
   D. Psychogenic pain
   E. Skin graft donor site pain

3. A 43-year-old man sustains a burn while working. He requires significant amounts of opioids, which were escalated rapidly. You are later consulted given concerns for opioid-induced hyperalgesia. Which of the following would be the least helpful for this condition?
   A. Clonidine

B. Dextromethorphan
C. Ketamine
D. Meperidine
E. Methadone

4. A 21-year-old female has severe pain following a burn injury to her leg. Which of the following would be the least helpful for management of her pain?
   A. Intravenous ketamine
   B. Intravenous lidocaine
   C. Intravenous methadone
   D. Transdermal fentanyl
   E. Pregabalin

5. When compared with benzodiazepines for sedation, which of the following can reduce mortality in critically ill patients by approximately 70%?
   A. Propofol
   B. Dexmedetomidine
   C. Fentanyl
   D. Ketamine
   E. Morphine

ANSWERS

1. **D.** Burns are classified by the following depths: first degree (epidermal), second degree (partial thickness), and third degree (full thickness). Partial-thickness burns can be classified further as superficial or deep. Superficial partial-thickness burns are characterized as painful and pink with a wet appearance and blistering. Epidermal burns are limited to the epidermis and are red and painful without blistering. Deep partial-thickness burns are pale or fixed red staining with poor capillary refill, possible blistering, and can be painful or painless. Full-thickness burns are leathery white or brown without blistering and sometimes with pain at the edges.

2. **C.** Burn pain can be characterized as rest pain (constant, dull, background), breakthrough pain (intermittent, short duration, rapid onset/offset, sometimes excruciating), procedural pain (short duration, greatest intensity, occurring with certain activities such as wound cleaning, debridement, dressing changes, hydrotherapy, and joint range-

of-motion exercises), and psychogenic pain (anticipatory pain without mechanical stimulation). Fentanyl is a potent synthetic opioid analog with rapid onset of action and quick redistribution from the central circulation, making it most useful for procedural pain.

3. **D.** Opioid-induced hyperalgesia is a possible consequence of rapid and massive opioid dose escalation. Medications that may reduce or even reverse this condition include methadone, ketamine, dextromethorphan, clonidine, and ketorolac. All of these are nonopioid analgesics except for methadone; however, methadone is a longer-acting opioid with N-methyl-D-aspartate (NMDA) receptor antagonism. Meperidine is a synthetic opioid agonist and, although it has some NMDA receptor antagonism, its long-term use is contraindicated because of accumulation of a toxic metabolite.

4. **B.** All of the options listed have been used for the treatment of pain; however, intravenous lidocaine would be the least helpful. There is a randomized control trial comparing intravenous lidocaine with placebo that showed decreased pain scores; however, there was no significant difference in opioid consumption or satisfaction. A systematic Cochrane review was unable to recommend routine use of intravenous lidocaine in burn pain management. (Wasiak J, Mahar P, McGuinness SK, et al. Intravenous lidocaine for the treatment of background or procedural burn pain. *Cochrane Database Syst Rev.* 2014;10:CD005622.)

5. **B.** Dexmedetomidine is a highly selective central and peripheral α2-adrenergic agonist. This results in reduced autonomic outflow by sympatholysis. Potential benefits include reduced pain intensity, morphine-sparing effects, anti-inflammatory effects, improved macrophage function, anti-apoptotic activity, reduced delirium, and reduced mortality. A study based on the MENDS randomized control trial showed approximately 70% reduction in mortality compared with lorazepam for sedation in critically ill patients. (Pandharipande PP, Sanders RD, Girard TD, et al. Effect of dexmedetomidine versus lorazepam on outcome in patients with sepsis: an a priori-designed analysis of the MENDS randomized controlled trial. *Crit Care* 2010;14(2):R38.)

Pain Management in the Emergency Department

75

QUESTIONS

1. All of the following contribute to undertreatment of pain in the emergency department (ED) **EXCEPT:**
   A. Fear of opioid adverse side effects
   B. Lack of ED pain research among populations at extremes of age
   C. Racial and ethnic bias
   D. Concern for medication costs
   E. Lack of emphasis on pain management education

2. Which patient is most likely to be undertreated for pain in the ED?
   A. A 5-year-old female with a sore throat and temperature of 101.2°F
   B. A 35-year-old male with an ankle sprain yelling for pain medication
   C. An 81-year-old (non-English speaking) female with abdominal pain and rectal bleeding
   D. A and C
   E. All of the above

3. Which analgesic is most commonly used in the ED?
   A. Morphine
   B. Ibuprofen
   C. Acetaminophen
   D. Fentanyl
   E. Meperidine

4. You are evaluating a 56-year-old patient with a 5-year history of prostate cancer. They arrive in the middle of the night, reporting severe right hip pain rated at 10/10. The ED staff refers to them as a "frequent flyer" because they repeatedly come in with severe pain and ask for a dose of intravenous (IV) hydromorphone. The nurse wants you to give them the pain medication and move on to the next patient. You should:
   A. Give them their usual dose of IV hydromorphone and discharge them
   B. Verify the patient's opioid use at home with an online prescription drug monitoring program and treat them with ibuprofen 800 mg by mouth (PO)
   C. Obtain a better history, order the appropriate laboratory tests and imaging studies to evaluate for metastasis or other sequelae of the cancer, and treat pain as appropriate
   D. Discharge them with instructions to call their oncologist in the morning to get a refill of morphine tablets
   E. Refer them to an addictionologist

5. A patient with metastatic hepatocellular carcinoma has been taking 10 tablets of oxycodone/acetaminophen 5/650 mg every day because the pain has been escalating. They rate their pain as a 9/10 in severity and state the medications decrease the pain to a 6/10. Laboratory and imaging studies are unremarkable. What would be the best way to titrate their dose of opioids for effective analgesia?
   A. Increase the frequency of oxycodone/acetaminophen 5/650 mg to every 2 hours
   B. Treat the patient's severe pain with IV opioids until the pain is well controlled; following this, adjust the patient's pain regimen to equivalent dosing of short-acting PO oxycodone and monitor for adequate pain control
   C. Treat the patient's severe pain with IV opioids until the pain is well controlled. Following this, adjust the patient's pain regimen to a long-acting PO opioid based on their IV consumption and provide short-acting PO opioids for breakthrough pain.
   D. Give the patient IV ketorolac and discharge them with oxycodone 10 mg
   E. Taper opioids until the patient is completely weaned

6. What would be an appropriate dose of IV morphine for an 80-kg patient in pain?
   A. 2 mg of IV morphine every 5 minutes until pain relief
   B. 8 mg of IV morphine, then 16 mg of IV morphine every hour until pain relief
   C. 8 mg of IV morphine, then 4–8 mg of IV morphine every 5 minutes until pain relief
   D. 8 mg of IV morphine, then transition to oral regimen until pain relief
   E. None of the above

7. You are evaluating a 23-year-old female who presents with severe vaginal pain caused by a Bartholin's abscess. She is extremely anxious because she will need an incision and drainage. You decide to provide minimal sedation for this procedure. Which medication would you use?
   A. High-dose ketamine
   B. Midazolam
   C. Propofol
   D. Etomidate
   E. Thiopental

8. What are the most common side effects seen with the use of ketamine for procedural sedation and analgesia?
   A. Respiratory depression, hypothermia, and myoclonus
   B. Emergence phenomena, laryngospasm, and tachycardia
   C. Bradycardia, agitation, and hallucinations
   D. Laryngospasm, wheezing, and malignant hyperthermia
   E. Hypotension, nystagmus, and nightmares

9. Why is meperidine being used less often in the ED?
   A. Potential risk for the accumulation of the toxic metabolite normeperidine, which can cause seizures and neurotoxicity
   B. Interaction with monoamine oxidase inhibitors, which can lead to serotonin syndrome

C. Cost of medication
D. A and B
E. All of the above

10. A patient is undergoing an ED procedure with sedation and is able to respond appropriately when lightly touched. Which level of sedation is being administered?
    A. Minimal
    B. Moderate
    C. Deep
    D. General
    E. None of the above

ANSWERS

1. **D.** A variety of factors may contribute to the undertreatment of pain in the emergency department. Research shows that some of the underlying factors are fear of opioid side effects, misuse and potential for addiction, and lack of emphasis on pain research and pain management education for medical providers. Medication costs have not been identified as a concern.

2. **D.** The term oligoanalgesia has been used to describe the underuse of analgesics for the adequate treatment of pain. Unfortunately, it occurs in a significant percentage of patients presenting to the ED. The recognized contributory factors are extremes of age and minority ethnic groups.

3. **A.** The majority of analgesics administered in the ED are opioids. Among these, morphine is the most frequently prescribed at 20%.

4. **C.** Prescription opioid abuse is a serious problem that affects patients who frequently visit the ED. The role of the ED physician is to obtain the proper history and examination and imaging studies to evaluate all patients appropriately and rule out life-threatening events. The online prescription monitoring programs are available to help clinicians verify the use of opioid analgesics and identify problematic requests. In this case, the patient's home prescriptions could be verified with an online prescription monitoring network, but their pain is severe and thus, ibuprofen 800 mg would probably be inadequate in relieving the pain.

5. **C.** This patient presents with an acute pain crisis and will benefit from titration of IV opioids to control the severe pain. Upon discharge, the pain will probably be better controlled on a long-acting PO opioid to avoid the waxing and waning in analgesic coverage that is associated with short-acting opioids. Short-acting opioids can also be provided for breakthrough pain. In addition, this patient is taking too much acetaminophen and would benefit from separating the opioid and nonopioid components to prevent hepatotoxicity.

6. **C.** Opioids can be safely titrated to treat acute pain crisis. The typical dose of IV morphine used in the ED is 0.1 mg/kg, with repeat boluses of 0.05–0.1 mg/kg every 5 minutes until pain relief is achieved. For this patient, an ideal starting dose would be 8 mg IV morphine, with repeat dosing of 4–8 mg/kg every 5 minutes.

7. **B.** The medications typically used for minimal sedation include fentanyl, midazolam, combinations of the two, and low-dose ketamine. Propofol, etomidate, and high-dose ketamine are used for moderate to deep sedation.

8. **B.** Ketamine is a dissociative anesthetic classified as an N-methyl-D-aspartate (NMDA) receptor antagonist. It is frequently used for procedural sedation to provide pain relief, sedation, and amnesia. Patients should be monitored for respiratory depression and possible laryngospasm (although rare). Patients can also experience an emergence reaction, which has been described as an unpleasant perceptual experience as they regain consciousness.

9. **D.** Many EDs have eliminated the use of meperidine because there are many other opioids with greater efficacy and fewer side effects. The most concerning side effect seen with meperidine is CNS toxicity resulting from the accumulation of its toxic metabolite, normeperidine. The clinical manifestations of CNS toxicity include mood alterations, anxiety, tremors, myoclonus, and seizures. Meperidine can also interact with monoamine oxidase inhibitors to cause serotonin syndrome. Accumulation of meperidine can be seen in patients with impaired renal function.

10. **B.** This patient is under moderate sedation, which is a drug-induced depression of consciousness in which the patient responds appropriately to verbal commands, either alone or with light tactile stimulation.

Pain Management in the Critically Ill Patient

76

QUESTIONS

1. You are evaluating pain in a patient who has recently been admitted to the intensive care unit (ICU). They are alert but sedated, intubated, and unable to communicate their level of pain. What strategy might you use to assess the patient's pain?
   A. Empirically treat based on what was administered in the emergency department
   B. Question the patient's family members about home pain medications and use this as a basis for acute conversion to parenteral medications
   C. In collaboration with the patient's nurse, work to identify nonverbal cues to pain severity and place a visual analogue card at the bedside for the patient to rate their own pain level
   D. Use the nursing assessment of pain severity as the sole basis of deciphering pain level
   E. Titrate parenteral medication until the patient is entirely sedated and unresponsive to any painful stimuli

2. An ICU patient is intubated, sedated, and unable to communicate their level of pain intensity. Their facial expression is grimacing, with partially bent upper limb movements, and they are actively fighting the ventilator. What would their sum score be on the behavioral pain scale?
   A. 6
   B. 7
   C. 8
   D. 9
   E. 10

3. You are evaluating pain in a patient who recently underwent emergent thoracotomy for a gunshot wound to the right anterior chest. After successful tamponade of the acute bleeding, the thorax has been closed, with two chest tubes in the right lateral chest wall draining serosanguinous fluid. The patient is sedated and minimally responsive, but showing significant nonverbal signs of pain, including facial grimacing and difficulty with ventilation. What strategy might you use to treat this patient's pain?
   A. Apply localized lidocaine to the chest tube and thoracotomy suture sites and ketorolac administration

B. Titrate parenteral opioids until an improvement in nonverbal signs of pain and ventilator compliance is achieved
C. Start an opioid patient-controlled analgesia (PCA) so that the patient may titrate their medication to achieve a reduction in pain severity
D. Place a thoracic epidural analgesia catheter for scheduled infusion of opioids and local anesthetics as tolerated
E. B and D

4. An opioid-naïve 48-year-old female patient is admitted to the ICU for severe diabetic ketoacidosis (DKA). She has resultant acute kidney injury (creatinine 2.6), and testing reveals that the likely precipitant of the DKA was acute cholecystitis. The patient is complaining of severe abdominal pain and pending surgery. Which medication should be used to treat this patient's pain?
   A. Ketorolac 30 mg IV
   B. Acetaminophen 650 mg PO
   C. Morphine sulfate 4 mg IV
   D. Hydromorphone 0.5 mg IV
   E. A and C

5. A 54-year-old patient presents to the hospital with worsening epigastric abdominal pain and severe dehydration. They are found to have metastatic pancreatic adenocarcinoma. The patient is admitted to the ICU for resuscitation, where they are continued on their home medications of transdermal fentanyl patch 25 μg and PO oxycodone 5 mg/acetaminophen 325 mg, which they have been requiring every 6 hours. Their clinical status improves, but they continue to have severe pain. Which treatment strategy should you use to treat this patient's pain?
   A. Continue 25 μg fentanyl patch and encourage as much oxycodone as needed until pain relief is achieved
   B. Start the patient on a hydromorphone PCA until pain is better controlled
   C. Schedule the patient for a celiac plexus block
   D. Schedule administration of morphine 2 mg IV every 2 hours as well as ketorolac 30 mg IV every 6 hours
   E. B and C

6. You are evaluating a patient who was preemptively intubated in the ICU prior to endoscopy for an esophageal variceal bleed. The patient's vital signs postintubation are as follows: T 98.7°F, RR 16, HR 47, BP 96/56. As the initial dose of succinylcholine wears off, the nurse asks about a potential drug for sedation that can be titrated appropriately. Which drug would be unadvisable in this setting because of its known side effect profile?
   A. Midazolam
   B. Dexmedetomidine
   C. Fentanyl
   D. Propofol
   E. All of the above are appropriate.

7. A patient has been transferred to the ICU postoperatively following the placement of a pericardial window for evacuation of a large malignant pericardial effusion. Intraoperatively, the patient had a thoracic epidural catheter placed and was administered a dose of local anesthetic. Which of the following is the most common adverse effect of administering a local anesthetic in this clinical scenario?
   A. Anaphylaxis
   B. Bronchospasm
   C. Hypotension
   D. Platelet dysfunction
   E. Local anesthetic systemic toxicity (LAST)

8. A patient presents with ureteral colic secondary to a large obstructing renal calculus in the mid-ureter. The patient has been on PRN IV morphine 4 mg every 4 hours and IV ketorolac 30 mg every 6 hours as needed for pain control. They are now on hospital day 3. After how many days has it been recommended to discontinue ketorolac?
   A. 2 days
   B. 3 days
   C. 4 days
   D. 5 days
   E. 6 days

ANSWERS

1. **C.** The presence of an endotracheal tube or the severity of the underlying physiologic process may prevent ICU patients from communicating with nursing staff or physician regarding their level of pain. In this case, you are giving the patient not only an opportunity to address their own pain if their clinical picture improves, you are also advocating for nursing staff to use nonverbal cues.

2. **D.** Based on the behavioral pain scale, the patient's facial expression is grimacing, which would give a score of 4. They are partially bent in upper limb movements, which would give a score of 2, and they are fighting the ventilator in respect to compliance with mechanical ventilation (score of 3). Thus, the patient's sum score would be 9.

3. **E.** Postthoracotomy patients derive special benefit from the placement of a thoracic epidural analgesia catheter. These catheters provide coverage of chest tube insertion sites and pain from surgical incisions. The thoracic epidural catheter can be used to infuse combinations of opioids and local anesthetics as tolerated. Local anesthetics can lead to hypotension and their addition is therefore based on the patient's hemodynamics. In addition, the patient will probably require parenteral opioids for postoperative surgical pain, which will also aid in sedation and increase ventilator compliance. Nonsteroidal anti-inflammatory drugs should be avoided immediately following surgery with significant blood loss. PCA can be helpful with postoperative pain; however, the patient needs to be coherent enough to use it successfully.

4. **D.** Despite significant evidence showing benefit with the use of parenteral nonsteroidal anti-inflammatory drugs for pain from cholecystitis, this patient has evidence of acute kidney injury and thus, nonsteroidal anti-inflammatory drugs are contraindicated. The patient is complaining of severe pain and thus, acetaminophen alone will not effectively treat this patient's pain. Secondary to the patient's acute kidney injury, morphine is also relatively contraindicated because it undergoes renal elimination. Thus, parenteral hydromorphone would be most appropriate because of reduced side effect profile with kidney impairment and the severity of the patient's pain.

5. **E.** Advising the patient to continue oxycodone/ acetaminophen when necessary may lead to exceeding the upper limit of acetaminophen (3 g daily), putting the patient at increased risk of liver injury. In the setting of severe and uncontrolled pain, PCA is an ideal strategy to optimize the patient's pain relief and give the patient autonomy over their pain management. It also allows reassessment and recalculation of the patient's new pain medication requirements, which can then be converted into oral formulation for discharge. The celiac plexus block is an additional modality of pain control because it can be used to block afferent sympathetic nerve fibers responsible for somatic and visceral pain secondary to tumor burden in the abdominal area.

6. **B.** Although all of the answer choices listed do cause systemic side effects, such as relative hypotension, dexmedetomidine has been specifically associated with increased rates of hypotension and bradycardia as compared with midazolam (Jakob et al.). According to this study, dexmedetomidine was found to be noninferior to propofol and midazolam in maintaining target levels of sedation in ICU patients who required prolonged mechanical ventilation and had a number of positive effects as compared to midazolam and propofol, but hypotension and bradycardia are limiting factors. (Jakob SM, Ruokonen E, Grounds

RM, et al. Dexmedetomidine for long-term sedation investigators. Dexmedetomidine vs midazolam or propofol for sedation during prolonged mechanical ventilation: two randomized controlled trials. *JAMA* 2012;307(11):1151-1160.)

7. **C.** Of the available choices, administration of local anesthetics should be most concerning for hypotension and ensuing poor end-organ perfusion. Given the restricted use of intravenous fluids associated with many thoracic surgical cases, the patient may arrive with relative hypotension that may be worsened secondary to the interruption of sympathetic tone.

8. **D.** Despite ketorolac being shown to have opioid-sparing effects, there are also associated adverse effects on gastric mucosal perfusion, platelet aggregation, and renal perfusion in those patients with suboptimal intravascular volume status. It has been recommended that ketorolac be discontinued after 5 days and used with caution in older adults.

QUESTIONS

1. Which of the following is associated with a higher likelihood of complementary and alternative medicine (CAM) use?
   A. Lower household income
   B. Attainment of a bachelor's degree
   C. Older age
   D. Less use of life-sustaining treatment
   E. All of the above

2. Which of the following is true regarding acupuncture?
   A. It is an effective antidepressant.
   B. Although it has a positive effect on chronic obstructive pulmonary disease, it does not have any significant effect on dyspnea associated with end-stage cancer.
   C. It is found to be helpful in asthma.
   D. A and C
   E. All of the above

3. Patients in the terminal stage of illness often experience multiple mechanisms of pain simultaneously (e.g., both nociceptive and neuropathic). Inadequate pain relief might hasten death via:
   A. Morbid effects of increasing physiologic stress
   B. Risk of pneumonia and thromboembolism
   C. Increasing myocardial oxygen demand
   D. All of the above
   E. Pain does not affect mortality.

4. Which of these pain assessment tools has been validated as a self-report instrument for pain intensity in patients with mild to moderate cognitive impairment?
   A. Visual analog score
   B. Numerical pain rating scale
   C. Pain thermometer
   D. DOLOPLUS
   E. All of the above

5. Patients in palliative care at the end of life frequently experience constipation, in part because of opioid therapy. Which of the following medications for opioid-induced constipation should be avoided in this patient population?
   A. Senokot
   B. Psyllium
   C. Lactulose
   D. Polyethylene glycol
   E. None of the above

6. Your patient is receiving high doses of morphine for chronic pain; subsequently, they develop myoclonus. Which of the following is the most appropriate statement regarding the initial treatment of this side effect?
   A. Clonazepam 0.5–1 mg should be administered by mouth every 6–8 hours.
   B. Lorazepam can be given sublingually if the patient is unable to swallow.
   C. Parenteral administration of diazepam is indicated if symptoms are distressing.
   D. Switch to an alternate opioid
   E. Any of the above

ANSWERS

1. **B.** Tilden et al. interviewed caregivers of deceased patients regarding the prevalence of CAM use in an end-of-life population and found that 53.7% of the deceased used CAM therapy. These individuals were more likely to be younger with college degrees and higher household incomes and were more likely to have used one or more life-sustaining treatments. (Tilden VP, Drach LL, Tolle SW. Complementary and alternative therapy use at end-of-life in community settings. *J Altern Complement Med.* 2004;10(5):811-817.)

2. **E.** Several researchers have found acupuncture to be an effective antidepressant. Studies show that acupuncture has a significant positive effect on chronic obstructive pulmonary disease, dyspnea associated with end-stage cancer, and asthma.

3. **D.** Pain can increase physiologic stress and reduce mobility, increasing proclivities toward pneumonia and thromboembolism, and increasing the work of

breathing and myocardial oxygen requirements. This can affect mortality.

4. **C.** The "pain thermometer" has been validated as a self-report instrument for pain intensity in patients with mild to moderate cognitive impairment.

5. **B.** Bulking agents such as psyllium should be avoided in debilitated patients, because these tend to increase desiccation time in the large bowel and debilitated patients can rarely take sufficient fluid to facilitate the action of bulking agents.

6. **A.** Myoclonic jerking can occur with high-dose opioid therapy. Cases of myoclonus have been reported in patients with renal insufficiency who are taking high doses of morphine, probably because of metabolites such as morphine glucuronide and normorphine accumulation. If myoclonus develops, switch to an alternative opioid, especially if using morphine. A lower relative dose of the substituted drug may be possible because of incomplete cross-tolerance. Benzodiazepines may be used for symptom management of myoclonus.

78 Pain Management in the Home: Using Cancer Patients as a Model

QUESTIONS

1. Which of the following is least concerning for a family member caring for a cancer patient at home regarding the administration of opioids at the end of life?
   A. Potential to give too much medication and overdose
   B. Knowing the correct dosage and administration of medication
   C. Cost effectiveness of the pain regimen
   D. Assessing the patient's pain level correctly
   E. Concerns for addiction and dependency

2. A distressed caregiver calls the on-call hospice nurse because their father continues to be in severe debilitating pain despite multiple attempts to make him comfortable. They are concerned that their father is actively dying and stayed up throughout the night managing his pain. What should the hospice nurse do next?
   A. Tell the caregiver to give a rescue dose of morphine and call again in a few hours to see if it was effective
   B. Address all of the concerns the caregiver might have regarding their father's care at the end of life and arrange a home visit to evaluate the patient
   C. Take note of the call and tell the case manager in the morning
   D. Inform the caller this is normal at the end of life and not to worry because their father has only hours left
   E. Provide reassurance

3. Which nondrug interventions would you recommend to a home cancer patient as strategies for pain relief?
   A. Massage using cold and hot pads
   B. Meditation and deep breathing exercises
   C. Prayer and imagery
   D. All of the above
   E. None of the above

4. You have a 52-year-old patient with metastatic pancreatic cancer who was recently discharged home from the hospital. They just enrolled in home hospice and you are evaluating them for severe pain. They say their abdominal pain escalated to a 10/10 on the numerical pain scale and they are not getting any relief with the use of the breakthrough medication because of frequent emesis. What could you do to control their pain?
   A. Insert a subcutaneous line and start a parenteral opioid infusion after a careful history and physical examination by the nurse to rule out causes of emesis unrelated to the terminal disease
   B. Send them to the hospital to be evaluated for a small bowel obstruction and insertion of a peripheral intravenous (IV) line.
   C. Double the dose of long-acting oral opioid and breakthrough dose
   D. Order an antiemetic and IV hydration by a peripheral line
   E. B and C

5. In the clinic, you meet a 40-year-old survivor of breast cancer who underwent a radical mastectomy 5 years ago, followed by chemotherapy and radiation. Now that she is in remission, most of her symptoms resolved, but she continues to experience an aching, shooting sensation on her anterior chest wall and shoulder. What is the best course of action?
   A. Explain this is a side effect from the chemotherapy and the pain will go away
   B. Recognize that she has a neuropathic pain syndrome and start her on a serotonin-norepinephrine reuptake inhibitor (SNRI), a tricyclic antidepressant (TCA), or gabapentinoids
   C. Consider disease recurrence and obtain imaging studies
   D. Recognize that this is a result of chronic inflammation and start her on a nonsteroidal anti-inflammatory drug
   E. Recognize that this is a sign of recurrence and start her on low-dose opioid medication

C. Patient and family fatigue, fears of addiction, lack of knowledge about pain management, failure to report pain, concerns regarding harm, and limited access to care hamper the ability to provide pain care at home. Studies show several caregiver concerns, as described in the answer choices. However, results did not show cost as a major concern for family members.

B. The hospice provider should address all the needs of the patient and the family members when evaluating distress. Caregivers often show distress when they lack knowledge about pain management and when they fail to recognize the stages of dying.

D. Nondrug interventions that patients should use to control their pain include massage using heat and cold and cognitive strategies such as relaxation techniques, imagery, meditation, and prayer, as appropriate. It has been shown that these strategies will help control their symptoms and also help the individual to regain a sense of control.

4. **A.** Insertion of subcutaneous lines for continuous infusion could be easily accomplished in the home hospice setting to reach the goals of therapy. This technique, also known as hypodermoclysis, requires minimal equipment and supervision and is less distressing than inserting a peripheral intravenous line.

5. **B.** Neuropathic pain syndromes are associated with neurotoxic chemotherapies, surgery (mastectomy or thoracotomy), lymph node dissections, and radiation therapy. These often result in chronic pain syndromes for cancer survivors. This patient describes having a chronic pain syndrome, specifically neuropathic pain with shooting, "lightning-like" pain, secondary to radiation and chemotherapy treatments. The best course of action would be to start her on a medication such as an SNRI, TCA, or gabapentinoid. Neuropathic pain has been shown to be less responsive to opioid medications.

79

The Health Implications of Disparities in Cancer and Pain Care: Unequal Burdens and Unheard Voices

QUESTIONS

1. When describing health disparities, a key theme is the concept of poverty's negative cumulative effect. What is being described by this?
   A. Multiple exposures to changes in age, race, class, health, and socioeconomic factors make individuals especially susceptible to pain secondary to the cumulative nature of the disparities presented to them.
   B. A sudden change in socioeconomic factors causes reduced exposure to health disparities.
   C. It is primarily a concept related to younger adults and white women.
   D. It is primarily a concept related to older racial and ethnic minority women.
   E. A and D

2. Consistent with the health disparity literature, which groups are particularly vulnerable to chronic pain's negative sequelae?
   A. Older adults
   B. Racial and ethnic minorities
   C. Women
   D. Impoverished individuals
   E. All the above

3. A 64-year-old woman shows up in your outpatient pain clinic for initial evaluation for her chronic low back pain. She has tried multiple providers previously and in the process, has tried many different analgesic approaches, including nonsteroidal anti-inflammatory drugs, and low- or moderate-dose opioids as well as gabapentinoids, with minimal response to her pain. Her primary care physician referred her to you and stated that despite it being an ongoing problem for years, she had not seen any medical professionals regarding the cause or potential treatment options. She describes her pain as chronic, worsened by daily activity, and so severe that by the end of the day, she cannot finish her job of housekeeping. When you walk into the room, the patient is hunched over, yelling, "This is the worst thing that has ever happened to me and today is the worst it's ever been! This is more pain than any human should ever experience!" What coping mechanism is the patient exemplifying?
   A. Poor information seeking

B. Passivity
C. Catastrophizing
D. A and B
E. B and C

4. Several studies have reported significant disparities in the treatment of cancer pain in racial and ethnic minorities. Which of the following factors contribute to these disparities?
   A. Poor physician assessment of pain
   B. Inadequate pain treatment, including decreased ability to obtain pain medications
   C. Significantly less access to complementary and alternative medicine
   D. Being in a geographic area consistent with a minority neighborhood
   E. All the above

5. You were evaluating a 64-year-old male with a history of recently diagnosed metastatic prostate cancer who was started on oral chemotherapy several weeks prior. He has been admitted to the intensive care unit for worsening chemotherapy-related esophagitis, decreased oral intake, dehydration, and septic shock from a urinary tract infection. During the discussion with his wife about his pain and his response to treatment, she describes that initially, her husband was coping with his new diagnosis and subsequent therapy with extreme fear of reporting his pain and worsening difficulty swallowing. He would often stay quiet and would not communicate whatsoever with the rest of his family. Similarly, he would try to work longer hours at his job as a fisherman, often coming home extremely late at night. His coworkers said that he was barely able to complete his work, despite minimal complaints of this nature. What type of coping has been described in the above example?
   A. Stoicism
   B. John Henryism
   C. Wishful thinking
   D. Religious coping
   E. A and B

ANSWERS

1. **E.** The pain literature focusing on the intersection between race, gender, and aging has primarily focused on younger adults and white women, whereas the concept of poverty's negative cumulative effect is often a problem of older racial and ethnic minority women. It is described as having multiple exposures over the life course that have a combined effect on health.

2. **E.** Consistent with the health disparity literature, older adults, racial and ethnic minorities, women, and impoverished individuals (primarily low-income racial and ethnic minority women) may be particularly susceptible to chronic pain's adverse sequelae.

3. **E.** The patient always describing her pain in harsh language but not seeing any medical professionals regarding the cause or potential treatment options is an example of inadequate information seeking. Her initial description, yelling, "This is the worst thing that has ever happened to me and today is the worst it's ever been!" is an example of catastrophizing. These maladaptive coping styles and poor adjustment influence the response to pain and are potentially detrimental to coping successfully with a pain problem.

4. **E.** The literature describes significant differences in the ability to discuss pain complaints when patients are ethnic minorities. These include physicians being generally more verbally dominant, engaged in less patient-centered communication, significantly less rapport building, and rating conditions as less severe with ethnic and minority patients. Similarly, racial and ethnic minority patients have been prescribed less potent analgesics and were significantly underrated concerning the WHO recommendations for managing cancer pain. The literature has also shown racial and ethnic minorities, specifically Blacks, use fewer complementary and alternative medicine techniques (including acupuncture) and significantly less manipulation, biofeedback, or relaxation training than Whites for chronic pain. Also, two pharmacy studies showed that pharmacies located in minority neighborhoods were less likely to carry opioid analgesics than those in nonminority neighborhoods.

5. **E.** The patient is clearly expressing stoicism, which often accompanies a belief that pain is inevitable and fear that reporting pain will be misunderstood by family and friends. The clinical vignette also highlighted John Henryism, which is characterized by actively coping with stressors by working increasingly harder against potentially insurmountable obstacles.

Clinical Trial Design Methodology for Pain Outcome Studies

80

QUESTIONS

1. A biotechnology firm begins testing a novel drug for the treatment of type 1 diabetes in a small subset of patients for a prospective randomized control trial under optimal circumstances. What step is the company at in the appraisal of its health care intervention?
   A. Efficacy
   B. Effectiveness
   C. Efficiency
   D. Initiation
   E. None of the above

2. An investigator's knowledge of patient assignment to different therapies is known as:
   A. Selection bias
   B. Performance bias
   C. Attrition bias
   D. Reporting bias
   E. Detection bias

3. A study of 30,000 patients examined in pain clinics between 2001 and 2008 finds that the most common chronic pain complaint in this population was low back pain. Which of the following best describes this study?
   A. Cross-sectional study
   B. Cohort study
   C. Case control study
   D. Nested case control study
   E. Population study

ANSWERS

1. **A.** Efficacy answers the question "Can it work?" and is the first stage of appraisal for a new intervention. These studies are usually done under ideal settings in a controlled population. Effectiveness answers the question "Does it work?" in a clinical setting and involves pragmatic trials in real-world settings. Efficiency answers the question "Is it worth it?" in terms of cost effectiveness and acceptability to patients.

2. **B.** Performance bias is a result of knowing the therapies to which patients are assigned. Selection bias results from differences between groups that exist other than the intervention itself. Attrition bias results from a difference in those who do or do not complete the study. Reporting bias results from a tendency to present only certain results (i.e., those that are statistically significant). Detection bias occurs when outcomes are differentially interpreted based on the assigned interventions.

3. **A.** A cross-sectional study determines the prevalence of disease at a certain period of time. A cohort study is a longitudinal study that examines a group of individuals over time. A case-control study is an observational study where two groups with and without an outcome of interest are compared based on a risk factor. A nested case-control study samples cases from an existing cohort. A population study examines a group of individuals from the general population with a common characteristic and answers a question that is generalizable to the whole population.

81 Ethics of Research in Patients With Pain

QUESTIONS

1. What is the meaning of the concept of "minimal risk" as it pertains to federal regulation of research studies?
   A. Risk is minimized as much as possible.
   B. Probability of death is <1%.
   C. Risk is less than alternative existing options.
   D. Probability and magnitude of harm is not greater than that encountered in daily life.
   E. Risk to the patient is minimized because of utilization of a therapy already FDA approved for a separate indication.

2. Informed consent has at its core the principle of respect for which of the following?
   A. Beneficence
   B. Justice
   C. Minimal risk
   D. Nonmaleficence
   E. Autonomy

3. Which of the following is true regarding the Belmont Report of 1979?
   A. Examined the results of withholding treatment in patients with syphilis to observe the progression of the disease
   B. Was the first document to address experimentation in children and others with limited decision-making capacity
   C. Declared that voluntary consent is absolutely necessary for all research involving human subjects
   D. Declared that subjects in a study should be protected from unnecessary physical and mental suffering
   E. Describes the basic ethical principles underlying the conduct of research: respect for persons, beneficence, and justice as it applies to research conduct

ANSWERS

1. **D.** "Minimal risk" as it pertains to federal regulations for research studies requires that harm does not exceed that encountered in daily life.

2. **E.** Informed consent at its core represents the principle of autonomy.

3. **E.** The Belmont Report describes the basic ethical principles underlying the conduct of research.

Postoperative Pain Management: Trends and Future Directions and Areas in Need of Investigation

82

QUESTIONS

1. All of the following are advantages of thoracic epidural analgesia in patients undergoing cardiothoracic-vascular procedures **EXCEPT**:
   A. Better quality of life and quality of recovery
   B. Decrease in pulmonary complications
   C. Decrease in cardiac dysrhythmias and overall cardiac complications
   D. Faster resolution of postoperative ileus
   E. Increased pain control

2. All of the following are associated with an increased incidence of postoperative delirium **EXCEPT**:
   A. Age
   B. Benzodiazepines
   C. Meperidine
   D. Regional anesthesia
   E. Postoperative pain

3. At what point can a diagnosis of persistent postsurgical pain (PPP) be made? This is a persistent pain state that occurs more than:
   A. 1 month postoperatively
   B. 2 months postoperatively
   C. 3 months postoperatively
   D. 6 months postoperatively
   E. 12 months postoperatively

4. The Opioid-Related Symptoms Distress Scale to assess symptoms related to opioid intake includes all of the following **EXCEPT**:
   A. Difficulty voiding
   B. Headache
   C. Uncontrolled pain
   D. Feelings of lightheadedness
   E. Fatigue or weakness

ANSWERS

1. **A.** Several systematic reviews in patients undergoing high-risk cardiothoracic-vascular procedures suggest that a decrease in pulmonary complications, cardiac dysrhythmias, and overall cardiac complications may be seen with perioperative thoracic epidural analgesia with a local anesthetic-based analgesic regimen. In patients undergoing abdominal surgery, the perioperative use of thoracic epidural analgesia with a local anesthetic-based regimen is associated with faster resolution of postoperative ileus. Despite the analgesic benefits of regional analgesic techniques, it is not clear whether this improved analgesia can be translated to improvements in some other patient-centered outcomes such as quality of life and quality of recovery.

2. **D.** One of the more significant complications for older patients in the perioperative period is the development of postoperative delirium. Although the etiology of postoperative delirium and postoperative cognitive dysfunction is uncertain, it is clear that a major risk factor is age, with a higher incidence of postoperative delirium with increased age. Certain drugs or classes of drugs (e.g., meperidine, benzodiazepines) have been associated with an increase in postoperative delirium. In addition, an increase in the level of postoperative pain has been shown to correlate with an increased incidence of postoperative delirium.

3. **B.** PPP, also known as chronic postsurgical pain (CPSP), is a persistent pain state which occurs more than 2 months postoperatively and cannot be explained by other causes such as disease or inflammation. The incidence of PPP ranges from 5% to 50%, and the mechanisms causing it are multifactorial. Potential mechanisms include inflammatory (release of inflammatory prostaglandins and cytokines) and neuropathic (sustained ectopic activity of injured nerves and changes in spinal inhibition and facilitation). Preoperative causes include psychological factors, presence of pain, genetic factors, gender, and age. Intraoperative factors include the type of anesthesia, surgical approach, and nerve injury.

4. **C.** The Opioid-Related Symptoms Distress Scale to assess symptoms related to opioid intake includes: difficulty passing urine, headache, feelings of lightheadedness, and fatigue or weakness.

83 Future Directions and Trends in Pain Medicine

1. Which of the following is true of epidural steroid injections?
   A. There is no evidence of benefit for axial low back pain.
   B. There is significant benefit for back pain associated with spinal stenosis.
   C. There is evidence of long-term benefit for extremity pain related to disk herniation.
   D. There is evidence of short-term benefit for axial low back pain.
   E. None of the above

2. A patient presents with burning, tingling, and lancinating pain. Which of the following would be considered a first-line treatment?
   A. Ibuprofen
   B. Morphine
   C. Duloxetine
   D. Celecoxib
   E. Nitroglycerin

3. Which of the following could be a potential target for pain related to disk herniation?
   A. Phospholipase A2 (PLA2)
   B. Interleukin-6 and -8 (IL-6 and IL-8)
   C. Tumor necrosis factor-α (TNF-α)
   D. A and C
   E. All of the above

ANSWERS

1. **A.** There is no evidence of benefit for axial low back pain with epidural steroid injections and only moderate short-term benefit for extremity pain associated with disk herniation. More research should be done to provide evidence of effectiveness.

2. **C.** Based on guidelines from several organizations, anticonvulsants, serotonin norepinephrine reuptake inhibitors, and tricyclic antidepressants are recommended as first-line treatments for neuropathic pain. Duloxetine is a serotonin norepinephrine reuptake inhibitor.

3. **E.** Disk herniation results in an increase of inflammatory cytokines including IL-6, IL-8, IL-1 beta, TNF-α, and PLA2, resulting in the production of prostaglandins. TNF-α inhibitors injected into the epidural space have shown some efficacy in treating pain related to herniation. All of the cytokines listed could serve as potential targets for future therapies.

Index